D0640801

THE DRUG TRIAL

THE DRUG TRIAL

Nancy Olivieri and the Science Scandal
that Rocked the Hospital for Sick Children

Miriam Shuchman

RANDOM HOUSE CANADA

Copyright © 2005 Miriam Shuchman

All rights reserved under International and Pan-American Copyright Conventions. No part of this book may be reproduced in any form or by any electronic or mechanical means, including information storage and retrieval systems, without permission in writing from the publisher, except by a reviewer, who may quote brief passages in a review.

Published in 2005 by Random House Canada, a division of Random House of Canada Limited. Distributed in Canada by Random House of Canada Limited.

Random House Canada and colophon are trademarks.

www.randomhouse.ca

Library and Archives Canada Cataloguing in Publication

Shuchman, Miriam
The drug trial : Nancy Olivieri and the scandal that rocked
the Hospital for Sick Children / Miriam Shuchman.

Includes bibliographical references and index.
ISBN 0-679-31084-3

1. Pharmaceutical ethics. 2. Drugs—Research. 3. Drugs—Testing.
4. Olivieri, Nancy. 5. Apotex Inc. 6. Hospital for Sick Children.
7. Pharmaceutical industry—Canada. I. Title.

RS100.5.S58 2005   174.2'951   C2005-901457-1

Jacket design: CS Richardson
Text design: Kelly Hill

Printed and bound in the United States of America

10 9 8 7 6 5 4 3 2 1

For my father

CONTENTS

I happened upon this story in the spring of 1998 before it made headlines. I was freelancing for CBC Radio, preparing a documentary on the drug industry's influence over medical research, and got referred to Nancy Olivieri. At first, people were willing to talk to me about Olivieri and her struggle with the drug company, Apotex, which had been funding her research, and I tape-recorded nearly all of my interviews. Later, many of my sources became wary of the tape recorder and of being identified. As a result, this book makes extensive use of off-the-record material.

Here's why. Many of the doctors and scientists who witnessed the events described here feared for their reputations if they were quoted, and some worried that they could be fired from their jobs or sued for libel. As I was conducting my interviews, it became clear that those fears were legitimate. The administration of the Hospital for Sick Children reprimanded some of the doctors involved; Apotex, the drug company that figures in this story, threatened to sue Olivieri; individual doctors at the hospital said they would sue other doctors for libel; Olivieri and a few of her closest supporters filed grievances and harassment charges against a series of hospital administrators; and Olivieri laid legal charges against Apotex, the hospital, the University of Toronto, the CBC and the *National Post*. Apotex subsequently countersued her.

Understandably, people began to think of the Olivieri-Apotex saga as a litigious environment, and doctors and scientists close to the story were reluctant to speak on the record or to be taped. In some cases, the same thing was true of Nancy Olivieri's patients and their families. Given the circumstances, I offered most of those I interviewed the option of speaking off the record, with the understanding that my publisher could contact my sources for fact-checking purposes.

One scientist explained his willingness to be interviewed by saying he'd recently heard Bishop Desmond Tutu speak. Tutu, winner of the Nobel Peace Prize and head of South Africa's Truth and Reconciliation Commission, had a simple message, which the scientist paraphrased: "In any disaster, there must be a telling of what happened in order for people to be able to move on. People have to feel that they've told their stories. There needs to be someone who says, 'Here's the story. It's not a simple one-sided story.'"

The story in this book was a disaster for the Hospital for Sick Children and for several of the physicians and scientists involved. It's also become a disaster for Canadians and Americans who have the blood disorder thalassemia, an inherited disease in which they can't manufacture their blood properly and need frequent transfusions to survive. But Olivieri and her supporters did not take part in the hospital's inquiry (known as the Naimark Review), and the inquiry sponsored by Canada's national organization of university faculty unions—the *Olivieri Report*—didn't hear from hospital and university administrators or company officials. Both efforts were viewed as partisan by one side or the other, and a journalist can be effective in that sort of vacuum. I've spoken with individuals on all sides of this dispute, and I owe you fair warning: it was a complicated process.

When I broke the story on the CBC in August 1998, I portrayed it as I saw it: a terrible tale of a drug company privately flexing its muscles and a brave woman blowing the whistle. The documentary I narrated that September was titled "For Profit or for Patients?" But in researching this book, I discovered new information that didn't match what I'd reported earlier, and as the pieces of the puzzle fell into place I had to discard the idea that this was the straightforward story of the machinations of a powerful company exposed by a whistleblower. That narrative line no longer held. I urge readers to keep an open mind and be prepared to re-examine their own prior notions of this scandal.

In August 1998, a story about a doctor named Nancy Olivieri grabbed headlines in Toronto. The articles stated that Olivieri had discovered serious problems with an experimental drug manufactured by Canada's largest pharmaceutical company, a Toronto-based generics manufacturer called Apotex. The drug at the centre of the scandal is a white tablet called L1, or deferiprone, intended for use by patients with the inherited blood disorder thalassemia. Olivieri planned to tell patients about the problems, as required by her hospital. But Apotex played dirty pool, ejecting her from their research program, cancelling the study she was running to test the drug and threatening her with court action if she went public. The scandal was in the news for months. And for four years, legal charges and personal accusations flew back and forth between Olivieri, the company and Toronto's Hospital for Sick Children, where Olivieri worked.

Parts of this story are well known. The CEO of the drug company Apotex is a billionaire alumnus of the University of Toronto, where Olivieri is a professor. At the same time that Apotex was funding Olivieri to test its drug on patients in a clinical trial, he was offering to put scores of millions toward university research facilities and teaching hospitals such as the Hospital for Sick Children, where Olivieri ran the treatment program for patients with thalassemia. The hospital and the university didn't step in to defend

Olivieri against the company's threats when they arose. Determined to tell her patients and scientific colleagues about her discoveries, she became a whistleblower, publicly accusing Apotex of suppressing her discoveries. She also blamed her home institutions for allowing it to happen because they didn't take up her cause. News of her plight shocked academics, and they sprang to her support. She has won medal after medal for courage.

In 1998, her hospital sponsored its inquiry to figure out what had happened; two years later, Canada's national organization of university faculty associations conducted its own. But the inquirers lacked the power of the coroner or the courts: they couldn't compel disclosure, ensure confidentiality or allow for appeals. John le Carré spoke to Olivieri and spun a fictional account of the events. Casting her as Lara from Leningrad, he wove her into *The Constant Gardener,* his recent novel about the human costs of Big Pharma's corporate greed. Yet the full story of the science scandal that rocked Canada is not as convenient as fiction, and it turns out to be far more shadowy than le Carré imagined.

This is a complex story about medical research and the rules that govern it. Those rules are science's moral code, the standards scientists live by and train under. Here are a few examples: "Don't lie about your work." "Don't steal someone else's work and claim it's your own." "Report your findings; don't bury them." The rules should be easy to follow, but in the fiercely competitive world of modern medical science, they're not.

In studies of new drugs, the research involves patients, so there are additional strictures: "Don't ask patients to volunteer for an experiment that's likely to harm them." "Report the serious side effects of an experimental drug." "Allow patients to drop out of an experiment at any time." The rules for research on humans are discussed in numerous places—the Belmont Report, the Declaration of Helsinki, the Nuremberg Code, National Institutes of Health

(NIH) regulations, Food and Drug Administration (FDA) regulations, Canada's Tri-Council guidelines. They're supposed to be enforced locally by hospitals and universities, and if violations are widespread, federal authorities at the FDA, the NIH or Health Canada can get involved, even to the point of shutting down research at a university.

Yet the rules for doing science aren't well understood, and newer rules about how to conduct research in an era of public-private partnership are still being hammered out, largely as a result of fiascos such as the one I am about to explore. The debacle of Nancy Olivieri and the pill to save thalassemia patients revealed every crack in the system. It is emblematic of what happens when the standards for scientists' behaviour and the lines of institutional accountability are unclear.

The saga also unfolded against the background of an ongoing debate over drug research. Those who want greater protection from risky drugs point to innocent victims killed by dangerous prescriptions and lay those deaths at the feet of profiteering drug companies or unwitting drug agencies that approved products too quickly. On the other side, people with rare diseases for which few treatments are available demand the right to decide for themselves how much risk to bear, and urge drug agencies to speed the approval of products in the pipeline.

But at its core, this is a story of scientific rivalry and revenge. "Good scientists will tell you that being a good scientist requires a very competitive spirit in this day and age," said a sociologist of science, Harriet Zuckerman, in the mid-1980s, around the time that L1 was discovered. "It isn't really clear what the causal relationship is. Maybe you have to be competitive in order to succeed, but maybe succeeding also helps you be competitive."

In the story of Nancy Olivieri and L1, highly successful scientists fought intensely for predominance over a tiny territory—the field of drug treatment for thalassemia. A pharmaceutical company got into the mix and the result was the scientific version of a Greek epic, with researchers battling over ideals, such as the well-being of patients and the integrity of their work, while simultaneously competing against one another for power and position. At first, Olivieri was the epic's heroine, telling the secrets of how her science had been thwarted by her enemies. The ferocity of the drug company's retaliation caught and held our attention. The truth, however, remained obscured until much later, when others emerged to tell the rest of the tale, speaking mostly in whispers to one another. To disentangle a whistleblower's moment from the legend that's grown up around her, we'll need to bring some of those other conversations into the open. Then we may begin to understand what happened here.

I

CHILDREN WHOSE BLOOD DOESN'T WORK

The story of L1 begins—and ends—with sick children. One of these children was Howard, who has suffered from the congenital blood disorder thalassemia for over forty years. Howard's mother first noticed that something was wrong with her son when he was a toddler in the 1960s in Hong Kong. He was jaundiced and sickly. His family soon emigrated to remote Northern Manitoba so that his dad could work with the mining company Inco. While his father learned about the substantial nickel deposit under the ground, his mother worried about how insubstantial her son was becoming. At four he was thin, pale, and underdeveloped for his age, so she took him to the local doctor. When she went for the results of his blood tests, the doctor told her to make the long trek south to Winnipeg. Howard needed to see an expert physician at the university hospital there.

It was an eight-hour drive, rewarded with bad news. Howard had a disease called thalassemia, almost unheard of in Manitoba. His parents didn't know anything about it, but they each carried a gene for it and they'd passed those genes on to their son. "This disease is one of the worst diseases there is," Olivieri told me when I was reporting on her story for CBC Radio in 1998. "It's long-term, it's chronic, it's never-ending . . . Many of the patients develop liver problems and heart problems, and many of them don't grow normally or develop normally."

A child with thalassemia is born without the necessary equipment to make his or her own blood properly. The child's body makes blood, but it's defective because the genes that direct a major step in blood production are mutated. The mutations in the globin genes interrupt the production of the hemoglobin molecule—the part of a red blood cell that carries oxygen. The result is malfunctioning hemoglobin.

Blood cells are produced in the bone marrow. Howard's marrow manufactured red blood cells, but they emerged small and pale, and most died before ever reaching his bloodstream. This left him with severe anemia, accounting for his ghostly pallor. There are many different defects possible in the hemoglobin molecule, and every different foul-up is coded by a separate mutation in the gene, but the bottom line remains the same: the child with thalassemia has blood that doesn't work. Mutated globin genes are so widespread among people of Mediterranean, Middle Eastern and Asian origins that thalassemia is the world's most common single-gene genetic disorder. Biologists have figured out that it's akin to sickle cell disease. In both conditions, the mutation causes severe anemia, yet simultaneously protects a person from contracting the most deadly forms of malaria. The so-called "malaria hypothesis" explains why people are more likely to carry the gene for sickle cell disease or thalassemia if they're from regions infested with malaria-spreading mosquitoes. But both parents have to carry a mutated gene in order for a child to inherit the disease, making it relatively rare in Canada.

Luckily for Howard, the physician in Winnipeg had studied hematology. He'd seen thalassemia before and had learned how the bone marrow and abdomen could be commandeered by troops of defective red cells. In the marrow, the defective cells lead a forcible expansion that deforms a child's bones. This is especially noticeable in the face, where pushed-out bones create distorting bulges.

Doctors used to describe children with thalassemia as having "rodent faces"—a cruel term meaning that they looked like rats. Their teeth stuck out because their jaws were deformed, and their foreheads looked odd because their nasal bridges were flattened instead of making a sharp angle. Their bones were also weak and easily fractured. In the abdomen, the surplus of defective cells collected in the liver and spleen, leaving them chronically enlarged. By the age of six or seven, a child with untreated thalassemia appeared misshapen, with a gargoyle face and thin legs and arms sticking out from a balloon torso that hid an oversized liver and spleen.

Howard was small and thin, weak and tired, but he wasn't yet misshapen or deformed. The Winnipeg doctor explained to his parents that transfusing him regularly with fresh healthy blood would give him back the energy and weight that had been zapped by his anemia and would also prevent fractured bones. The doctor recommended frequent blood transfusions, as often as every month or two.

The family returned to their northern outpost, where the local doctor did what he could to learn more about Howard's rare condition. At one point, the doctor gave Howard's dad some articles about thalassemia from medical journals. He pored over them at the dinner table and then wrote the author of the articles—an American doctor by the name of David Gordon Nathan—to ask for advice.

Nathan was a professor at Harvard Medical School and a specialist in thalassemia. He was then about forty years old and had treated many patients with the disease, becoming quite close to some of them. He wrote back to Howard's worried father to say that the care his son was receiving in northern Manitoba was exactly what would be recommended in Boston. It was the most up-to-date treatment available.

Years later, Nathan described how frustrated he'd been by what he could offer patients like Howard in the 1960s. "By the time these children reached the age of 15 or 16, half of them were dead," he wrote in the journal *Pediatrics*. "And they were all dead before the age of 25." He continued, "The children felt they had no future. They were on a death course, and they knew it, and there was nothing anybody could do about it. This was the state of affairs in 1970."

Howard was doing better than many with thalassemia, and on his steady regimen of fresh blood he grew to look so healthy that his family was able to keep his disease a secret. Unfortunately, the very transfusions that put colour in his cheeks were steering him toward an adolescence and adulthood plagued by disease, for every transfusion was inexorably raising the iron level in his body.

Iron is essential to life. It's loaded into prenatal vitamins, infant formula and cereals to ward off iron deficiency in women and children. But to physicians who treat thalassemia, iron is the agent of death. Their patients must depend on blood transfusions to survive. Over time, the transfusions raise their iron levels to a point that's higher than they can process and iron clogs their vital organs, including the heart and liver. Despite advances in care, individuals with thalassemia can still die in their twenties or thirties, victims of the heart or liver problems caused by an overabundance of iron. In Howard's case, iron already clogged his liver and heart, and also affected his pancreas, causing diabetes.

In Britain, academic pediatricians had faced this problem in the 1960s as they cared for hundreds of children and teenagers with thalassemia whose families had fled war-torn Cyprus for North London. At first, London doctors gave their young patients frequent transfusions, but they found that within a few years the older ones began getting sick from iron overload. When the doctors heard of new medications that might be able to clear out the iron, they began testing them.

The one that seemed to work best was an injection-only drug called Desferal. It attached to iron and pulled it out of a child's body through the urine. But very large quantities of Desferal had to be injected several times a week to achieve this, and these bolus injections were painful. A large-bore needle had to stay jabbed into a child's muscles for minutes at a time. The pain and discomfort were more than some of the younger children could bear. Desferal was enormously expensive as well; its manufacturer, the Swiss drug firm Ciba-Geigy, said the price tag was due to its complex mode of production.

Desferal cemented Ciba-Geigy's reputation as an innovative firm. The company's chemists used the new abilities of chemical engineering and microbiology to grow live fungus in the labs, extract an active chemical agent and isolate it. Then they fermented it, using techniques that were brand-new in the 1960s, and followed that by concentrating, crystallizing and purifying the product into an injectable drug.

Yet some British doctors weren't convinced that the benefits of the drug were worth its costs—in dollars or in their young patients' pain. There was no proof that Desferal would save lives, and children hated the shots. At London's Hospital for Sick Children on Great Ormond Street, physicians argued against using the drug until there was better evidence that it worked. In 1966, they embarked on a study to compare children with thalassemia who received Desferal injections with those who didn't. But a pediatrician working in North London, Dr. Bernadette Modell, wanted every child with thalassemia to get the shots. As a young doctor in training, she'd seen too many children die of the disease and now, as head of her hospital's thalassemia program, she prescribed Desferal to all of the patients.

Modell and the Great Ormond Street doctors were dealing with a classic medical tension. Do you tread the conservative path until it's clear that a new treatment works? Or do you test a new idea, hoping to improve the lot of your sickest patients? In medicine, conservativism has a certain comfort. It's predictable, whereas the unknown can be disastrous. But the outcome of conservative practice for thalassemia was well known: young patients would do well until their teenage years, when they were destined to grow sicker and face early death. Based on preliminary reports, Modell was convinced Desferal was their route to survival and she went ahead and used it while her colleagues across town held back.

By 1972, it was clear that children who got the drug were living longer than those who didn't. Long-term studies such as the one from Great Ormond Street showed that the drug protected children with thalassemia from liver damage. The doubters had the irrefutable proof they'd been waiting for. Most children with thalassemia in London began getting Desferal shots five days a week, and the same regimen was put in place in cities in Italy and Greece that were home to large numbers of children with thalassemia. In Boston, David Nathan jumped on the Desferal bandwagon too. He later wrote of one of his patients that the boy disliked his shots "intensely," but Nathan went ahead with the regimen of daily injections. "David really cared about these families and wanted their treatment to be great," says Darlene Clark Sallan, the nurse in charge of the thalassemia program at Boston Children's Hospital during the early 1970s.

It's not that doctors in Canada didn't care, but few of them knew much about the new drug. In fact, thalassemia was such a rare phenomenon among Canadian children that most doctors knew very little about it at all. In 1973, Howard and his family left Manitoba for the Toronto suburb of Mississauga, but his treatment didn't change. Once a month his mother took him to the local hospital, where the nurses called him Howie and got him to smile and laugh as he waited for the bags of blood to arrive for his transfusion.

Around the same time, a Greek Cypriot family immigrated to the southwestern Ontario city of Kitchener with a two-year-old daughter who had thalassemia. She continued to get regular transfusions as she had in Cyprus, but her doctor also prescribed injections of iron—the girl had anemia, and most children with anemia are iron deficient. He told the girl's parents that she required supplemental iron to stay healthy. It wasn't until the family went home to Cyprus for a visit that they learned from a pediatrician there that the iron injections, combined with the iron the girl was getting with each transfusion, would slowly kill her.

In Scarborough, just east of Toronto, an Italian mother whose four-year-old daughter had thalassemia told the girl's doctor that they would be visiting Italy soon. The doctor warned them about a new drug for thalassemia that was being tested there. He said it was unproven and advised them to ignore what they heard about it. The new drug, of course, was Desferal.

Italy made Desferal shots available to most of the country's thalassemia patients in 1975. Australia followed suit the same year. In 1976, when the Food and Drug Administration (FDA) approved Desferal in the U.S., the drug essentially had the seal of approval from the largest drug agency in the world. The following year, its use was heavily promoted by an editorial in the *New England Journal of Medicine*.

David Weatherall, the author of the editorial, was an Oxford professor and author of the first comprehensive medical textbook on thalassemia. A scientist who broke new ground in the genetics of thalassemia, Weatherall wasn't the sort to advocate early use of a new drug. But Desferal was no longer new, and his editorial left no wiggle room. He wrote that the standard of care for patients with thalassemia had changed. Their treatment couldn't be limited to frequent blood transfusions; they had to be on Desferal too.

In Toronto, as immigrants arrived from Europe, Asia and India, the numbers of children with the disease rose. Typically, they'd be sent to Peter McClure, then the head of diseases of the blood at the Hospital for Sick Children. McClure routinely pulled out the stops to save children's lives, but when it came to patients with thalassemia, his determination was undercut by a dearth of expertise. In the late 1960s, after examining one-year-old twin girls with thalassemia, McClure told their Greek parents to consider heading home. "If you're here, we'll do what we can," he said. "But back in your country, the experience with this disease is much bigger."

At the time, Sick Children's in Toronto was known primarily for its size—it was the largest children's hospital in the world. But studies such as those that focused on leading-edge drug treatments weren't happening in Toronto yet. Then, under a savvy chair of the board named Duncan Gordon, things began changing at Sick Children's. "Gordon knew more four-letter words than anyone else on the board—maybe that's why he ran the place," said one doctor. But Gordon also had a vision. Senior partner in a powerful Toronto accounting firm, he intended to turn the hospital into a great scientific institution. For research manager, he recruited Aser Rothstein, a scientist who'd spent twenty years in Rochester, New York, running a project for the U.S. government on the hazards of radiation. For funding, Gordon tapped the Sick Kids' foundation, where eighty per cent of the endowment was earmarked for research.

From the outset, in 1972, the millions at Rothstein's fingertips surpassed the amount available for research at any other Canadian hospital. His ability to hire scientists was limited only by the amount of lab space available. That wasn't much of a limit at first, since the hospital had just completed a new wing and Gordon had turned the entire area over to research. "We could recruit people from anywhere," Rothstein says, "from the States, from England, from Germany, wherever the best people were." He outfitted their labs, paid for their assistants and generally did what it took to get them to come. "He built a floor—we got a whole extra floor!" says Lou

Siminovitch, who later became director of research at Toronto's Mount Sinai Hospital.

Rothstein had recruited Siminovitch to build up genetic research at Sick Children's, and soon his new floor was filled with young scientists who wanted to use the novel technology of recombinant DNA and needed the space and equipment to do it. Landing junior faculty with the skills to isolate and identify individual genes focused the hospital on forward-looking science and opened a highway between the Hospital for Sick Children and the prestigious medical schools of the United States. Harvard and Johns Hopkins University, especially, lost a series of rising stars to the new kid on the block in Toronto.

The hospital began to catch up to its contemporaries. In infectious disease, Sick Kids went from two part-timers to five full-time staff. Cardiology grew to include seven heart specialists. And hematology grew from a one-man performance to a four-man division. In 1978, the hematologists were invited to collaborate on a Desferal study with doctors at Boston Children's Hospital. "Boston needed larger numbers of patients," explains hematologist Melvin Freedman. "We had them and they didn't." The study involved a new pump system for delivering Desferal. Invented by Richard Propper, a young doctor in Boston, and Dean Kamen, a college drop-out who went on to become a millionaire inventor, the pump was a lot less painful than the original intramuscular needles. It seemed to work, but it still needed testing in a clinical trial. The news that doctors at Sick Kids were inviting kids with thalassemia to join a study reached the Scarborough mother who'd been told to ignore what she heard in Italy. She volunteered her daughter Josie for the research, and the eight-year-old flew to Boston with her dad to learn about injecting Desferal via the pump. But Howard's pediatrician in Mississauga didn't hear about it.

Over the next few years, the Italian community in Toronto nearly doubled. In 1982, when Italy won the World Cup, two hundred thousand soccer fans poured out onto the stretch of St. Clair Avenue known as the "Corso Italia." As traffic ground to a halt, Torontonians discovered that their city now claimed the largest Italian community outside Italy. That same year, the Hospital for Sick Children finally developed its own Desferal program and Howard's doctor signed him up.

By this time, the pump was the preferred method. Half-inch-long needles were inserted just under the patients' skin and taped down. The needles were attached to bulky pumps that sat on their abdomen or thigh and permitted large doses of Desferal to drip in slowly overnight as they slept. Sick Kids had a four-day course to teach patients and their parents how to mix the drug with sterile water, draw it up into a syringe and fill the pump, then inject it under the skin. Howard was a teenager and went alone. He'd been keeping things from his parents and his doctor. He was frequently short of breath and occasionally he would pass out. "I'd be walking and then it was as if my eyes were closed for a few seconds and I'd fall," he remembers. "It was as if someone had pushed me." Howard's heart, under its burden of iron accumulated from fifteen years of monthly blood trans-fusions, was failing him.

Melvin Freedman examined him when he was admitted, as did a young physician who was assisting Freedman, a resident in hema-tology named Nancy Olivieri. The two doctors tapped on Howard's abdomen and discovered that his liver and spleen were both enlarged. They listened to his heart and lungs and got a chest X-ray to confirm their suspicions of congestive heart failure. They did blood tests and discovered that his liver was near the point of cirrhosis. His pancreas wasn't functioning well either: he had diabetes. Iron had choked off his vital organs.

Howard's stay at Sick Children's turned into an attempt to save his life. The cardiologists prescribed digoxin and amiodarone, a new drug that was still experimental, to prevent a heart attack. The endocrinologist began managing Howard's diabetes with insulin. And the young doctor in training, Nancy Olivieri, co-ordinated everyone's efforts. But as Howard's doctors busied themselves consulting the specialists in different services, Howard was left to guess at what was going on. Lonely and confused, and far from the nurses in Mississauga who had become his friends, he called his pediatrician and demanded an explanation. The doctor visited him in the hospital and spoke honestly: Howard was dying from iron overload, but there was a chance he would make it. After a few weeks, he discovered he'd turned the corner when he was moved from intensive care to the hospital's hematology wing.

He didn't have a lot of company and looked forward to his occasional visits with the young doctor assigned to his case. She was extraordinarily attractive, with a petite, perfect figure, a circle of blonde curls enveloping her face and a wonderful, warm smile that seemed to mock him and welcome him into her inner circle at the same time. As far as he could tell, she wasn't much older than he was. In fact, Olivieri was twenty-seven, but Howard wasn't alone in thinking she looked younger than her age. A professor who worked with her that year thought she had a way about her that made her seem fragile and vulnerable. Howard sensed, correctly, that she wasn't a full-blown doctor yet.

Olivieri had completed a residency in internal medicine in Hamilton and a specialty fellowship in hematology-oncology in Toronto. Now she was at Sick Children's for extra training in sickle cell disease and thalassemia—two of the diseases caused by abnormal hemoglobin production. As the resident, she let down her guard a little more than the staff doctors. Howard thought Olivieri and Freedman were night and day as they moved through the hospital wards. With her youth, her high energy and her enthusiasm, Olivieri virtually flew in and out of patients' rooms. She spoke so quickly that Howard couldn't follow her, and neither could Freedman from what Howard could tell. Her words just seemed to bubble over, a fountain of exuberance. He loved watching her. Frequently, she shot him a sideward glance paired with raised eyebrows and a caught-you-in-the-act sort of smile. And she seemed to be always hovering about, checking his lab tests, reading his medical chart or arranging for him to be seen by specialists.

Freedman, with his seniority and more pacific nature, was quiet most of the time. One patient described him as "stoic." A parent of another patient recalled him as "knowledgeable but cool. It was not easy to have a rapport with him." Many of the families addressed Olivieri by her first name, but would never dream of referring to her supervisor as "Mel." Like Howard, most felt immediately comfortable with Freedman's younger assistant. "We had the utmost confidence in Dr. Olivieri," one mother said. Her daughter was diagnosed with thalassemia as a baby and started on Desferal as a preschooler. "She was so tiny, she had to be poked three or four times sometimes, because they had such a difficult time finding veins," her mother recalled. "But if . . . Dr. Olivieri told her she had to do something—have a needle, or try to be very still—she would do it." In appreciation, the mother knit a sweater for Olivieri. In turn, Olivieri found special trinkets for the child.

"She was very caring and also very careful . . . your typical picture-perfect TV-program doctor," was how the patient's mother described Olivieri. Her daughter said that when she was a child in the hospital, Olivieri "made a horrible day so much better because she wasn't just a doctor, she was a friend." Another patient thought of her as "very loving towards her patients."

Howard concluded that Olivieri had saved his life. "There are three things I think I owe my life to after age nineteen," he said,

"Nancy Olivieri, Desferal and amiodarone." He left the hospital after half a year on the wards. At home he found that knowing where to stick the needle and how to attach it to the pump didn't make the drug easy to take. In fact, it was a constant annoyance. When he took the needle out each morning, the site was terribly sore. He couldn't imagine having to stick himself again that same evening. "It was like a seeping wound," he said later. "To be quite frank, it looked like I had urine spots on my shirt. It was disgusting, hot to the touch, throbbing, painful."

Until this point, Howard had managed to keep his disease secret from most people, including his friends. He didn't want his buddies asking why he had spots on his shirt or ugly bumps and swellings on his lower abdomen in the places where he'd injected himself. He hated how sore he was and he hated the pump itself, which sat heavy and thick, pressed against his skin. He wanted to drop it out his bedroom window. Doctors in Athens and London had heard similar complaints from their teenage patients. They'd tried giving Desferal by mouth, but those attempts failed. The drug wouldn't work unless it was injected.

Study after study showed that Desferal was changing the face of thalassemia. It prevented liver and heart disease and kept patients alive. But it worked only if patients took it regularly. Parents could hold down a four-year-old or convince a nine-year-old to have his shots, but many teenagers and young adults skipped their shots for days, weeks and months at a time. They needed a solution that didn't involve an injection.

2

THE MAKING OF A SCIENTIST

Thalassemia was a disease Nancy Olivieri had known her whole life. When she was growing up in Hamilton, Ontario, almost any child with the disorder was a patient of her dad's.

Nancy's medical training differed markedly from her father's. Fernando Olivieri, whom everyone called Red, was a pediatrician and a generalist, while Nancy trained in adult medicine and was on her way to becoming a specialist. But they were alike in a lot of ways. Red's young charges found him bubbly and energetic. Similarly, Howard and many of the young people Nancy Olivieri cared for in the early 1980s described her as "hyper." And patients of both physicians became deeply attached to them.

Red kept a photo in his office of his five daughters. If Nancy, the second eldest, had ever found time to decorate her tiny office space at Sick Children's, she might have tacked a picture of him in between the rows of sticky reminder notes she posted above her computer monitor. She often told people that it was Red who'd inspired her to be a physician. "She idolized her father," said one friend. "She was enamoured of him," said another.

Her mother had a graceful elegance, friends said, that comple- mented her husband's high-strung nature. Victoria Olivieri was a former physiotherapist who made the household rules, kept the peace and attended school functions. But it was Red who coached

8

Nancy to excel in school and in life. Later, she would rarely mention her mum. "Her father was the good guy," said one friend. Another friend said she seemed disappointed in her mother, adding, "She didn't think much of someone who made a career out of looking after children."

When Nancy was small, the Olivieris lived in Hamilton's east end, in the Italian neighbourhood where Red himself had grown up. But the Olivieri girls didn't attend school there. Their mother sent them to the Loretto Academy in the city's west end. It was a strict Roman Catholic girls' school housed in an imposing Victorian building. Classes were small, classrooms were old and decrepit, and many of the nuns who taught there were elderly. The girls wore dull blue dresses with white collars and the school's initials monogrammed on their sleeves. They risked dismissal if they were caught being dishonest or skipped school. But the Loretto sisters stressed education as much as discipline. Nearly all of their graduates went on to college or university, often at Hamilton's McMaster University or the University of Toronto.

After school and on weekends, the nuns offered private piano lessons for an extra fee. Nancy and her sisters became accomplished amateur musicians. In the school's 1965 yearbook there's a photo of the three older Olivieri girls seated on a piano bench in their pinafores after winning medals at the Kiwanis competition and the Canadian National Exhibition. Sixth-grader Nancy is in the middle, with an open smile and wavy hair. Anne, in the eighth grade, is on one side, with the same hair but a less confident smile. On the other side is black-haired Margot, with the toothy grin of an excited third-grader.

The three girls looked remarkably different in the black-and-white photo, and even more different in real life—Anne with her father's bright red hair, Nancy, a strawberry blond, and Margot with her pitch-black bangs. Friends recall them vying with one another at school, and Nancy's younger sisters admit to fighting with her over their toys. But they also remember Nancy's strong efforts to guide them through their school life, as if imitating her father and the mentoring he was giving her.

Her dad treated Nancy differently from her sisters, apparently, and so did her teachers. Of the three older Olivieri girls, it's Nancy whom people from Loretto recall as "a perfect little doll," "very sweet" and "full of life." Olivieri later accepted a journalist's description of her as "a straight-A nerd," but the "nerd" part was a little off, since she always had a circle of friends at school. The "straight-A" label was also misleading. Her high-school grades were in the high seventies and low eighties.

After a few years, her parents moved the family to "the Mountain"—the part of Hamilton where most of the city's doctors lived. It was really the outcropping of the Niagara Escarpment, but it offered its residents stunning views, with the added benefit of being directly behind the major hospitals. But the Olivieris were very protective of their daughters, and a friend of Nancy's from the Mountain said the girls never became part of the neighbourhood social life.

Following graduation, Nancy headed for the University of Toronto, where she did her pre-medical studies, returning three years later to Hamilton and the new experimental medical school at McMaster University. It was a small school where one friend says Nancy became known as a "funny, comical person." She stayed on at Mac to train in internal medicine, and the three years of residency brought a marked change. In what seemed to be an effort to look more mature, Olivieri slimmed down and began dressing more professionally. Her new look was accompanied by a change in demeanour. She became more serious and focused. Her professors saw her as conscientious. One said of her, "As a trainee, her conduct was exemplary . . . We gave her outstanding reviews because she was superb." A fellow resident described her as driven.

During residency, Olivieri applied to spend a year at Toronto's St. Michael's Hospital. Once there, a friend said later, she was "very smart but actually a little bit insecure and intimidated by the whole thing." He thought she had trouble adapting to the larger medical arena of Toronto, and said "she seemed to undervalue herself, constantly apologizing for how little she seemed to know," and presenting herself "in this soft, understated sort of way." Yet, in his view, "she didn't realize how much medicine she knew, and she led the team very well." When she completed residency, she managed to conquer her fears of the larger university. Though the hematologists in Hamilton pressed her to continue her studies there, she decided to do her specialty training in hematology at the University of Toronto. With its multiple teaching hospitals, the U of T was on its way to becoming the largest medical school in North America.

Perhaps because of her relationship with her dad, Olivieri seemed to understand better than most doctors just starting out how crucial a role a mentor could play in her career. She thought highly of doctors she studied under at the Toronto Western Hospital, such as Michael Baker, the chief hematologist there, and worked to build relationships with them.

However, Olivieri spent a year at the Toronto General Hospital during her hematology training, and she let people know she had little respect for the senior hematologists there. Faculty at the General said that they viewed Olivieri as energetic and enthusiastic but lacking in interpersonal skills. At the completion of her time there, a Toronto General physician told her that her behaviour at times surprised him because of the strife it generated. "Are you calling me a flake?" she replied. Subsequently she told Michael Baker about the criticisms she'd received and he duly informed the Toronto General's hematologists that Olivieri refused to accept their evaluation. From then on, it seemed, wherever Nancy Olivieri went, she had both protectors who were charmed by her behaviour and detractors who criticized her.

The final year of her fellowship was spent at Sick Children's, where she raced ahead of Mel Freedman on the thalassemia service. She was the first doctor the patients saw when a crisis brought them into hospital. "I know these patients very well," she said. She knew them so well that if you gave her a patient's name, she could tell you their date of birth and just about everything else about them, since she'd seen them—or their medical records—so many times.

Melvin Freedman was her immediate supervisor, but her mentor at Sick Children's was Freedman's boss, Alvin Zipursky. Zip, as his colleagues called him, had chaired pediatrics at McMaster before stepping down to become head of hematology at the larger medical centre in Toronto. In Hamilton, he'd been friendly with Red Olivieri and he'd known Nancy as a child. Zipursky thought she was a terrific resident. She'd performed well in her patient care duties and she was already starting to do research, acting as the liaison between Toronto and Boston for the Harvard-run trial of the Desferal pump.

Zip complimented her on her work and encouraged her. He and his wife were quite close to her, having her over to their house several times. Zip told Nancy that he wanted her back in his department as a faculty member, practising and teaching at Sick Children's, but that she needed further training. He wouldn't hire her until she'd done a stint at "the bench" by apprenticing in a scientific laboratory. It was what most young doctors interested in university jobs were hearing at the time. He thought she should learn molecular biology, the basic science that would enable her to help figure out the different genetic mutations that caused thalassemia. In a molecular biology lab, Olivieri would master cutting-edge techniques that only a few physicians at Sick Kids knew, which would improve her chances of obtaining a faculty appointment at the university.

Zipursky began working to find her a spot in a productive laboratory and helped her apply for a training grant to cover the costs. She thought she should go to England; he advised Boston, where she already knew some of the clinical thalassemia specialists through her liaison work on the Desferal studies.

Olivieri agreed to head to Harvard for training in a lab headed by hematologist and geneticist Stuart Orkin. Orkin rode the crest of the molecular biology revolution during the mid-1970s, just as that field was exploding with its new-found ability to clone genes. By the late '70s, his lab at Harvard had identified several different mutations responsible for various forms of thalassemia.

In Cambridge, Massachusetts, where Harvard had its undergraduate campus, the mayor held public hearings on gene-splicing, and the town imposed a moratorium on the new genetic research in 1981 because of its presumed dangers. Orkin was in Boston at the medical school, which had set up its own committee to review the new genetic science. But he and his lab partners weren't violating the school's policies and were able to carry on using gene cloning and DNA sequencing to study the way that genes control the body's production of hemoglobin. A few years later, their discoveries would open up the possibility of preventing thalassemia entirely, because knowing the specific mutations made prenatal testing possible. When the test predicted a high likelihood of the disease, parents could choose to terminate the pregnancy. In the Mediterranean, especially Greece and Sardinia, parents began making that difficult choice, and the rates of the disease started to decline.

When Olivieri joined them, the molecular biologists in Orkin's lab were continuing to tease out further mutations in the globin genes. Initially, she spent most of her time just staying afloat. She'd been eager to be at Harvard because of the opportunities there, but she had no advanced degrees in a scientific field, and as a Canadian-trained physician, she had less laboratory training than her

American counterparts. PhD scientists often view MDs as incompetent at science, and Nancy Olivieri's limited science background left her even more vulnerable to being caught on the wrong side of that divide.

"As long as she didn't cause any problems, it was fine," was Orkin's view, according to one person from the lab. Orkin was willing to let her learn, but he wasn't going to start from scratch to teach a doctor how to do science. Olivieri didn't cause problems, but she didn't shine. Orkin and his collection of graduate students concluded that molecular biology—and bench science generally—wasn't her forte. A scientist who knew her in Boston explained, "It's not unusual for somebody who's clinically trained to come into a lab and find they don't get much out of it. Some do well, some don't. She was not a person who was cut out to have a bench career in research." It wasn't meant as harsh criticism; Olivieri was a physician whose strengths lay elsewhere.

After she'd been at Harvard nearly a year, Olivieri was still floundering. "It wasn't where her life should have been," says an individual who observed her in the lab. It must have been unsettling for her, but she faced her tasks in the lab head-on. One of her roles as a research fellow was to design her own research project. She had some genetic information from Canada on a family with thalassemia, and she approached an MD-PhD student working with Orkin, Alan Michelson, about using the information as the basis for a study. She made it clear to him that she was grateful for his help, and he realized that her information might allow them to discover an unidentified mutation in one of the genes for hemoglobin. He sought Orkin's permission to coach her in her project.

Orkin wasn't sure that Olivieri would succeed, even with Michelson's assistance, but he misjudged her determination and tenacity. Together with her new lab partner, Olivieri cloned and sequenced the DNA of the Canadian family. The result was just what they had hoped for: they discovered a new thalassemia mutation. Olivieri presented the finding at a pediatric research meeting in California and got her name on several papers based on work she did in Orkin's lab. But her paper with Michelson was the one she was first author on. It came out in September 1987, in the specialty journal for hematology, *Blood,* with a suitably scientific title—"An Alpha-Globin Gene Initiation Codon Mutation in a Black Family with Hemoglobin H Disease."

Determination aside, Olivieri seemed to realize that she was better at clinical medicine, and she began spending time on the hematology wards at Boston Children's Hospital, making rounds with the doctors there. She got a warm reception and began contributing to discussions of patients' problems. Over time, she built a mentor relationship with David Nathan as she had with Zipursky and Baker. Soon, Nathan and his staff were involving her in their ongoing clinical research projects to assess the patients' progress on various treatment protocols.

She also stayed in close contact with Zip and let him know about the research projects she was participating in at Harvard. He visited her when he was in Boston, and during her second year Zip offered her a job caring for the thalassemia and sickle cell patients at Sick Kids, together with her former boss, Mel Freedman. She flew home to interview for the position, meeting the hospital's research director, Aser Rothstein, for the first time.

Rothstein by now had spent more than a decade building a research empire at the Hospital for Sick Children. "The house that Aser built" was a hugely successful research institute that served as a model for other hospitals throughout the country. Its major impetus was in genetics, and Olivieri was interested in studying the genetics of thalassemia and sickle cell disease. To Rothstein, it was a perfunctory meeting. He had a traditional view of science, one that perpetuated the MD vs. PhD rift. Looking over her c.v., he saw Olivieri as a clinician interested in doing research, not as a laboratory-based investigator.

Like many female physicians of her generation who embarked on careers in academic medicine, Olivieri was hired on the hospital's clinical side. Though she would be on faculty at the University of Toronto, she would be expected to spend the bulk of her hours with patients and students. She wouldn't have protected time to do research the way a laboratory scientist would. With the projects she'd attached herself to in Boston, she might have climbed the academic ladder as a clinical scientist, but clinical research didn't carry the same weight as bench research. At the Hospital for Sick Children, the doctors who studied patients rather than molecules generally didn't have access to Aser Rothstein's phenomenal resources.

Olivieri had done what Zip had advised. She'd apprenticed herself to a molecular biology lab, and she considered herself a scientist. She had authored several articles, she had ongoing collaborations with doctors at Harvard and she was returning to Canada to help lead Toronto's thalassemia service. In July 1986, she began her new job. Olivieri intended to see patients and do research, and the families of children with thalassemia who had known her before she'd gone to Boston were thrilled about it. A member of the clinic staff said, "The sun set and rose on this individual as far as these families and these kids knew."

3

THE ORIGIN OF A DRUG

Howard saw Olivieri during the first few months she was back, in
1986. The years in Boston had changed her, he thought: "She had this
aura of being a lot more confident, this air of being so much more competent and knowledgeable." In the clinic, her first mission was to get the
patients to take Desferal regularly. She pressed Howard about his
missed shots, and he resented it. He was now a man in his twenties, and
he didn't want to be told what to do. "That's never worked on me," he
said. "I do what I want. I have my own mind." The fact that Desferal
was the only drug that could keep him alive over the long term didn't
necessarily mean he would take it. Patients with similar attitudes about
Desferal were stumping thalassemia specialists worldwide.

When people with a rare disease are desperate for new treatments, there's a science establishment that ensures that the search is
on. In the U.S., the establishment involves the National Institutes of
Health in Bethesda, Maryland, the major source of U.S. government
funding for medical research. Even before Howard contemplated dropping his pump out the window, hematologists at the NIH had been
leading the charge to find a drug to replace Desferal. They'd held discussions with Nathan and other leaders in the field, and they'd allocated
money for the effort. The money was announced in RFPs (requests for
proposals) that let scientists throughout North America know that
finding a better drug for patients with thalassemia was a fundable goal.

In the 1970s and the early '80s, the idea that a team of scientists could design a drug using the tools of biotechnology was still new. Scientists seeking a pill for thalassemia typically used one of two conventional methods. Either they went through hundreds of molecular combinations until they found one that gave them the reaction they were looking for, or they identified something close in nature and tried to copy it. The human body evolved with a system for hanging on to its iron because the body needs the mineral to survive. Now scientists were looking for a way to eliminate iron. They thought that by testing thousands of compounds they would find the right one—the compound that would attach to iron in the right form and bring it out of the body in urine or feces.

At the University of California in Berkeley, a biochemistry lab was focusing on soil and the bacteria that live in it. More than 100 million bacteria are found in a teaspoon of soil—some give a garden its earthy smell while others take in iron from the soil. The iron-grabbing species produce chemical compounds to accomplish their mission, and the Berkeley scientists hoped to emulate the bacteria in a test tube and produce the same compounds, much as Ciba-Geigy had replicated the work of a fungus in developing Desferal.

British chemist Robert Hider joined the Berkeley project for a year while he was on sabbatical, and got hooked. He returned to Essex University in England, where he was a lecturer, intent on finding compounds that worked better than the ones he'd tried in the United States. He applied for funds from the British Technology Group (BTG), an arm's-length agency of the U.K. government set up to help academic scientists develop their ideas into profitable products. When his grant came through, he phoned a graduate student at Essex who had done his master's thesis on the biochemistry of hemoglobin, George Kontoghiorghes.

Kontoghiorghes was a Greek Cypriot who had let professors know that he wanted to work on something connected to thalassemia, the disease so devastating in his homeland and he jumped at the chance to join Hider's search for a drug. He'd grown up in Cyprus in the 1960s, one of three boys in his extended family who were about the same age. His two cousins both had thalassemia. One died at seven, the other at nine. Cyprus now delivered high-level care to its thalassemia patients, but they still died in their teens and early twenties, and many of Kontoghiorghes' friends had lost children to the disease. The frequent funerals and the potent images from childhood fed his passion for curing thalassemia, and Hider's call galvanized him into action.

Kontoghiorghes began by following up on leads provided by Hider. Whenever he found himself in a blind alley, he went to the university library and began flipping through the large bound volumes of chemical abstracts. If an abstract looked interesting, he requested the original paper via interlibrary loan. When it arrived, he read it carefully, searching for chemical formulas that might somehow grab onto a molecule of iron. Then he used those formulas to synthesize compounds in the lab. He went through the same process numerous times, combing through published papers, synthesizing chemical compounds and testing them to see if they attached to iron. It was arduous work, and none of his attempts were successful.

After several months of fruitless effort, Hider heard from another lecturer at Essex that a compound called maltol, a fruity-smelling chemical used as a flavour enhancer, could bind to iron. "This gave us the idea to look for related nitrogen compounds," Hider says. Renewing his search, Kontoghiorghes found a set of abstracts on a veterinary drug called mimosine that had been studied in the mid-1970s in Australia, Japan and Taiwan. He was convinced he had finally found the right direction.

Mimosine was isolated in an Australian veterinary laboratory by chemists seeking a replacement for clipping shears. When sheep and goat farmers fed mimosine to their animals, the animals shed their fleece. The drug worked because it prevented the animals' hair follicles from producing DNA. Specifically, it attached itself to enzymes involved in DNA synthesis. The enzymes turned out to contain metallic elements and Kontoghiorghes and Hider deduced that mimosine might be capable of attaching to iron.

The veterinary drug wasn't hard to come by. Kontoghiorghes and Hider found they could purchase it from a chemical manufacturer, and they began making compounds related to it. In biochemical terms, the compounds were "ligands," since they would bind to other molecules such as iron. Kontoghiorghes tested the compounds, and soon they had seven chemicals that could bind to iron. He was overjoyed, and not just because his doctoral work was succeeding. Beatrix Wonke, a London thalassemia expert, explained, "When you are a Cypriot, you see a little island with so many children dying. And then suddenly, as an analytic chemist, you find something in a test tube! And this could change the world!"

Kontoghiorghes numbered the compounds from one to seven, calling them "ligand 1," "ligand 2" and so on, referring to them in shorthand as L1 through L7. He described the compounds at a meeting in Japan in 1981, and the description formed the basis for his doctoral thesis.

The next step was to test the compounds further to see if any of them could be used as a drug, but as chemists, Hider and his colleagues couldn't do that alone. They needed to collaborate with a physician, and they had to act quickly because the race to replace Desferal with a pill was building. They were up against several teams already, including the chemists at Ciba-Geigy headquarters in Switzerland. Desferal was now Ciba-Geigy's fifth leading product, earning the company US$400 million annually. Rather than risk losing that market, Ciba-Geigy was putting its own research and development funds toward the search for a pill.

Hider described the situation to his sponsors at BTG. The British funding agency was designed to stimulate public-private partnerships, but it also functioned as a patent and licensing agency. BTG's lawyers did the legwork of applying for a patent on the ligands, and the patent—a limited one—came through in 1982. As Hider explained, "The difficulty with the L1 patent was always that it was not a new compound. It had been made by others and all we could do was patent the medical use of the compound." Hider and Kontoghiorghes then assigned BTG their intellectual property rights. If one of the ligands succeeded as a drug, BTG would license the patent to a private company for development, and if the drug wound up on the market, BTG would return part of the profits to Essex University in the form of royalties. The university, in turn, had agreements with Hider and Kontoghiorghes.

Though this sort of arrangement was still relatively unusual when Hider and Kontoghiorghes entered into it, it would become increasingly common over the next decade. In the U.S., the Reagan administration was embarking on an economic strategy that directly involved university-based scientists. The way to stop losing jobs to other countries, the Reaganites said, was to harness the profit-making potential of professors' discoveries. They argued that many scientific inventions lay hidden away in the back recesses of American university laboratories, unpatented and underdeveloped. To move inventions out of the ivory tower and into the marketplace, the government had to encourage it. In 1980, Congress took a first step in that direction: the Bayh-Dole Act, also known as the Patent and Trademark Amendment Act, a law that encouraged universities to turn their professors' research into patents. Patents in hand, a university could invite private companies or investors to commercialize the results, and the university would benefit via royalties on the invention. Essentially, Bayh-Dole laid out new duties for university scientists—they were supposed to invent things that could turn a profit for American investors.

The door was open between academia and industry, said MIT professor Charles Weiner. "Virtually overnight, academic biologists never before involved with industry have become consultants, advisors, founders, equity holders and contractees of new biotechnology firms or new divisions of multinational corporations," he wrote in 1986. Al Gore accused Congress of selling the tree of knowledge to Wall Street. Similar concerns could be heard at U.S. universities, where some academics argued that once industry arrived on campus with its for-profit ethos, they would lose the freedom to research any scientific question, no matter how basic. Yet over the course of the next decade, Congress would pass more than a dozen pieces of legislation aimed at restructuring U.S. science and technology policy in order to move ideas into the marketplace.

The debate that raged in the 1980s over professors and their sponsors foreshadowed a chaotic environment for science on both sides of the academia-industry divide. U.S. lawmakers had assumed that the products of academic research would translate into high-tech jobs and boost the economy. First, however, the new laws boosted the financial status of universities. With federal dollars for science dwindling, the industry funds promised by Bayh-Dole were a windfall. Partnerships sprung up, linking major research institutions to multinational pharmaceutical companies, and small teaching hospitals to local entrepreneurs. The media spoke of a technology transfer boom and a patent craze; the role of the universities was to keep it booming and crazy. Buildings designed to house joint university-industry research were constructed with industry funds; campus development officers wooed private companies for research grants and outright gifts; universities created centres to support professors' entrepreneurial activities; and technology transfer offices were set up to systematically turn discoveries on campus into patent applications. These efforts had measurable results: the amount of private dollars flowing into academic science rose steadily, as did the rate of university filings at the Patent Office.

But old codes of conduct no longer applied, new standards hadn't been written, and behaviour began to break down. In 1986, Harvard researcher David Blumenthal revealed publicly what scientists knew privately: biologists were beholden to their corporate benefactors. In a survey, 24 per cent of life scientists at major universities said that they couldn't publish their research results without the consent of their commercial sponsor, and nearly half acknowledged that industry sponsorship undermined their intellectual exchange of ideas with colleagues. Though it wasn't clear how scientists or their sponsors were supposed to behave, free and open inquiry was a basic tenet of universities, and it, at least, had been upended. Over the next few years, American universities began to experience the other side of the boom—disputes in court with professors who were patent holders, battles with federal agencies over contracts with Big Pharma and the emergence of a cadre of whistleblowers who feared that the various confidentiality and do-not-publish clauses they were asked to accept as a basic condition of research funding were placing the public at risk.

In Britain, the debate was more muted because the door hadn't opened quite as wide. BTG was a path through which professors connected with industry, but it had been around for decades and wasn't the focus of new worries. George Kontoghiorghes said he hoped BTG would "take the thing forward, that it would be a fast-moving way of getting a drug." Bob Hider appreciated the agency's support and was sure its funds would help when he and Kontoghiorghes went looking for a physician. They started with Bernadette Modell, the London thalassemia specialist. By this time she had left medical practice to become a public health scientist, and drug development wasn't her line of work. When they explained what they wanted, she referred them to Ernest Huehns, a physician at London's University College Hospital who had experience studying animal models of thalassemia. Huehns readily agreed to work with the team from Essex.

Kontoghiorghes headed for London and soon began testing the ligands in cell cultures in Huehns's lab. The work went well, and he moved on to mouse and rabbit models. In mice, he was able to show—to his own satisfaction—that one compound in particular increased the excretion of iron significantly. It was the first ligand, L1.

Despite his productivity at University College, Kontoghiorghes began to feel unhappy about his status as Huehns and Hider's post-doc, and he resented their ties to BTG, with its focus on L1's potential as a profitable drug. BTG had advised them to keep information about L1 private until they could get a company interested in commercializing it, but Kontoghiorghes thought that dictate was blocking the drug's development and undermining his scientific career. He was friendly with leaders of the U.K. Thalassemia Society, fellow Cypriots whom he often talked to—in Greek—about their family members with the disease. "I explained to them that I couldn't publish with the situation in University College Hospital and Essex," Kontoghiorghes says. "And they said the only way to move forward with this is to forget all about it and start publishing all the materials you have at hand." They arranged for him to speak with a solicitor about his situation.

Fifteen years later, doctors from Harvard would argue that universities need to adopt explicit safeguards around partnerships with industry to ensure that academia's most vulnerable and dependent members, namely students and post-docs, are able to publish their results freely and without delay. But those sorts of safeguards weren't even being thought of when Kontoghiorghes pleaded for the right to make the findings on L1 public. He expected Hider and

Huehns to persuade BTG that he needed to publish his work. But they didn't, and he later claimed they took credit for work he'd done—for example, by putting Hider's name first on the L1 patent, instead of his. "Dr. Hider was not involved with the invention of L1 itself," he said in an interview. Hider describes himself as the drug's lead inventor and wrote me, ". . . many academics in my position wouldn't even have included George on the patent."

Hider wasn't as keen as Kontoghiorghes about the drug. Certain aspects of the L1 molecule bothered him. As the senior and more experienced scientist on the project, he worried that L1 could cause free radicals—highly reactive molecules that catalyze chemical reactions, injuring cells and interfering with DNA. Huehns and others in the lab agreed with him. They wanted to send the experimental compound out to a commercial toxicology lab for further evaluation, and they also planned to test other compounds and compare them to L1. "We felt that L1 was not the best compound, and we wanted to make a better compound," says Hider. But Kontoghiorghes didn't think they needed to involve commercial labs, and he disagreed with his partners that a different compound could work better.

The team began to fall apart. They'd begun by racing against other scientists to find a pill for thalassemia; now they were competing with one another for control of their project, and the politics were intense. Reflecting on that period of his life, George Kontoghiorghes says, "Unfortunately, in the academic world, there's a lot of infighting." In this case, after several months, Hider let Kontoghiorghes know that the British Technology Group would soon discontinue funding his salary through the university. The drug-discovery whiz kid was losing his job.

Kontoghiorghes was incensed, but he was also resourceful. He told the U.K. Thalassemia Society about his unemployed status, and the Society promised to pay for his continued work. With funds in

hand, Kontoghiorghes left University College Hospital for its nearby rival, the Royal Free Medical School, where he got a spot in a
hematology lab and continued to test L1. He also began writing
papers to describe his tests of L1 and the other ligands. He says he
was following the advice he received in his meeting with the solicitor. But he was also trying to protect his claim to a drug that, in his
view, he'd discovered.

"Scientists today don't make discoveries, they publish papers,"
medical historian Joel Howell of the University of Michigan
quipped in an interview. Historians and philosophers of science
write treatises on the process of scientific discovery, of course, yet
Howell's brief point is actually a serious one: when a scientist
doesn't author a paper on a research project it's almost as if the scientist never did the project in the first place. Papers aren't only a
way for scientists to communicate their findings, they're a major
tool for seeking status. The person whose name comes first—the
lead author—gets the most credit.

Kontoghiorghes was first author on two papers he wrote about
L1, but he acknowledged some of his collaborators, attaching
Hider's name and the names of one or two other scientists he had
worked with onto the manuscripts. Then he submitted one to a biochemistry journal. In the fall of 1984, he wrote Hider about the
papers and sent him copies of them, but his former supervisor found
"a number of difficulties" with both. Hider took the unusual step of
withdrawing one paper from the journal it had been sent to, the
Journal of Inorganic Biochemistry, and he wrote Kontoghiorghes that "as
senior author," he also didn't want to submit the second manuscript.
He objected to the way the papers were organized and to the order
of the authors, writing Kontoghiorghes, "We should adopt the normal procedure of the authors being presented in alphabetical order."

Normal procedure at the time was unclear. Sometimes the person who had done most of the work came first and the senior

author came last; in other cases, the first named author was the person who'd had the original idea. Authorship disputes became so common over the next decade that, by the mid-1990s, journal editors had begun to hash out clear rules for scientists to follow in assigning who came first, second and last in a list of authors of a scientific paper.

At the Royal Free, Kontoghiorghes was working under Victor Hoffbrand, its renowned chair of hematology. The author of over three hundred journal articles and textbook chapters, Hoffbrand had built his department into the academic powerhouse of hematology in Great Britain. Now, Hider sent him a copy of his correspondence with Kontoghiorghes, and Huehns also spoke to Hoffbrand about it, yet Hider said later that Hoffbrand barely responded to them. Asked about it years later, Hoffbrand recalled that he felt "that it was sort of a matter between them and Kontoghiorghes."

Less than six months later, Kontoghiorghes wrote a letter about L1 to the editors of the *Lancet*, Britain's leading medical journal, saying the drug showed "no apparent toxic effects in animals." He was the letter's sole author, though he credited the U.K. Thalassemia Society for its support. In Essex, Hider read Kontoghiorghes' letter to the editor and scowled. The younger man hadn't credited Hider or Huehns, even though his letter seemed to refer to experiments they had collaborated on. He didn't mention their institutions or BTG either. "Kontoghiorghes was publishing the work of others without giving them credit," says Hider. Kontoghiorghes disputes the claim, saying that because of his conflict with Hider, he didn't publish data they had gathered together. "We disagreed on everything, basically," he told me. "So I did the work with different animals . . . at the Royal Free and I published as soon as I had the results."

Hider and Huehns wrote Hoffbrand again. "We have just seen the letter from Dr. G. Kontoghiorghes," they began, and proceeded to name all the individuals they felt should have been co-authors of the letter to the editor. They asked Hoffbrand to write the *Lancet* "setting the record straight," but Hoffbrand continued to view it as a situation that didn't involve him or his department. He also felt supportive of some of Kontoghiorghes's arguments and wrote Huehns, "George seems to have done research over many years with no publications to show for it. He is extremely insecure about this and in having no permanent post and having to rely on grant applications for support." Hoffbrand thought that a letter to the editor "may be more excusable than unacknowledged articles," and urged Huehns to contact Kontohgiorghes.

Over the next two years, Kontoghiorghes published studies showing that L1 was non-toxic when tested in cell cultures, safe and effective when used in rabbits and similar to Desferal when tried in rats. In the end, the only scientific publication that would ever include his name together with Hider's and Huehns's would be the abstract for his first presentation in Japan in 1981. Hider exchanged letters with Hoffbrand in 1986 and 1987, complaining that the names of several students had been left off Kontoghiorghes's papers, and Hoffbrand replied that he was encouraging Kontoghiorghes to get together with Hider and Huehns "to get published jointly all the work that was done before George joined our department." But he also couldn't understand the arrangement Hider had with BTG, and wrote him, "I find it quite difficult to get a coherent message about why work performed up to five years ago has not been properly published."

At the time notions of scientific misconduct were vague. Failure to give credit where credit is due is a scientific wrong, but in the mid-1980s, few institutions had procedures for responding to those sorts of allegations. (Today, nearly all do.) Hoffbrand didn't refer Hider or Huehns to the dean of his medical school, or to any other office, where they could formally charge Kontoghiorghes.

The courts could intervene to protect a scientist's intellectual property, but Hider didn't sue. Though he held the patent on L1 along with Kontoghiorghes, the patent applied only to the use the ligands, not to the ligands themselves. At the Royal Free, Kontoghiorghes essentially circumvented the patent by publishing a new, unpatented formula for making L1. The new method was simpler and cheaper, and Kontoghiorghes published it in two different chemistry journals, thereby placing it in the public domain and devaluing its commercial potential. Long before the idea of "open access" to science was popular, Kontoghiorghes was already thwarting the motive behind agencies such as BTG. He wasn't interested in profiting from his formula; he wanted it to be used.

Hider's only recourse was to let other thalassemia researchers know his version of what had happened between himself and the younger researcher. As every experienced scientist knows, spreading that sort of story has a certain power. In Boston, for example, David Nathan took Hider's side in the dispute; in his 1995 book about thalassemia, he described George Kontoghiorghes as "unwise and impetuous" and cast aspersions on Hoffbrand. Soon doctors at the Royal Free Hospital were also questioning Kontoghiorghes about his claims, and his answers didn't quash their concerns. In one case, a senior hematologist who was collaborating on animal studies of L1 became worried when rodents on the drug began to salivate heavily. "I don't know what it signified," says Hoffbrand, "but it may have signified that it tasted awful to the animals." It needed to be investigated and explained because it could be a serious side effect, but when the hematologist raised his concerns at a research meeting, Kontoghiorghes retorted that there was nothing wrong with the animals.

Hoffbrand acknowledged to others that he thought Kontoghiorghes was "a difficult character," but he attributed the young man's difficulties to his intense commitment to the work.

Hoffbrand's friends say that he tried to place limits on Kontoghiorghes but felt he had to be diplomatic. Kontoghiorghes was enthusiastic about L1, but he could also be forceful and aggressive. Hoffbrand didn't confront Kontoghiorghes directly, one friend says, because he couldn't tolerate a shouting match.

In the end, Hoffbrand responded to worries about the zealous young chemist by taking the time to review the data on L1 himself. The chair found no evidence of serious toxicity, so Kontoghiorghes kept on testing the drug. Soon he was urging Hoffbrand to let him test it on humans, and in 1986, Kontoghiorghes and Hoffbrand took the first step toward human studies, applying to the British Department of Health and Social Security for permission to test an experimental drug. The federal authorities issued a certificate permitting human testing of L1 at the Royal Free, and when Kontoghiorghes and Hoffbrand approached their hospital's ethics committee, the committee allowed the request to go forward. Bob Hider was aghast when he learned that a human trial was being considered, since, in his view, the necessary toxicity studies—carried out in several species of animals—hadn't been done.

The research subjects were three men in their seventies and eighties with a cancer of the blood called myelodysplasia. All three required multiple transfusions to survive and, as in thalassemia, the transfusions overloaded their bodies with iron. Hoffbrand, an expert on their disease, thought the men had very few treatment options. Kontoghiorghes gave the trial participants their gelatin capsules of L1 once a day before breakfast. On the second day of the trial, Hoffbrand visited one of the patients on the ward. By the side of the man's bed he saw a large flagon of brown fluid. As soon as he spotted it, he knew L1 was working. Iron was the only product that could have discoloured a patient's urine so dramatically and so quickly.

The team measured the amount of iron each patient excreted and published the results in the *Lancet* in June 1987. "This preliminary study demonstrates the efficacy . . . of . . . L1 in man," they wrote. Now they were ready to test the drug on patients with thalassemia. But before they began, the doctor in charge of the Royal Free's thalassemia clinic, Beatrix Wonke, said she wanted to test L1 by taking it herself. Wonke said later, "You can't just give patients anything." She thought L1 was bitter and awful-tasting. Kontoghiorghes agreed it was bitter, having tasted it himself. "The drug could have been killed there and then," he said. But it wasn't. Instead, says Wonke, the researchers were "very careful to put it in capsules in such a form that the patients didn't have to taste it."

During the spring and summer of 1987, four thalassemia patients who weren't very good at taking their Desferal started on L1. When the patients came into the Royal Free for their regular transfusions, Kontoghiorghes collected samples of their blood and urine. By the fall, he was tabulating the data. There was no question in his mind that L1 worked.

The best place to present new findings about treating thalassemia is at the annual meeting of the American Society of Hematology, the major professional organization in the field. Nancy Olivieri had been attending the meeting since the early 1980s, when she began her hematology training in Toronto. She and her colleagues referred to the organization by its acronym. "I'll see you at ASH," they'd tell each other. The annual meeting was always in December and usually in a warm spot.

In December 1987, before an audience of about two thousand hematologists in San Antonio, Texas, including Olivieri and Melvin Freedman, Kontoghiorghes presented a paper with the marked before-and-after contrast that he was so proud of: a bright yellow slide showing a patient's urine before ingesting L1, and a red slide showing the patient's iron-filled urine after. Though these patients had received only a few doses of L1, the drug clearly pulled iron out of the body. The paper was published in the *British Medical Journal* that same month. It concluded that L1 was "highly effective" and "without obvious toxicity short term." Among doctors treating thalassemia, word was spreading quickly that L1 worked. Patients could avoid all-night-long injections and just take a capsule, or a few capsules, instead. They also heard that L1 had clear advantages over Desferal: it could be supplied for less than half the price and without the extra cost of the pumps.

Suddenly, George Kontoghiorghes was spending a lot of his time on the phone, talking to physicians as well as patients and their families. "I was receiving inquiries from all over the world," he recalls. The chemist said he offered to collaborate on studies with doctors from other hospitals who wanted to use the experimental drug and he told them how to make it, explaining that the process was available to anyone because he had published it. Doctors in India and Europe began putting patients on L1. For Kontoghiorghes, winning the race to replace Desferal meant making L1 available as widely and as cheaply as possible. He intended to be generous with the invention—a generosity that dovetailed neatly with his disagreements with Hider and Huehns. As doctors in India and Europe began making L1 and giving it to patients, they chipped away at Hider's claim to the drug as his intellectual property.

Victor Hoffbrand began to get worried. Though he thought L1 was safe, it was an experimental chemical compound, approved by British authorities only for use at the Royal Free Hospital in London. Yet apparently Kontoghiorghes was telling doctors who wanted to collaborate with him how to make the drug for use in patients. Hoffbrand said, "This was a risky business, with a drug that was barely ethically approved and barely licensed." It was especially risky since Kontoghiorghes himself wasn't a doctor. Kontoghiorghes contends that the only way he worked with doctors from India or Europe was in research collaborations, and he adds, "I never gave the drug to any clinician without getting permission from their ethical committee copied to me."

To prove a drug's value, doctors have to do more than test it in a handful of patients. Drug research is governed by a three-phase system. After pre-clinical testing in animals, an experimental compound is moved into human trials. The first phase is an initial study involving a small number of patients who take the drug for a short period of time. The aim is to check for side effects and to figure out the size of dose to use in order for the drug to be effective without causing serious problems. Phase 1 studies also give researchers an opportunity to study what happens to the drug once it's ingested—how it's metabolized, how much of it gets into the blood and how much of it is excreted. Phase 2 trials involve more patients taking the drug for a longer period to assess its long-term effectiveness and safety. Phase 3 studies can include even greater numbers of patients in trials aimed at deepening the understanding of the drug's safety and effectiveness at different dosages or in different settings.

A drug usually won't be submitted for licensing to the drug regulatory agencies until all three phases of study are completed, and Kontoghiorghes's colleagues at the Royal Free thought they were still completing the first phase. With tensions mounting, the Royal Free group agreed to run a long-term clinical trial along the lines of a Phase 2 trial. Kontoghiorghes wanted to be in charge of it, but some of the hematologists collaborating on the work didn't think non-physicians were qualified to run a clinical trial.

Hoffbrand thought he could contain the conflict by planning two papers at the trial's outset: a scientific paper with Kontoghiorghes as its lead author and a separate clinical report with a hematologist's name in the lead spot. That way, a hematologist in the department could run the trial but Kontoghiorghes would be assured of being first author on one of the papers.

Kontoghiorghes was worried about getting credit for his work, but he also wanted a say in designing and running the L1 trials, and Hoffbrand didn't offer that. Though the junior partner went along with the plan for collaborating with the hematologists, he wasn't as comfortable at the Royal Free as he had once been.

In the early winter of 1988, Hoffbrand flew to Toronto for a week-long stay as a visiting professor in hematology at the University of Toronto. Some of the talks he gave involved his research on the treatment of leukemia, but he also spoke on L1. Nancy Olivieri was in the audience, listening closely. The new compound had caught her interest when she had heard Kontoghiorghes speak at ASH. Now, at a restaurant dinner to fete Hoffbrand, Olivieri asked Melvin Freedman to introduce her. Later, Olivieri sat at Hoffbrand's side, peppering him with questions; her excitement about the new drug was unmistakeable.

After the dinner, she asked Hoffbrand if she could send someone from Toronto to learn more about L1. He said he'd welcome it, so she followed up with a phone call to Kontoghiorghes, who told her he'd be happy to show one of her assistants how to make L1 in the lab. Kontoghiorghes explained later, "All this information I had I used to give to everyone, because I thought the only way to go forward with the drug was for hematologists to work with it."

Kontoghiorghes had been trying to move forward with the drug from the time he and Hider had first begun looking for a chemical that would bind iron. But their progress had faltered amid professional jealousies and personal distrust. L1 thus began its unusual course, bouncing from University College, where it entered animal studies, to the Royal Free, where it made its debut as an experimental drug for humans, and from there to India and Europe, where it was eventually used both inside and outside of experimental protocols. Kontoghiorghes gave out information about the drug for free, but the stories surrounding L1 engendered suspicions. With clinical trials in thalassemia patients scheduled to begin, the pill was already dogged by controversy.

There wasn't much else on the horizon, however. In the spring of 1988, BTG co-sponsored a workshop with Ciba-Geigy to discuss promising alternatives to Desferal. Several different compounds were being tested in the U.S., the U.K. and Europe, but none of them had been subjected to formal toxicity studies, and testing them in humans seemed a long way off. Moving a product beyond small laboratory studies was simply too expensive. Governments weren't willing to pay the costs, and the drug industry wasn't interested either.

The doctors treating thalassemia were intensely interested, though. And George Kontoghiorghes's unpatented formula for making L1 was already published and available to anyone who wanted to try it—including Nancy Olivieri.

4

PUTTING TOGETHER HER TEAM

Olivieri's first year back in Toronto wasn't easy. Zipursky had arranged for her to have the spot she wanted, with clinical responsibilities for thalassemia and sickle cell patients and research space in a lab. But on her own, away from the support structure of Orkin's lab and the tutelage of Alan Michelson, her laboratory projects didn't always go as she'd hoped. Yet, buoyed by her previous successes, she was presenting at all the major meetings and her work from Boston was being published in important journals. In 1986, she was first author on a paper that put the fledgling thalassemia program in Toronto on the map. "Our reputation began to spread nationally and internationally," says Mel Freedman.

The paper stemmed from Olivieri's clinical experience in Toronto. The mother of one of the thalassemia patients had called in a panic, worried that her child was going deaf. The four-year-old girl had been turning her head sideways while watching television, so that one ear was aimed at the set, as if she could hear in that ear. By the next morning, it seemed as if she couldn't hear at all. Olivieri had the girl examined by the hospital's hearing specialists and told the mother to stop giving her daughter Desferal.

Freedman and Olivieri had been experimenting with higher and higher doses of Desferal, hoping that early, intensive use of the drug would give young patients a better chance for the future. As one thalassemia nurse put it, it was the philosophy of "some was good, more must be better." Hematologists in Boston and other major centres were also using high-dose Desferal on their thalassemia patients. The higher doses appeared to have certain benefits, but they were also more likely to cause side effects. There had already been reports that the drug caused blindness, which meant it could be toxic to the brain. In that case, Desferal might be linked to the little girl's hearing loss.

Inquiring among the patients, the clinic staff quickly learned of several other young patients with possible side effects. In one family, a five-year-old girl went nearly blind in one eye four months after starting on Desferal. Two months later, her three-year-old sister also had serious vision problems. Both girls then developed hearing difficulties and became clinically deaf. Olivieri and Freedman determined that it was the Desferal and that the drug probably was neurotoxic at high doses. Nearly eighty patients were being treated with monthly transfusions and nightly Desferal injections through Sick Children's thalassemia program; the doctors arranged for all of the patients to be tested by neurologists, ear, nose and throat specialists and eye doctors. They also got in touch with Ciba-Geigy, and the company provided funding to support their investigations.

Olivieri took the lead in writing up the results of these tests, and the report was published in the *New England Journal of Medicine* in the spring of 1986. Interviewed by the *Toronto Star* when the study came out, Freedman said, "This drug, prior to our discovery of its toxic side effects, was felt to be one of the safest drugs in the pharmacy, so we tried to improve the iron removal by escalating the dose." But as they reported in the study, the higher doses led to visual loss or deafness in thirteen of eighty thalassemia patients. The problems were most serious for the youngest children—the group whose parents had been the best at making sure the drug was administered every night. Though the doctors stopped the drug, resuming it only at lower doses, several young patients were left with permanent damage. Three of the girls had hearing loss, and one remained blind in one eye.

Olivieri and Freedman established firmly that high doses of Desferal should be avoided due to serious toxicity. Their adroit handling of the situation went beyond protecting their young patients. By sounding the alarm about high-dose Desferal and backing it with solid research, they ensured that doctors everywhere were more careful with the drug. Their article in the *New England Journal of Medicine* set a world standard and would be referred to repeatedly by physicians treating thalassemia. As its first author, Olivieri raised her profile in a way that was crucial for her career. She had published a paper that would change practice in her small field.

She was beginning to build a name for herself as a rising star in Boston and Toronto, and that helped her solidify her close relationships with several of the major players in her area of research. In Canada, Olivieri was close to a few leading hematologists, including Baker and Zipursky. In the U.S., she'd worked to maintain her friendship with David Nathan, who served on the editorial board of the *New England Journal of Medicine* and reviewed grants for several agencies that funded research in thalassemia. Olivieri had grown close to Nathan by working in his division and through her ongoing collaborations with his department, but officially she wasn't his student—she didn't spend time in his lab or train clinically in his department. That turned out to be a mark in her favour, for Nathan wasn't obliged to excuse himself from peer reviewing her papers or grant applications as he might be if she'd been his doctoral or post-doctoral student. "I wasn't Nancy's mentor," he told journalists and journal editors. That meant he could recommend her and her work freely. From time to time, he would put in a good word for her and his influence was such that his praise could go a long way to boost her reputation.

Olivieri won support from such men as Zipursky and Nathan, but other prominent doctors found her hard to deal with. In Toronto in the summer of 1986, Nancy Olivieri's initial interaction with her new boss—Sick Kids' chief of pediatrics, Bob Haslam—was so off-putting that he recalled it years later as if it had just happened. Haslam had just arrived at Sick Kids after spending eleven years as chair of pediatrics at the medical school in Calgary. He met Olivieri when she appeared at his door to discuss a research grant and asked him to sign off on her grant application. Haslam told her he would read it as soon as he could. She responded that he didn't need to read it, just sign it—and soon, please, because she needed to mail it that night. Sick Kids, like almost all teaching hospitals, required doctors to have the approval of their department head before studies were carried out. Some department chairs might sign off on proposals in a pro forma manner, but Haslam said he couldn't put his name on something he hadn't read. He told her he would read it, sign it and take it to the post office himself to be sure it made its deadline. Olivieri asked him again to simply sign the proposal.

Haslam had plenty of experience with the grant-writing process from his time as department chair in Calgary and before that as director of a renowned treatment centre at Johns Hopkins University, and again he insisted on reading Olivieri's grant. Finally they agreed that he would read it at home that night and bring it back to the hospital the next morning. In the future, he told her, it would expedite the process if she gave him a few days' notice.

Olivieri had already been talking to David Nathan about the test of L1 she wanted to undertake with the patients. She said she thought she could do a better human study of L1 than the group in London, and he agreed with her. Despite his deep reservations about the drug, Nathan had come to think that it deserved another chance in a new environment.

She also raised the idea of testing L1 with Freedman, whose own energies were focused on his research on bone marrow transplantation. If a matching donor could be found, marrow transplants offered a possible cure for a small number of patients. But the risks were high. More than one child got worse after a marrow transplant, or died. Freedman agreed to support Olivieri's project to study the new drug.

And Olivieri had a new mentor at the hospital, Gideon Koren, a faculty member in clinical pharmacology and toxicology. Gidi, as she and everyone called him, was a native Israeli who had immigrated to Canada in the early 1980s. In Israel he had been a practising pediatrician as well as a performer who was heard frequently on the radio, telling children's stories and singing funny songs. In Canada he became a star in the new field of pediatric toxicology.

Koren had arrived in Toronto to do a pharmacology fellowship just as Sick Kids was emerging from a scandal involving the deaths of more than thirty babies on the cardiac ward. Police charged a young nurse with homicide, saying she'd poisoned the babies with injections of the heart drug digoxin. But the nurse was found to be innocent, and teams of investigators then descended upon Sick Children's to figure out just what—or who—had claimed the children's lives. Gideon Koren, while still in training, got the attention of his colleagues by helping to develop a better method of detecting digoxin in the body.

His training finished, he went on staff at Sick Kids. Within a few years, he had a hospital-wide reputation as a doctor who was pioneering the study of the effects of medications on children. In addition to his experience designing drug trials, he was expert at the specialized techniques required for determining how quickly a drug entered and filtered out of bodily fluids (an area known as pharmacokinetics) and at toxicology. It was in that context that Nancy Olivieri first approached him looking for research guidance. What she found, according to several observers, was close counsel and mentoring.

Olivieri admired Koren's research expertise, while he, like Zip and Nathan before him, thought she was a wonderful person to work with. In the late 1980s, shortly after she won a major grant from the Medical Research Council, Olivieri and Koren attended the annual retreat sponsored by the hospital's Research Institute. During dinner, Koren stood behind her chair, describing her to some of the others in "abjectly admiring" tones, according to one scientist who was there. He seemed to hover over her, said the observing scientist, "as if she was some sort of a princess and he was personally responsible for her presence among us."

He was often in her office, and she was in and out of his, though the two environments couldn't have been more different. Hers was a messy cubicle. To get to her desk, he picked his way over piles of file folders, manuscripts, books and trashcans. He might wait, perched on a table if there was no empty chair, while she answered her "bell-boy"—her name for her frequently buzzing pager. Visitors to Olivieri's office often smiled when they described it. "She had books and stuff piled everyplace and she was looking for her lunch from two days ago," said a staffer with the thalassemia program, recalling a meeting with Olivieri in 1989 or 1990. "She was living out of her office." Koren's workspace was larger and neater. His carpeting was visible, for one thing, and his secretary took his calls. But both Olivieri and Koren were self-deprecating. The hematologist and the pharmacologist laughed at each other's jokes, flirted openly, praised one another's work and appeared to be devoted friends. "They were together all the time," said one person who worked with Olivieri. Her insecurities persisted, and she seemed to need the praise Koren offered. "She needs constantly to be told that she's brilliant and right, as opposed to believing it herself," said one former friend. It was natural that Olivieri would ask Koren for help studying L1.

Inviting Gidi Koren and Mel Freedman to work on the project with her was relatively easy as both were men she saw frequently.

But to study L1 properly, Olivieri talked herself into the labs of the
other scientists she needed as collaborators, skilfully presenting
her project in ways that made it difficult for them to turn her
down. She would be studying a drug that bonded to iron, so she
needed someone on her team who understood the complexities of
how iron was metabolized in the body, preferably a chemist or biochemist. After hearing from another Sick Kids doctor about Doug
Templeton, an MD-PhD who taught in the university's department
of clinical biochemistry, she phoned him up, introduced herself and
set a time to meet.

"I've heard you can measure iron," she said when they got
together. Then she explained her ideas for testing L1. The drug
could pull iron out of the body—the group in London had shown
that. But Olivieri needed to be able to measure exactly how much
iron it brought out. Templeton groaned. From a scientific point of
view, he told Olivieri, iron wasn't interesting. "What's there that's
new to be discovered about it?" he asked rhetorically.

She answered him head-on. The drug she wanted to experiment
with was new, and the disease she'd been dealing with for the past
five years, thalassemia, would be new to his lab. As they sat at his
desk, Olivieri told him more about why the L1 project was important and kept asking him questions. When he mentioned that one of
his post-doctoral students had worked out a mathematical technique for separating iron from other elements, she got especially
excited and asked for a copy of the paper. She told him she thought
the work he and his group had already done on iron could be crucial to the L1 project.

Ciba-Geigy was putting money into research on thalassemia.
The company's liaison in Canada would be coming to Toronto, and
Olivieri thought Templeton should meet him—the company might
be interested in funding him to study the biochemistry of iron. Soon
Templeton was being drawn in despite himself. He began attending

meetings Olivieri had put together at Sick Children's on Monday mornings, where she, Koren and Freedman were all present.

Though he had spent most of his professional life in the lab, Templeton was trained as a physician and he could act as a translator between bench scientists and dyed-in-the-wool clinicians such as Freedman. The group Olivieri had brought together was trying to hammer out answers to a whole series of questions: Which patients should be eligible for the study? Should it just be thalassemia patients, or could patients with other forms of anemia also be included? How long would they keep the patients on L1? Koren thought that it would depend on what they found out about the length of time the drug stayed in the body. What was the chemical nature of iron in iron overload? This was Templeton's area of expertise, and he was soon fired up, leaving the Monday morning sessions with a sense of momentum. "Everyone was excited," he says.

Olivieri needed one more collaborator—someone who could make the drug. She spoke to some chemists doing research at the hospital. Did they know anyone who could prepare a drug from a chemical formula? Sure, said one woman, and described the U of T lab where her husband, an organic chemist, was doing his post-doctoral fellowship. Olivieri found the lab and dropped by to meet the professor who was head of it. She took along a copy of George Kontoghiorghes's paper describing how to make L1. "It turned out to be a very easy preparation," says U of T chemist Robert McLelland, who found that he and his students could concoct the drug using the equipment they already had in the lab. As McLelland explained later, "We did L1 because it was so easy. If it had been a long multi-step process, it just would not have been feasible in our department."

Nancy Olivieri said, "Bob McLelland said he could do it and Bob did, and he did this largely free of charge for many months." First, though, McLelland wanted to clarify the patent situation. He was reassured once he spoke directly with George Kontoghiorghes. "You know, do you mind us making the compounds?" McLelland began. Kontoghiorghes, in fact, was pleased to hear that the drug was to be made in North America.

Now that McLelland had agreed to make L1, the team needed government approval to test it on humans. Like George Kontoghiorghes and Victor Hoffbrand in Britain, they had to give the Canadian authorities a persuasive rationale for experimenting with an unproven drug in patients. Olivieri met with representatives of Health Canada's Health Protection Branch and explained that she planned to offer L1 to thalassemia patients "who do not have Desferal as a therapeutic option" because they had developed toxic reactions to it or wouldn't take it. Olivieri said that if she couldn't give certain of her patients L1, they would be dead within five years.

The Canadian authorities had the right to refuse permission to use the drug or they could ask for further proof that L1 was safe before allowing it to be tested on humans. Olivieri hadn't run the drug through any animal experiments, but she hoped to get around the federal requirements for animal testing by referring to the studies that George Kontoghiorghes had done in rodents. In September 1988, the regulators at Health Canada's Health Protection Branch allowed her to do that, giving her the nod to go ahead and offer the drug on a "compassionate basis" for patients who didn't have an alternative. Olivieri later told the *Globe and Mail* that Ottawa granted permission because "if you don't use something, these patients are going to die."

To pay for the study, she turned to the agency that funds the bulk of the country's research, the Medical Research Council (MRC, now the Canadian Institutes of Health Research), and wrote a formal research proposal to test L1's effectiveness in patients. She was successful and the funds were to begin in July 1989. The next thing she needed was a grant to pay for basic science investigations of the drug. She and Templeton were wondering about some of the same questions that had concerned Hider. For example, they wanted to know whether the drug would affect the formation of free radicals since that could lead to toxic reactions. They wrote a proposal to observe L1 in the lab in cultured cells and sent it off to a small Ontario-based funding agency—Physicians' Services Inc., or PSI. To their surprise, it was promptly rejected, perhaps because PSI was interested in studies in patients, not in cell culture.

The two rewrote their proposal and sent it off to the MRC and the Heart and Stroke Foundation, organizations that were likely to fund basic science. "Both funded it," Templeton said. "And then Heart and Stroke heard about MRC, so Heart and Stroke went down a little on the award." A slight decrease in one of the grants didn't dampen the group's excitement. The L1 project would involve research in patients and in the lab, and it now had stamps of approval from two outside agencies and the federal government. It was late in the fall of 1988, and the idea of bringing the drug to Canada was no longer an abstract notion.

Nancy Olivieri had returned from Boston intending to do research. Now she not only had a project that ignited her passions, she was the project leader, a striking accomplishment for a doctor with junior stature in the world of scientific research and no advanced degree. It was an especially unusual feat for a young woman in medical science, a field still heavily dominated by men. The rest of the team that Olivieri assembled to work on L1 was male and senior to her, but she was the driving force.

5

RECRUITING THE PATIENTS

The patients Nancy Olivieri spoke about in Ottawa were easy to spot in the clinic. There was a Saudi Arabian man in his early twenties. He'd become nearly deaf from Desferal at seventeen and had to have his dose reduced significantly. There were the two sisters from London, Ontario—the girls who as preschoolers had become partially blind and deaf after being treated with high-dose Desferal—and a boy whose leg bones were deformed by another side effect of Desferal. He had been started on night-long infusions of Desferal as a baby, but the drug turned out to be harmful if it was given to children under age three because they hadn't been transfused for long enough to develop an overload of iron in their organs. Italian researchers who studied Desferal's toxic effects on bones determined in 1988 that the drug interfered with critical iron-dependent enzymes and attached to other trace elements when it was used in young children, resulting in a syndrome that looked like rickets, with stunted growth and weak, stiff joints. Howard was also eligible for the study, since by this point he had completely stopped taking Desferal. He says he endured "five years of Desferal bumps and swelling and various complications" before giving up on the drug. A teenager named Paula was in the same situation as Howard; she'd stopped using Desferal after getting hives and a swollen leg in reaction to her shots.

The young people with thalassemia had all gotten to know each other through a patients' group that a few of them had organized. They would meet in a room on the first floor at Sick Kids, pull the chairs around in a circle and talk. Some of them were too old to be treated at Sick Kids any more. A clinic for older thalassemia patients had been set up at the Toronto General Hospital in 1987, and patients were now expected to graduate to the adult hospital by their late teens or early twenties.

In the spring of 1988, Nancy Olivieri gave a talk to the patients' group. Josie, the girl whose family had been warned against Desferal, was in the audience with her parents. She was in her last year of high school now and was enormously impressed by the presentation. The talk was being held in a lecture room at Sick Kids, but there was a problem with the microphone, so Olivieri moved out from behind the podium and shoved the mike aside. Leaning against the lectern, she spoke to the patients directly. "That gave me a gut feeling about her, that she was a good person," Josie said.

The hospital's research ethics committee approved Olivieri's study plan for L1 that fall, and she began asking patients to join up. She planned to run several tests of the drug, including one pitting L1 against Desferal to see which brought more iron out in the urine, and another comparing two different doses of L1. Olivieri referred to the various tests as a "pilot study"; the federal authorities knew it as a compassionate use arrangement. The Sick Kids team expected L1 to be safe, based on the published animal data from England, but they were using it in patients who had no alternatives; even if it turned out to have risks, the risks could be justified. Since the drug had never been tested before in Canada, they were starting small, but if the pilot project went well, the next step would be a longer-term study that could go on for months or even years.

Olivieri's patients heard about the research in meetings at the hospital, such as the one in early 1989 that Josie attended. When

Olivieri finished speaking, Josie raised her hand. One of the things she wanted to know was the molecular structure of L1 so she could show it to her chemistry teacher. Olivieri drew it for her on a piece of paper.

Olivieri approached her afterwards and said, "You seem really interested in this stuff." In fact, Josie hoped to go to medical school. She'd even done a science project using a slide of her own blood, setting up the blood smear under a microscope and guiding her classmates as they tried to visualize her defective red blood cells. At the end of that conversation with Nancy Olivieri, Josie had landed herself a summer job doing research at Sick Kids.

Patients who agreed to be in the study comparing L1 to Desferal were admitted to the hospital's research unit in twosomes, right after their regularly scheduled transfusions. Then they were randomly assigned to receive either Desferal in standard overnight infusions, or L1 three times a day. They had to submit to blood tests every other day and to continuous collection of their urine for the week they were hospitalized, and they had to agree to return to the research unit the next month and go through the same process on the other drug. Though Howard was a likely candidate for L1, he declined when Olivieri asked him to participate; he wanted no part of another hospital stay, even a short one. But many of the others whom Olivieri approached were very interested.

A woman in her early twenties had always been excellent about taking Desferal, even to the point of having injections seven days a week when the doctor asked her to. But she was frustrated because all her injection sites were now sore and red. "One thing about the needle," she said. "I would get hives, but even worse than hives—they'd look like little balls almost, all over my body." One day she got a call from the hospital. "Dr. Olivieri, just by fluke, happened to call me. She was asking me about something else but then she was like, 'Are you interested?' She was telling me that L1 was coming out . . . And I said, 'Sure, I'm interested.' And she said, 'Well it means that you'll have to come in the hospital for three weeks and do a lot of tests.'" Preferring a hospital bed to further injections, the young woman signed on to the study.

So did a twenty-year-old man who'd spent his teenage years unable to hear properly due to a toxic effect of Desferal. Whenever the doctors tried to increase his Desferal dose, his hearing loss got worse, but he didn't want to use a hearing aid. Andrea, the girl from the Kitchener area who'd been on extra iron until her mother spoke with doctors in Cyprus, was now a teenager. She and Josie were paired for the comparison test.

McLelland's lab made the drug, the technicians hand-weighing the powder and personally carrying it to the pharmacy at Sick Kids, where it was turned into capsules. Andrea and Josie were supposed to be taking six or seven capsules, three times a day. While McLelland was fine-tuning the drug's production, Templeton was analyzing the patients' urine and feces, attempting to quantify the amount of iron they contained. Koren was doing the pharmacokinetic analysis, working with a technician in his lab to determine how long L1 stayed in the body and whether it was changed chemically (via the process of metabolism) while it was there. After a while, Templeton determined that there wasn't any need to keep assessing patients' stool, because it didn't contain very much iron, so they revised the study to eliminate that step.

At the L1 project meetings on Monday mornings, the research team reviewed the numbers. It seemed as if L1 removed iron from the body, but not as quickly as Desferal. Olivieri decided to increase the dose and see if it made a difference. At the higher dose, L1 worked as well as Desferal, and the incidence of side effects appeared to be low. A few patients complained of nausea, but that was all. By the spring of 1990, they'd gathered enough data to complete the pilot study, and that March, Olivieri presented the findings at a meeting of the Cooley's Anemia Foundation in New York City. Now they were ready to enter patients into a long-term study.

Olivieri referred to her long-term study as the "compassionate use" trial, since the federal authorities had approved it on a compassionate basis. The team hired a data manager and they asked one of Koren's residents, an emergency room physician from Michigan named Christine Hermann, to take on the task of following the subjects who'd enrolled in the pilot study. Olivieri spoke to her patients about continuing to participate, and they were willing volunteers.

By the fall of 1989, Hermann was managing six patients; a year later, Olivieri would write the MRC that twelve patients had agreed to enter a long-term trial of L1; and later still, the number taking L1 on a compassionate basis would grow to twenty-one. Hermann became quite close to one of them—the young woman with the hives like little balls. After starting on L1 she'd wanted to stay on it, and the doctors had continued to provide her with the pills after the pilot study ended.

Josie had been consistently good about her nightly Desferal injections and she hadn't suffered from the side effects that others had experienced. Howard would tell people that she was "one of those ideal thal patients" because she never skipped a night on her pump. But the pill was easier to take and she, too, remained on it after the study ended. The two sisters from London also went on L1, as did another teenager named Shy-Rose, a Blue Jays fan who preferred to spend her evenings at ball games rather than at home hooked up to a pump.

If anybody had been looking over Olivieri's shoulder—a member of the hospital's Research Ethics Board or staff from the Health Protection Branch—the observer might have raised some questions. Patients who were rigorous about taking Desferal weren't officially supposed to be on L1. The authorities had okayed the use of the drug in patients who weren't doing well on standard therapy and had no alternatives, but Josie and some of the others to whom the drug was offered were doing well on Desferal, and that meant there was no justification for exposing them to the potential risks of an experimental pill.

Olivieri was in the conundrum that frequently confronts physicians who do research on their patients: she served two masters. As a doctor, she was supposed to act in her patients' best interests. In keeping with the "First do no harm" adage of medical practice, she was obliged to protect patients from any unnecessary risks, including the risk of an untested drug. But as the director of a drug study, she had to look out for her research. In any study of human subjects, half of the work is enrolling patients. If enough patients don't sign up, the results aren't meaningful and the paper describing the results won't be published in a leading journal.

During the late 1990s, the rules about protecting patients became stringent. An American scientist faced the threat of being banned for life from conducting clinical trials because he tested a therapy on patients who weren't strictly eligible. But Olivieri wasn't officially running a trial—she was operating under the rules of a compassionate-use drug program.

Later, in presentations and journal articles about her study, she described its subjects as patients "in whom [Desferal] treatment was failing" or for whom Desferal "was not a therapeutic option." As far as other scientists could tell, the Toronto L1 patients were "unwilling or unable to use Desferal," because that's what Olivieri said.

Soon Josie was sharing an occasional laugh with Paula and a few of the other young women who'd joined up. For Josie, the easy camaraderie that had developed among the thalassemia patients was one of life's high points. Her friend Andrea was no longer around; she'd returned to Cyprus with her family. Josie had started to date another thalassemia patient, and she and her boyfriend spent some of their weekends hanging out with fellow patients. Occasionally that meant visiting the hospital, including the time when Howard had a car accident and wound up on the orthopedic service.

By then Howard was twenty-four. Leaving work, he drove the wrong way on the entrance ramp to one of Ontario's 400-series highways and slammed into a wall. He spent weeks recovering. Josie thought the accident must have been alcohol-related. His iron-clogged liver was less able to clear alcohol from his system than the liver of a normal twenty-three-year-old. Howard himself blamed his diabetes. He'd been diabetic since the age of nineteen, but he'd never been good at making sure he always had a snack on hand. The day of his accident, he missed lunch. He knew he needed something to eat, so he got in his car to head to a restaurant. He had no recollection of what happened after that.

Josie and her boyfriend, Alex, made another trip to the hospital in the fall of 1989. This time, they went to see Biagio, who had grown up with Alex, their mothers talking in Italian as the boys waited for their bags of blood to arrive or lay receiving their transfusions. Both were avid hockey players. Neither of them was religious about taking their Desferal shots, and Biagio seemed to be the unlucky one. At twenty-one he was suffering from severe heart failure. Josie knew to look for him in the cardiac care unit, but when they got there they discovered he'd died the night before. It was the first of many early deaths for their close-knit group.

Many of the patients and their families showed up at Biagio's funeral. For a few of the mothers, it was a tearful reunion. They sat side by side in the funeral home, whispering to one another and fearing for their children's lives. Seeing a member of the clinic staff walk in, one mother burst into uncontrollable sobs. The patients sat together in the back, reeling from the sight of Biagio's hockey jersey and sticks in the open coffin. "We're like a little family," explained a female patient, and Biagio was a renegade whom they all admired. "He wanted to live at risk and knew his consequences, but I think he also believed that it was never really going to happen to him," said the clinic nurse. "And I think that everybody thought he was infallible, and when he wasn't infallible, they all realized they weren't."

Could L1 have made the difference for Biagio? Had it been available sooner, would it have kept him alive? The nurse thought he would have been able to take a pill. If similar thoughts haunted Olivieri, she didn't share them with her patients. She was on a mission to help people like Biagio—young men and women who wouldn't inject themselves with Desferal but might be willing to take a pill instead. She'd completed a pilot study and had begun a long-term trial; she couldn't speed the process up.

6

A TOXIC DRUG?

It was Bob Hider's group in London that sounded the first alarm: L1 was toxic to mice. They made the discovery public in the *Lancet* in the summer of 1989. In some mice, the drug knocked out virtually all of the white blood cells, leaving the animals unable to fight infections. The drug also took a swipe at platelets—one of the primary clotting agents contained in blood. If the mice taking L1 began to bleed for any reason, their blood wouldn't clot properly. Some of Hider's mice had a bad physical reaction: severe sweating. It was most likely a symptom of damage to their bodies, possibly to the immune system.

Hider's group wanted their report to serve as a warning to Victor Hoffbrand and the group testing L1 at London's Royal Free Hospital and to Nancy Olivieri and her collaborators in Toronto. "The finding of potentially serious toxicity in animals is important because L1 is being given to man in the UK and in Canada," they wrote. "It would appear prudent that its use be curtailed."

The second alarm came a few weeks later and was a lot worse. Hoffbrand got a call at home from his hospital's senior resident. A twenty-eight-year-old L1 patient was in the Accident and Emergency ward at the Royal Free. "She has no neutrophils," the young doctor told Hoffbrand, referring to the white blood cells that protect the body against infections. Hoffbrand said, "You mean she has no red cells." He explained that the young woman was born with a very rare condition, an anemia in which patients are unable to make red blood cells. The disease is known as red cell aplasia or Diamond Blackfan syndrome, and patients who have it require frequent transfusions to survive.

The resident interrupted him. "No, I mean she has no neutrophils," he said. As a result, a mild infection that had given her a sore throat and fever earlier in the week had now spread throughout her system, poisoning her bloodstream. She was in septic shock, a condition that could quickly become fatal.

Hoffbrand was horrified. His patient's problem was the same one that Hider's group had described in the mice they'd dosed with L1: not enough white blood cells to prevent infections. That problem had never been seen in humans. Among more than twenty thalassemia patients at the Royal Free who were taking L1, the side effects had been limited to occasional stiff joints. Two of the patients who had stopped using L1 had died less than two months later, but they were sick from iron overload and there was no evidence that the drug had harmed them. Yet now his patient was hovering between life and death after nearly a year on L1.

The doctors stopped the drug immediately. In three weeks the patient improved enough to be moved out of intensive care. Her white blood cell count began to climb, and she slowly recovered. Hoffbrand and Kontoghiorghes wrote up what had happened and sent it off to the *Lancet*. They wanted to be sure that doctors using L1 knew it was capable of destroying a patient's white blood cells. Meanwhile, Kontoghiorghes ran new tests of L1 in animals. This time his rat studies showed that L1 significantly decreased the number of white blood cells. So there it was. In mice, rats and humans, L1 caused a life-threatening side effect.

In Boston, David Nathan was becoming vocal about the dangers of L1. His negative opinion would prove costly for the drug. As Johns

Hopkins hematologist George Dover later put it, "David Nathan was and is one of the most powerful figures in hematology in the country, if not the world." Nathan's group was collaborating with scientists from Ciba-Geigy on another pill to replace Desferal, but it was a completely different molecule from L1 and they were testing it on monkeys, not humans. In Nathan's view, that was a crucial difference. In July 1989, he had published a paper advising doctors working on any new drug that attached to iron that they needed to experiment on primates before moving into human trials.

Nathan saw the near-fatal experience of Hoffbrand's patient as confirmation that the research on the drug at the Royal Free was irresponsible. "They just went right into human studies," he said later. "They did no animal studies and there had never been sufficient animal data." He wrote of them later that they had "exposed patients to unwarranted dangers." Around this time, Nathan began to harbour similar doubts about Nancy Olivieri's work, becoming "sort of verbally and visibly cautious about Nancy" as she became more and more associated with L1, according to George Dover.

It wasn't merely the limited testing in animals that bothered Nathan; it was that L1 could threaten the goals that had been achieved with Desferal. He'd been Desferal's major champion in North America—"It was his operation that had put Desferal on the map," says Dover—and he was proud of the steady increase in survival rates for patients with thalassemia and of the decreased rates of heart disease now that Desferal was standard treatment. He didn't want to take the risk that it would be replaced by an oral drug that didn't work as well. "David did not want anything coming down the pike that would take Desferal off the map," Dover explains. "Many of us interpret David's stance to be sort of cautious about [L1] because he didn't want to raise patients' expectations that they could stop taking Desferal now." The bottom line for Nathan was that despite Desferal's serious side effects, such as blindness, deafness and stunted growth, it hadn't killed anyone; on the contrary, he had published numerous papers showing that many patients—those who could take it and stay on it— owed their lives to it.

It can't have been easy for Nancy Olivieri to discover that, after initially giving her the green light, Nathan now disapproved of her choice of a research project. Dover suspects it was quite difficult. "David can be very impressive and certainly intimidating when he wants to be, and all of us have felt his ire when we've wound up on the other side of an issue," he says. Ire was not what Olivieri was used to from Nathan.

He wasn't the only one with reservations about L1. At the *Lancet,* where the first articles on the drug had appeared, editors grew cautious. The journal consulted with hematologists and decided that human clinical trials of the drug ought to stop. In October 1989, the *Lancet* ran an editorial declaring L1 "too toxic for further development." By then, clinical trials of L1 were already in progress on three continents. In addition to Olivieri's studies in Canada and Hoffbrand's in the United Kingdom, L1 was being used experimentally in Holland, Italy, Switzerland and India. The *Lancet* editorial didn't trigger a country-by-country review of clinical trials using L1, though, because most countries left further monitoring up to the researchers themselves.

In Canada, Olivieri had required the approval of the Human Subjects Review Committee (later called the Research Ethics Board) at Sick Kids to get started, but now that her trial was in progress, the board wouldn't monitor it unless Olivieri specifically requested them to. It was the way things were done. Throughout Canada, ethics boards at teaching hospitals approved research but didn't keep tabs on it. Researchers were required to file annual reports with their hospital ethics board, but there was no active surveillance by the boards of what was happening in a given field or on a particular project. The following spring, Olivieri described her continuing studies of L1 to the hospital ethics board, which wrote back in July 1990 to say that the project was "ethically acceptable."

The week that the *Lancet* editorial appeared, Olivieri doctors were arriving in London for a symposium on L1, organized by George Kontoghiorghes. The doctors working with the drug accepted that it had risks, but they thought a risky treatment was justified given the severity of thalassemia and iron overload. The issue with toxicity, they argued, was to manage it. Olivieri and the others ran frequent blood tests on their patients to detect any drop in blood counts before a patient ran into problems. Beatrix Wonke, clinic director in the Royal Free's thalassemia program, said, "It was a question of seeing young people die, or trying out a new drug in a very cautious setting." Like most of Olivieri's patients on L1, Wonke's research subjects were teenagers and young adults who refused to take Desferal or had experienced bad side effects.

Olivieri and her team were putting together a grant proposal to the Medical Research Council to fund their long-term study of L1, a three-year project that was supposed to enrol thirty patients. Their proposal detailed the hazards of Desferal and was unambiguous about the potential value of L1. It made no mention of the *Lancet* editors' dismissal of the drug as "too toxic," nor did it discuss Hider's warning against testing L1 in humans.

"An alarming accumulation of reports have now provided evidence that serious toxicity is associated with long-term use of Desferal," it said, listing vision problems, kidney failure, severe pulmonary syndrome and stunted growth among Desferal's side effects. L1, as described in the grant proposal, sounded safer. When given to iron-loaded mice over a period of one year, it produced "no obvious harmful effects"; rats on L1 developed swollen adrenal glands but "No clinical correlates of these changes can be detected."

Some rats on L1 had declines in white blood cell counts, and "in one lab," some mice on L1 also had declines in white blood cell counts, but those rats and mice received higher doses of L1 "than that received by patients" and the toxic reactions in the mice were "unsupported by two other laboratories." The grant said the dose that was high enough to kill 50 per cent of animals exposed to a drug—a figure used by toxicologists called the LD 50—was lower for Desferal than for L1, meaning the older drug was more lethal to animals than the experimental one.

When it came to safety in humans, the proposal noted that an L1 patient of Hoffbrand's had experienced a sudden drop in white blood cells but "the role of L1" in that patient's problem was "unclear" and no similar problems were "reported in any other of the 120 patients who had received L1. . ." The proposal concluded that the L1 studies published so far did not "permit conclusions regarding L1 in terms of safety of L1." Olivieri submitted her application to the MRC on November 1, 1990.

Later that month, she flew to India for a meeting of L1 researchers in Bombay. "Oral pill to prevent thalassemia" was the headline in the local *Indian Express*. Adding up all the patients in L1 trials around the world, someone calculated that more than 130 patients were taking it. In India, nearly half the patients on L1 were suffering from joint pain and stiffness—the side effect that had been seen in the Royal Free patients. Some of the Bombay physicians feared that the joint problems could have dangerous implications; they thought L1 was disrupting patients' immune systems and causing arthritis.

Within a few months, it looked as if their fears were realized. An eighteen-year-old Indian boy died while taking L1. First he developed muscle aches and pains. His doctors thought he had lupus, an arthritis-like disease that results from a problem with the immune system. They took him off L1 and gave him steroids, the standard treatment for lupus. But in February 1991, he had a heart attack and couldn't be revived. The Bombay physicians were also treating a twelve-year-old girl with L1. When they checked her blood tests, she also showed early warning signs of lupus. "In our opinion, trials of L1 should be halted," the Bombay group wrote in the *Lancet* in a report on the boy's death. That winter, Hoffbrand's team hospitalized another L1 patient in London for her complete loss of white blood cells.

David Nathan now worried openly that L1 was deadly. He began telling people that the pill was "finished" because it was toxic and he was certain that if researchers proposed a study of L1 in the U.S., the FDA would turn them down because the drug wasn't proven safe for human use. But Olivieri disagreed. She was convinced the FDA would approve L1 trials. She discounted the doubts despite their source, because she viewed the trials in India with skepticism. In her opinion, the alleged dangerous side effects didn't necessarily implicate L1. Even the fatal case of lupus in the eighteen-year-old boy could have been caused by something else. She thought it was the process for making L1 in India that was the problem, not L1 per se. She told Doug Templeton that the Indian researchers were seeing complications "because their drug was not as pure as other people's." And she wrote a letter to the *Lancet* editors explaining that in her ongoing trial in Toronto, twelve patients were taking L1 and none of them had lupus.

Olivieri wasn't ready to cast L1 out. She didn't want to lose any more of her patients to the same lousy circumstance that had felled Biagio—a life-saving drug so cumbersome and unpleasant that the average teenager or young adult would simply avoid it. But she did take precautions. She added further tests to her L1 trials to show if a patient was running into problems, and she began speaking to patients about L1's toxic side effects. She advised three of them to stop taking L1. Josie recalls her telling them, "You were the ones who were good with your Desferal beforehand so you can go back to it and, as your physician, I have to tell you that you should go

back on Desferal, because there's this risk, this unknown, with L1."
Frightened by the news of L1's toxic side effects, Josie switched back
to Desferal. But the two other young women Olivieri spoke to
declined to return to nightly injections. They stayed on L1. One of
them got anxious after Olivieri spoke to them because she thought
Olivieri would force her to stop L1. "I was really upset," she said. "For
me, anyway, there was no reason to get off of it." She was so worried
about having to return to Desferal that she tried bargaining with
Olivieri, telling her, "I'll even sign something and I'll take full responsibility if something happens to me [on L1]." Eventually the patients
did sign consent forms to document that they'd been warned about
L1's toxic effects.

Olivieri didn't always give patients a choice. If they weren't
doing well, she made sure they went back on Desferal. Paula, a
patient who got hives on Desferal, worsened on the pilot study of
L1. Olivieri took her off the pill and returned her to intravenous
Desferal. Helen was also forced off the drug because her liver
enzymes went up, a sign that she could be suffering from liver damage. But the other patients who were taking L1 seemed fine, and
more patients were joining them. Howard started on L1 now that
an in-patient stay in the hospital was no longer part of the study. So
did a younger man named Corrado. Like Paula, Corrado often
broke out in hives within hours of injecting himself with Desferal.

At scientific meetings and in medical journals, the Toronto L1
group reported that in many of their patients, the pills were working as well as Desferal for removing iron buildup and that their
patients weren't having the sorts of side effects that had been
reported elsewhere. In the *Lancet,* doctors testing L1 in Bombay and
London had been describing joint problems in their patients. That
wasn't happening in Toronto. Olivieri had mentioned in her letter
to the *Lancet* editors that while joint pains had been seen in Bombay
patients on L1, "In striking contrast, none of the 12 patients receiving

a similar regimen of L1 therapy in Toronto for up to one year have had similar complaints."

In February 1991, after the death in India and the second hospitalization of an L1 patient in London for agranulocytosis—the potentially fatal loss of white blood cells—Olivieri wrote again to the hospital's Human Subjects Review Committee. "Last week, I had the opportunity to speak with my colleague Prof. A.V. Hoffbrand," she began, and then described Hoffbrand's thalassemia patient who'd experienced dramatic white cell loss on L1. She told the board that Hoffbrand's group had reported similar problems, eighteen months earlier, in a patient on L1 who had Diamond Blackfan anemia. She said the role of the drug in the earlier case was "confused" because of the patient's primary disease, and "furthermore, in vitro studies conducted at that time on the patient's bone marrow were inconclusive." An American hematologist argued in the *Lancet* that Diamond Blackfan anemia wouldn't cause patients to lose white blood cells and that such a loss was more likely a harmful consequence of taking L1. But Olivieri wasn't sure the drug was the problem.

Her letter to the ethics board referred to the drug's toxic effects on Hoffbrand's patients as "this potential toxicity of L1." Like her November submission to the MRC, her February letter to the board didn't say that the University College group had deemed the drug's toxicity too great to take it to human clinical experiments and didn't mention the 1989 editorial in the *Lancet* that declared the drug too toxic for human use. However, Olivieri's collaborator Gideon Koren was the head of the ethics board at the time, and she may have relied on his knowledge of L1's problems to flesh out the situation for the rest of the board members. Since she was prescribing L1 for compassionate use and not for a conventional clinical trial, her obligations to the board were unclear.

In her letter she wrote, "These patients should be informed of the occurrence of agranulocytosis in the British study, and should be offered a choice as to continuation of L1." But, she pointed out, patients who went off "the only existing alternative" to Desferal would be choosing "to withdraw from all chelation therapy, the fatal consequences of which must be reemphasized to each patient." At the end of her letter, Olivieri said she had updated the information forms she was giving to patients in her trials and she enclosed the revised form. The board responded by agreeing that she needed to provide appropriate information about the drug to study participants.

That summer, two years after she'd first started working with L1, she went to the FDA's drab headquarters in Rockville, Maryland, to present her results. Before a panel of FDA chemists, pharmacologists, toxicologists and medical officers, she ran through her slides, explaining that in her patients, L1 worked nearly as well as Desferal. Dr. Stephen Fredd, the FDA official with jurisdiction over drugs for thalassemia, listened to her presentation carefully. Fredd had been at the agency throughout the AIDS era and had been affected by the protests of AIDS advocacy groups, which argued that people with AIDS were paying with their lives for the status quo at the FDA. As the FDA waited for clinical trial data on newly developed drugs, patients with AIDS were suffering. They pleaded for quicker drug approvals, asserting that in the face of a terminal illness it was up to an individual patient to decide how much risk to bear. "People felt, 'How can someone be asked to wait ten years for a life-saving drug?'" said Fredd. "There was a sense that we had to speed things up but also that you've got to weigh safety versus benefit." The risk vs. benefit equation had always been calculated at the FDA, but safety got top billing. Now benefit was seen as equally important.

Before AIDS, the philosophy at the FDA was one forged in the 1960s by thalidomide: keep the public safe from harm. New rules implemented during the late 1980s required the agency to approve drugs faster, and certain new drugs intended for people with life-threatening diseases were becoming available for use before final testing and review were completed. Academics called it "a consumer-rights orientation" to drug regulation, since the push for less testing and quicker drug approvals came from consumers and patient advocacy groups. In FDA publications, officials explained that a separate standard for drugs intended to treat immediately life-threatening diseases was justified by the different risk-benefit considerations involved. It was in this context that Fredd listened to Olivieri and the other investigators at the meeting describe their data on L1.

He hadn't met Olivieri before, and she struck him as a serious researcher, and he was particularly impressed by the results from her clinical trial. He understood that L1 already had been associated with dangerous side effects in human and animal testing, yet he thought it was worth testing further. Olivieri and some of the others believed the dangers might be due to the formulation of the drug used in India; a different formulation might be less toxic. "Part of what Olivieri developed in Canada is part of what made us think we could go on with the drug," Fredd said. "She wanted to see whether the problems in India would repeat themselves." When the researchers were through, Fredd addressed the group. He accepted that in a different formulation, L1 might be more suitable for human use, and asked to see proposals to test L1 in clinical trials. The agency was looking for a randomized study pitting L1 against Desferal and a long-term study of the drug's toxicity, he said. But researchers would first have to present a formulation that was up to FDA standards. Those standards are spelled out in a long list of technical requirements for the production process that an academic lab would find impossible to meet.

Olivieri viewed Fredd's words as marching orders. "The FDA . . . said we believe your data but we need three things," she explained later. She hoped to come back eventually with all three: a study to compare L1 with Desferal, a toxicity study and a way to produce L1 according to the agency's standards.

She flew in and out of meetings in Europe and North America presenting her data. In November 1991 she spoke on the drug in France. The week she gave her talk, many of her patients back home were at yet another funeral, for Paula. In the spring of 1991, Paula had married another thalassemia patient in a full church wedding; now, six months later, she was dead. She hadn't done well in the L1 trial, but all her close friends knew she had not been very disciplined about her injections. Her husband said later, "She couldn't do the Desferal."

In December, Olivieri presented her results in the U.S. at ASH. More and more, it was her name that was associated with L1. She was a superb speaker and was usually chosen to present during the plenary session of whatever meeting she was attending. At ASH meetings, Olivieri "was really the Queen Bee" in discussions of L1, said Beatrix Wonke. Back at home, though, her colleagues were less aware of her rising reputation. In Toronto, her L1 research was spotlighted for the first time in the spring of 1992.

Her team had published a case report about a twenty-nine-year-old thalassemia patient who refused to take Desferal. After nine months on L1, his level of iron was substantially reduced. The article's take-home message was that L1 was as effective as infusions of Desferal and much easier for patients to take. "Our report is the first to present evidence in humans for L1-induced reduction of iron in the liver and heart," Olivieri wrote. She'd managed to achieve primacy in the field even though the London group had published their trial results two years earlier, because that group had only tracked iron excreted in the urine and through the iron-related blood test known as serum ferritin, while Olivieri used liver biopsies and magnetic resonance imaging (MRI) to measure the actual concentration of iron in her patient's vital organs.

Her case report appeared in *Blood,* a specialty journal typically read only by hematologists. But Sick Kids put out a press release about the paper and offered to arrange interviews with the researchers and their patients. Subsequently, the *Globe and Mail* headlined its article, "Pills replace pump ordeal. Drug for blood disorder 'going to save many patients.'" The quotation in the headline came from Nancy Olivieri, who told the *Globe* that L1 was "going to save many of the patients who could not tolerate the old treatment." Olivieri had invited some of her patients to come to the press conference. She introduced journalists to Shy-Rose Virani, now an eighteen-year-old poster child for L1. "It's been wonderful for me," Shy-Rose told the reporters. *The Globe and Mail* reported, "The only side effect Ms. Virani has noticed is a reddish colour in her urine—visible proof that iron is being expelled."

One week later, Olivieri attended an NIH-sponsored symposium in Gainesville, Florida, that drew many of the L1 researchers. Animal studies discussed at that Florida meeting confirmed what was already being seen in human clinical trials. Doctors at the NIH had run the pill through a standard toxicity study at a commercial lab in New York State in 1991. At the highest dose—eight times what Olivieri was giving to patients—the dogs died, while at lower doses (still about twice as high as any humans were receiving) the dogs' growth was slowed and their blood-cell counts dropped. Scientists in Switzerland at Ciba-Geigy had tested L1 on monkeys, dosing them with more than three times the level the Toronto patients were receiving. More than a third of those animals died, and the drug seemed to have a specific effect on the monkeys' white blood cells. A summary of the conference concluded there was "a delicate balance between safety and efficacy for L1."

Drug tests on animals don't always predict accurately what will happen in people. The results are reliable only if the animal model is a good replica of the human situation. Researchers testing L1 had attempted to develop dog and monkey models of a thalassemia patient developing a chronic buildup of iron, but the animals hadn't actually undergone the years of transfusions the patients had and didn't have the same load of iron in their organs. Some L1 researchers thought the animals weren't the best models for studies of L1, and though she had tested it on dogs herself, Olivieri seemed to be in that camp.

She accepted that L1 didn't work in every case and had toxic side effects; she'd taken some patients off it and urged others to consider stopping it. But overall, the evidence she and others had gathered convinced her that L1 could replace Desferal in some cases. She'd defended the drug in the correspondence pages of the *Lancet,* at the FDA and at ASH, and she had exclaimed over it to newspaper reporters in Toronto. Amid reports of L1's dangers, Nancy Olivieri's tenacity kept her plugging away. There was a controversy surrounding L1, but she intended to continue studying the drug.

7

WORKING WITH A RISING STAR

Nancy Olivieri had taken over the management of the thalassemia and sickle cell anemia clinics from Mel Freedman, and was now the director of the largest thalassemia program in North America. As a result of the large number of patients she was responsible for and of her rising reputation, she was invited to participate in many of the other major studies in the field. She was working with an Israeli scientist to test erythropoietin, a new product of genetic engineering that could boost a patient's production of red blood cells, and she was participating in an NIH-led multi-centre study of hydroxyurea, a new drug for sickle cell disease. She was looking at other possible uses for L1—others had suggested it could be used as an anti-malaria drug and she was testing it in adults infected with malaria in Africa while also giving it to breast cancer patients in Toronto to see if it could block the toxicity of chemotherapy drugs.

Toronto's ethnic diversity made it a rich territory in which to study the genetic roots of thalassemia, and Olivieri was collaborating on gene research with the doctors who ran Ontario's provincial screening laboratory for genetic blood disorders, searching for new mutations of the beta-globin gene that could cause various forms of the disease. Between 1992 and 1994, she and her colleagues at the provincial lab found seven novel mutations in Greek, Italian, Irish, Jamaican, Laotian, Filipino and Bangladeshi thalassemia patients.

Olivieri also networked with leaders of Toronto's black community to try to improve early detection of sickle cell disease. "Nancy got people to these meetings and there was kind of an excitement that we were finally going to do something for these kids," recalls one Toronto doctor who worked closely with the sickle cell patients.

But her scientific and clinical successes didn't translate into increased personal stability. Instead, she was more stressed. The mother of a patient Olivieri began treating in the early 1980s says that when she first met Nancy Olivieri, "I saw this beautiful human being, this warm human being," who was "very high-energy, very high-strung." The mother used to tell her, "It's all the chocolates that you eat." But then, the mother says, Olivieri "changed a lot who she was." The change came during 1991 and 1992. Olivieri "started to be too busy to talk, too busy to stop, and I felt she was very sad," the mother says. "She would be eating junk food . . . She didn't have time for a meal. You could see that this person is not doing well."

The pressure that Olivieri was experiencing wasn't only professional. She had been dating Alan Bernstein, a tall, good-looking scientist with black wavy hair. When Olivieri began spending time with him, he was second in command of research at Mount Sinai, recently divorced and clear about his scientific priorities. "If a medical researcher is not looking for a gene and doing molecular-biology work, they are nowhere," he told a Toronto reporter in 1990. Olivieri didn't see eye to eye with him about medical science and, as it turned out, the couple also diverged widely on other issues Olivieri held dear. Bernstein's liberal Jewish views were at odds with her Catholic upbringing. In the end, they broke up.

Over the next two years, Alan Bernstein dated other women and then remarried. He was promoted to head of research at Mount Sinai and was on a fast track to becoming one of Canada's most successful and visible scientists. Meanwhile, Olivieri's colleagues and friends worried about her. More than once, her remarks had a ring of hopelessness to them.

"You know, I'm really concerned about Nancy," one hematologist at the hospital told another. "I'm worried she might do something. What should we do?" The second physician admitted that he was equally concerned. Two hematologists pulled aside one of Olivieri's non-medical friends at Sick Kids and asked her whether Nancy was all right. The friend said she thought Olivieri's "stress level [was] at a peak" and that she'd asked Olivieri how she was doing. "You're losing weight, you don't look like you're getting sleep, you're flying to this country and the next all within two hours, you know—are you okay?" She said that Olivieri hadn't offered much explanation.

The pressure of being in the research spotlight had a spillover effect on her work. Olivieri was known in the hospital as rude, funny and quick to use profanity. Listening to her could be like sitting in on a session with a comic. But she was often highly critical of those around her, and her repartee could go too far. There were times when it seemed as if she forgot that she wasn't in the privacy of her own home but in the eighth-floor conference room or in the clinic seeing patients. Her temper would flare and, at those moments, she seemed unable to control her words or her tone.

As a hematology resident, she seemed to have painted the Toronto General Hospital black and the Toronto Western Hospital white. Now, as a faculty member, she reserved her black paint for several of her residents, nurses and secretaries. The residents discovered that Olivieri counted them as "in" or "out." "There was nobody that was just okay," said one of her residents. "Everybody was either wonderful or terrible. It was black and white. And usually when she switched, that was it. You could go from her 'in' group to her 'out' group, but you could never go back."

Even the residents who counted themselves in Olivieri's "in" group say she had good days and bad days. "If she was in a good mood, everyone could be joking and it would be fine," said one resident. "Then, other times, she'd just be snapping and biting people's heads off. You never knew what to expect. But as soon as you came in, you could look at her and you'd know, 'Okay, got to be on guard today.'"

Olivieri had delegated a number of research-related responsibilities to the residents. They didn't always carry out their duties according to her standards, but in the early years of the L1 research she could cope with that. Now, when residents did things differently than she would have or disagreed with her, she was intolerant. "She used to stand up in these meetings and berate them," said one person who sometimes attended the L1 meetings. Said another, "She has a rough, fierce anger . . . If some of the fellows didn't have the answer, she'd jump on them." For some residents who came to these sessions, "it was their hour or two hours from hell."

Medicine's stereotypes allow for male surgeons who are intimidating. There's no similar stereotype for a female hematologist, and Olivieri may have suffered from sexism. Janet Bickel, a U.S. expert on women in medicine, says that few academic women over forty escape being described as "difficult" by their peers. Yet Olivieri wasn't described as merely "difficult." During the early to mid-1990s, those who saw her interact with her residents and hospital staff say that at times she showed no consideration for the people she supervised.

Doreen Matsui and Mati Berkovitch were two of Koren's residents. Assigned to the compassionate use trial, they both attended the Monday research meetings. In the fall of 1992, Matsui was in her final fellowship year and held the position of chief fellow on the pharmacology service. Her junior colleagues were fond of her. One described Matsui as "a very fine person, delicate, very polite and gentle." Two of the residents teased her that she was "the world's most law-abiding fellow." They'd awarded her the moniker one day when she refused to walk through a hospital corridor on which a sign was posted saying, "Patient area: please do not use as a thoroughfare." Staff doctors and residents took it for granted that constraints on their time trumped a patient's need for quiet, but Matsui respected the sign and made the residents with her use a different route. In the Monday research meetings, Olivieri often insulted Matsui. Occasionally the young woman broke down in tears while the meetings were in session.

The thalassemia and sickle cell nurses also reported troubles with their boss. They saw the patients at their monthly visits for transfusions, taught them how to use Desferal, pressed them to stay on their medications, got to know their families, went to patients' homes or had them to their houses and, in some cases, became lifelong friends. "You saw them take their first steps and you heard about it when they had their first kiss and you knew about their first drinking night," said a nurse. "You were very intimate with these individuals." Many of them said that Olivieri had trouble acknowledging the difference the nurses made in patients' lives. Some of the clinic staff recalled a story from the early 1990s, when one of the thalassemia nurses worked closely with the hospital's medical engineers to determine which pump would work best for the patients using Desferal. The project took nearly a year, but before the nurse could present her assessment of the issues surrounding the pumps, Olivieri told her that she didn't care—all that mattered was getting the drug infused into the patients. Olivieri's comment, which she repeated several times, made the nurse think her time and effort had been for nothing.

Several nurses found it extremely stressful to work with Olivieri. They remember angry outbursts and door-slamming, and found her unpredictable behaviour extremely hard to deal with. One former nurse couldn't stop shaking while describing the experience of working alongside Olivieri. "I was so scared to death of her," the nurse said. "At the end, I cried every night because I am not a confrontational person." Another said it was difficult to talk about her time as Olivieri's clinic staff, explaining that "I'm still struggling here because it elicits a lot of emotional feeling." The encounter they feared most was Olivieri's clinic meeting on Thursday afternoons. As nurses described the patients seen in clinic that week, Olivieri would ask questions about lab work or vital signs. As with her residents, the nurses' answers didn't always meet her standards. Under greater personal and professional stress, she seemed less able to keep her frustrations in check.

Olivieri was described by her nurses as "putting them down, just making them feel like totally useless, hopeless people," said one doctor. "She would be really, really rude to them and use really bad language . . . ." Said another physician, "There was a kind nurse who loved the patients . . . Nancy was unkind to her, and this woman would be in tears." The physician had tried to speak to Olivieri about it. "She's doing her best. Don't ride her so hard," the physician said. But it wasn't clear that Olivieri understood how painful her words could be to another person.

Some of the nurses talked to nursing supervisors about Olivieri and some supervisors spoke to their own supervisors about Olivieri's behaviour, but nothing changed as a result, and the nurses in the thalassemia program began to speak with their feet. During the early to mid-1990s, Olivieri's clinics developed a high turnover rate. Howard describes it as "a revolving door of staff who've been working with her, for her, whatever." And the nursing supervisors found they were facing a new problem: if one of Nancy Olivieri's nurses was sick or on holiday, it was hard to find a substitute.

Olivieri's secretaries also complained. In earlier years, Olivieri had shared her clerical staff with other hematologists. Now she had her own secretary, but she seemed unable to provide a stable work environment. She had three secretaries in relatively quick succession, none staying for a full year. Patients sometimes referred to Olivieri as their own Murphy Brown. Melvin Freedman, her supervisor when she was in training and one of the original members of the L1 research team, was now her division head and spoke to her about some of the questions that the nursing and clerical staff were raising. Olivieri defended herself, telling Freedman that as a program head she believed her needs at the hospital weren't being met.

She told friends she had to fight "for secretaries, for paper clips, for everything." As one friend described it, "She was asking for more and more resources and she wasn't getting them. That created a dynamic where she had to be really aggressive just to make a name for herself." Freedman, as division head, was the one holding the purse strings.

Years later, scientist John Dick contrasted his situation to Nancy Olivieri's. Dick was a molecular biologist in the hospital's Research Institute with a successful and growing research program. If he needed resources for his projects, he says, he'd visit the director of the Research Institute, geneticist Jim Friesen. "I'd sit down with Jim and say, look, we need to do this, we're in competition with a California biotech company. I'd explain and I'd get grant support, technical support." In time, the hospital gave him a more spacious lab. "Just in general I became a player," he says. "I was somebody who was asked for their opinion on things." By the early 1990s, Olivieri was receiving substantial attention in her field. But at Sick Kids, Dick says, the difference between their situations was stark. "Nancy and I started at Sick Kids around the same time and I was supported from the very beginning and Nancy, I think, was not," he explained. "Nancy had to achieve her success by just fighting and getting whatever she could for herself." Too often, what she could get was less than what her scientific workload warranted. A friend who visited her laboratory at Sick Kids in the late '80s was surprised at how underequipped it was. "She didn't have pipettes or tubes or Styrofoam boxes to mail samples in," the friend recalls. She didn't always have the clerical assistance she needed either. In 1989, with the compassionate use study of L1 steadily enrolling patients, Olivieri needed a full-time assistant to do filing, data entry and other tasks associated with a clinical trial. Instead, she had secretaries who could not take on all the extra work.

Olivieri shared her caseload with clinical associates—pediatricians who saw thalassemia and sickle cell patients in clinic twenty-five hours per week. But Olivieri didn't see this as special support. In her view, the hospital was already obliged to hire an associate, since her award from the Medical Research Council directed her to devote 80 per cent of her time to research. She thought Freedman and the rest of the administration were failing to respond to her needs. Some of her friends thought she was judging Freedman too harshly, but they couldn't get her to change her mind.

Over time, her relationships with her clinical colleagues also began to deteriorate. Some complained that she no longer covered for them when they were away, but they had to cover for her because she travelled so often. Freedman and Mark Greenberg, the division chief for oncology, raised the issue of Olivieri more than once with their boss, chief of pediatrics Bob Haslam. In the spring of 1992, the concerns of the division chiefs and the complaints from the nurses built to a crescendo, and Haslam began an investigation. Following hospital protocol, his office scheduled meetings with about twenty nurses and physicians who worked closely with Olivieri, including her residents, and documented the conversations that took place.

"As you know, everybody is a little unhappy up there," Haslam began one such interview with a physician who worked alongside

Olivieri. "She's a difficult person," the doctor replied, adding, "There isn't any way you're going to change her." Haslam asked if there was anything happening in Olivieri's clinical program that was putting patients at risk. The doctor didn't think so.

Once again, sexism can't be ruled out. In a field such as medical research, where women are so few in number, a female scientist can be harmed by the fact that she stands out. Everyone knows her and, what's more, they know every mistake she's made. Though the complaints against Olivieri were real, they could have stayed on people's minds more because she was female.

Worried that she could be fired, Nancy Olivieri campaigned vigorously for herself among hospital staff she'd worked with over the years. "You know, I'm really being screwed here," she told one doctor. After explaining her predicament, she asked if he would please talk to Haslam about her in a positive way. She sought out nurses she'd worked with and asked them to speak up about her ability to get along with them. She met personally with physicians to warn them that the chief might contact them, and she wrote her own detailed response to Haslam's investigation, which formed part of the written record.

She also talked about her worries with cancer specialist Bob Phillips. In Phillips, Olivieri had found another caring mentor. He was well known to Canadian cancer researchers, and he provided Olivieri with what he later described as moral support and psychotherapy. Frequently, she asked him to review her grant applications or write her a letter of recommendation. Now, as Haslam tried to systematically determine what had riled the nurses, Olivieri told Phillips she feared she might lose her job. As she saw it, her division heads considered her a fractious character, always stirring up conflict, but the real problem was the environment in her division. She thought her bosses could be investigating her as a way of retaliating for her efforts to get the resources she deserved, but it wasn't clear where she could go to complain about it. Phillips was concerned for her and decided to act on her behalf.

One of his closest colleagues at the hospital was Jim Friesen, the chief scientist at the Research Institute. Long before either Friesen or Phillips came to Sick Kids, both were department chairs at the University of Toronto. Phillips ran medical biophysics; Friesen ran genetics. The pair had a relationship spanning two decades. Phillips left the university for Sick Kids in 1986 to head up cancer research; Friesen arrived at the hospital the following year as the new director of the Research Institute. When Bob Phillips turned to Jim Friesen to share his worries about the investigation Nancy Olivieri was facing, Friesen listened carefully.

Both men were aware of the profound differences between the personnel policies they'd grown accustomed to at the university and the nature of the investigation at Sick Kids that they feared had Nancy Olivieri in its crosshairs. At the university, structures for resolving disputes with employees were more transparent, and employees—including faculty—had unions to take their side in conflicts with the administration. But at the teaching hospitals, the administrations devised and enforced their own policies, without outside oversight. Hospital faculty had appointments at the university, but they weren't members of the faculty union, and hospital administration officials were beholden only to their boards. This outmoded, authoritarian structure was especially entrenched at Sick Kids, where the hospital's original constitution dictated a clear separation from the university. Sick Kids physicians felt helpless to counter administrative decisions they disagreed with, and there were always one or two stories circulating of doctors who had argued with the administration and paid a price.

Worried that the hospital's structures for investigating doctors were open to abuse, Friesen decided to pay a visit to the hospital's chief pediatrician. If anyone needed further evidence of the inbred nature of Canada's scientific elite, the connections between Phillips, Friesen and Haslam offered it. Friesen's and Haslam's families had grown up together on the prairies of Saskatchewan, and the two had known each other personally for decades. It wasn't hard for Jim Friesen to give Bob Haslam his two cents on the ongoing investigation of Nancy Olivieri. "Look," he said, "this is really unfair." He proceeded to explain to Haslam what he understood from Bob Phillips about the battles Nancy Olivieri was involved in and the real reasons her division heads were looking to find fault with her. He was using the old boys' network, and Sick Kids had no rules against that.

Olivieri also spoke to her staff about the investigation at the regularly scheduled meetings. "If they want a war then they're going to get it," she said. Then she announced that anyone who had anything to say should "say it now, before going into Dr. Haslam's office" and said she thought people were saying things about her that were "very slanderous." To one person who attended, it sounded as though she was putting her staff on notice, letting them know they could be accused of slander if they said negative things about her to her chief.

Haslam proceeded with his interviews and information-gathering. In the end, hospital administrators met and spoke about how to rectify the situation, and Haslam wrote Olivieri a letter laying out the department's expectations concerning her relationships with her staff. The nurses heard that her campaign to protect her job had been successful. Like Olivieri herself, the nurses didn't know where else they could turn.

In her stressed state, Olivieri's mood took a nosedive and she began to have run-ins with research collaborators. Doug Templeton said she got "quite pissed off" with him because he refused to add her name as an author to a paper that came out of his lab. Based on a complicated project by one of his post-doctoral students, the paper involved observations of L1 in cultured liver cells.

Olivieri couldn't understand why her name wasn't on a paper that was ostensibly about L1. Templeton said it was simple: there were only two names on the paper—the post-doc's name came first and his second—because they were the ones who had contributed directly to the research. Adding extra authors would dilute the credit the post-doc got for doing the work, and anyway, the paper wasn't going to appear in a medical publication; they intended to submit it to a chemistry journal. But it wasn't simple to Olivieri. She spoke sharply about it, then wrote a letter to Templeton that was harsher still. The biochemistry professor stuck to his guns, and for a time their relationship became more distant.

Olivieri's residents remember the days when she could be charming and gracious. When a resident completed his term, she would hold a dinner in his or her honour and invite everyone on the service. In the late 1980s, the dinners had been at Olivieri's small house in the Annex neighbourhood in Toronto. She'd serve lasagna in the winter, or do a barbecue in the summer. In the early '90s, she was busier and gave up on the home-cooked meals, but took her residents out to a restaurant. She'd always give a going-away present—usually a large and expensive medical text, such as the latest edition of *Nelson's Pediatrics,* the pediatrician's bible.

Her appreciation didn't temper her harsh judgments of residents, but it made the criticisms easier to bear, as did her laughter when she let them in on what she thought of others in the hospital establishment. Exchanging her work shoes for one of the two or three pairs of sneakers beneath her desk, she'd run with the residents from their offices at Sick Kids to a meeting at the Toronto General up the street. She always knew the quickest route—out this back door, through that alleyway, in through a little-used side entrance. Along the way she'd tell stories about people she referred to as "idiots" and "jerks"—the men and women who controlled her division and ran her department at the hospital. She had no end of four-letter words and a steady stream of witty characterizations of those she perceived as her enemies. It was a way to let her residents know that, really, she was on their side and that they were her co-conspirators in her fight against everyone else.

On one morning like that, when Olivieri was in a good mood, Doreen Matsui and Mati Berkovitch filled her in on what was going on with Howard. The patients were generally glad to be taking capsules instead of the nightly injections, and so was Howard. But he'd complained to Matsui and Berkovitch about the study's many requirements. In addition to his weekly blood tests and his monthly transfusion, he was now booked for appointments with multiple specialists. He had to have MRI scans of his heart, MRI and CT scans of his liver, scans of glands and a needle biopsy of his liver. Some of the tests had been added on since the study began because Olivieri had decided she needed more data on the patients in order to fully document the effects of L1. Howard thought that many of the tests were for research purposes and had nothing to do with his health. He told the doctors he wasn't going to go for "these added-on tests." Patients could skip some tests, of course, but that could weaken the findings—if the numbers declined, the study might not be able to show if the drug made a difference.

Olivieri conveyed her view to Howard by way of the residents. "They said, 'Well if you don't go for the tests, you know, you're not going to get any more L1,'" Howard said. "So once my L1 supply ran out, I didn't go to refill it." And he would not return to the only alternative—"Definitely not Desferal because I just basically gave up on Desferal." As a result, Howard was taking nothing to prevent iron from building up in his organs.

Olivieri tried to talk to him about it while he was in the clinic for his monthly transfusion. She sought him out and read him the riot act, reminding him that he'd stopped taking Desferal several times already. As a result, he'd developed problems caused by iron overload, including diabetes. He needed to take L1, and that meant doing the tests—all the tests.

"Look," he said, "I'm not a guinea pig. I agreed to a certain number of tests. But if you change the research, you've got to tell me. You've got to ask me about it, and I'll take it from there." Olivieri explained why each test was necessary. But Howard, who now worked in a lab processing medical tests, wasn't persuaded.

Olivieri was concerned—she wanted Howard on treatment for his iron overload—but she was also blurring the line between a proven therapy and an experimental trial. Doctors are free to cajole or plead with their patients to take a treatment, but a scientist studying human subjects doesn't have that same latitude. Patients who volunteer for clinical trials are always free to withdraw, yet Olivieri was telling Howard that he had to take the tests required by her study and couldn't drop out. Her interaction with Howard was typical of the way she communicated with study subjects, according to her staff. "Patients were ordered to do things if they were in studies," said a staff member with the thalassemia program during the 1990s. "[Olivieri] had strict guidelines when she did a study and if you signed on that bottom line, you had to come in and you had to do those tests." All drug trials make demands on the trial participants; the difference in this case was that the patients were desperate for the drug. Since most of them didn't want to return to Desferal, the thought of losing L1 was enough to make them undergo the many tests. "There was a bit of that bullying going on," explained Josie, "pressure on patients to comply with the protocol."

Another patient said that during her years on L1, she underwent many tests for the trials even when she was unwilling, because she knew the drill if she refused: "It's like, 'Well, then I guess you're not going to [have the test]. Then it's too bad, then you can't go on the drug.'" The young woman didn't want to take Desferal so she did the tests, but she felt she "really had no choice" in the matter. I asked what she thought would happen if she refused one of the tests. "If I said no?" she replied. "Then they would say, 'Well I'm sorry, then you can't get on this drug.' I'm sure that they would say that . . ."

Howard wasn't using Desferal and he wanted to take L1, but he wasn't willing to do the tests.

"I'm not doing it," he told Olivieri. "It's a free country."

"I don't scare easily," he said later, recalling the interaction. "I'm pretty stubborn. She's pretty stubborn too, so we butt heads."

In the end, it was the residents who got him back on the drug. Each month he stayed off L1, Doreen Matsui made a point of finding him when he showed up for his blood transfusion. She didn't want to lose Howard to the devastating effects of iron overload, and she hoped L1 could protect him. "You here to start bugging me again?" Howard would ask whenever he saw her. But the smile on his face belied his words.

Then Mati Berkovitch sat down with him. Berkovitch chatted with Howard for a long time—about life and living with thalassemia. "Howard, we want you back on L1," the young doctor said finally.

"What about the tests?" Howard asked.

Berkovitch waved his hand. "Forget about the tests." Howard says he began taking L1 again because of Berkovitch's assurance that he could refuse tests if he wanted.

As project leader, Olivieri was relying on Matsui and Berkovitch to do exactly what they'd done with Howard—to keep close tabs on the patients in the clinical trial. She had too much on her plate. Though she'd survived Haslam's investigation, it had underscored the sharp contrast between how she was treated at Sick Children's and how she was received in her field, where her profile as an academic was rising. She resented the difference and was especially annoyed that the hospital wasn't giving her more resources for her clinical commitments or her research. The research situation was dire. As Howard returned to L1, the study he was taking part in was acutely short on cash.

8

APOTEX TO THE RESCUE

Keeping a busy clinical trial group afloat is a bit like running a small business, and Olivieri was constantly struggling to give her trials the financial stability they required. "Nancy was fractionated," said a doctor who worked in her clinic in the early '90s. "She was writing too many grant applications." Nancy Olivieri's constant need for funds wasn't uncommon. Researchers in some medical fields spend as much as 40 to 50 per cent of their time writing grants, yet most of their applications are rejected. If Olivieri was short a few thousand, she could call on the leaders of the local thalassemia foundation, all of whom were parents of her patients, and they would often help her out, but that wasn't enough to forge ahead on several different studies at once, as she wanted to do. She had to expand her financial base.

In the fall of 1991, Olivieri's team at Sick Kids had applied to the Medical Research Council for further backing of the L1 project, proposing a randomized trial comparing L1 with Desferal. The subject matter was vitally important and Olivieri had unique qualifications for studying it, but it was turned down, a simmering disappointment. The only MRC funding she had for the work on L1 was billed as a "terminal grant"; it was scheduled to run out in 1993. Once again, Olivieri had faced peer review at the granting agencies and come up short, but this was different than her rejections in the

1980s. She was no longer just starting out—she was a leader in L1 research. Hoping the MRC might still reverse its decision, she contacted David Nathan, and despite his concerns about the dangers of L1, he wrote the agency on her behalf. That brought the response that Olivieri could resubmit her grant application, taking into account the comments of the MRC reviewers.

One of the MRC reviewers had suggested she collaborate with a drug company and reapply for a grant under the MRC's university-industry program, and she began to consider that. It was practical advice—eventually, Olivieri would need an alliance with a drug company in order to bring L1 to the market—but it was also political. The federal government was brokering a deal with Big Pharma to invest $200 million in academic research, and the Medical Research Council's industry program would be one of the beneficiaries. In the U.S., the process of private-public collaboration that had begun with Bayh-Dole in 1980 had led to an explosion of activity transferring discoveries from one arena to the other; now Canada hoped to get in on the action. From Olivieri's standpoint, the MRC's reviewer was echoing what she said the FDA's Stephen Fredd had already told her: partnering with industry was the crucial next step.

Money wasn't all she needed from industry. Her team had been concentrating its efforts on showing that L1 could work and was safe enough to use in patients, but that's only a small part of developing a new product or drug. They also needed to increase their production capacity, and that's the purview of a drug company. Companies spend months or years perfecting a process for mass-producing a new medication while meeting the complex requirements of the regulatory agencies. University labs, such as the one Olivieri had been using, could not function on that scale.

McLelland's lab on the U of T campus was still making L1 for the study patients, as it had been since 1989, but the patients' needs had accelerated. McLelland had taken on an assistant chemist, who had developed a better procedure for purifying the drug, and the lab could now churn out 50,000 grams of L1 over the course of a year—hundreds of thousands of capsules. But each capsule still had to be hand-weighed and hand-carried to the hospital. Knowing of Olivieri's grant rejections, McLelland kept making the drug but told her it was a short-term solution. They needed a drug company to step up.

Olivieri was counting on Ciba-Geigy. In Europe, it had taken the first steps toward developing L1 by signing an agreement with BTG, the British agency, and licensing the patent from them. Though L1's molecular structure remained unpatented, BTG's right to develop it for medical use was protected legally in Europe and the United States. Now Ciba-Geigy had acquired those rights, and its toxicologists were studying the drug in rats and monkeys. Olivieri hoped that when the company began clinical trials it would turn to her as a collaborator, but Ciba-Geigy hadn't yet made any moves in her direction. Toward the end of 1992, waiting for Ciba-Geigy was becoming frustrating, since her grant funding would run out soon.

That December at ASH, the Toronto group revealed that some of its patients on L1 had developed joint pain. Howard's knees hurt and were swollen; Corrado had similar complaints. Berkovitch and Olivieri had examined them thoroughly before sending them on to Sick Kids' arthritis specialists. In the end, three of sixteen patients developed serious pain and swelling in their knees and one had similar symptoms in his hands. All three of the patients with joint pain had immunological abnormalities that showed up in their lab tests—abnormalities that hadn't been present when they had started taking L1. Though the patients remained on L1, it was a serious adverse effect. Berkovitch took the lead on writing up and presenting the findings.

Hearing Berkovitch, hematologists from London were annoyed. Earlier, Nancy Olivieri had discounted the reports of joint pain from London and Bombay, writing the *Lancet* to say her patients didn't have that problem. "Until she saw the side effects, they didn't exist," said Beatrix Wonke. She thought Olivieri had jumped the gun by sending her letter to the *Lancet* without waiting to see if her patients developed the same toxic effects on L1 as patients elsewhere. At the Royal Free, doctors began to worry that Olivieri's reports on the drug were unbalanced. "The good effects were overemphasized and the bad was underemphasized," Wonke explained later.

Doctors in Bombay openly accused Olivieri and other L1 researchers of "inconsistencies and omissions in published trial reports." In a letter to the editor of the *Lancet,* the Indian doctors said Olivieri's group had been specifically leaving out data on immunological abnormalities in her patients. The implication was that she had tried to make L1 sound less risky than it was. Researchers are always free to publish certain data and not others, but they aren't supposed to select data in a way that could misrepresent their findings.

In March 1993, Ciba-Geigy scientists in Basel wrote to all the researchers studying L1, including Nancy Olivieri, to announce that they were cancelling further plans for the drug. The company had completed a series of animal experiments, testing L1 in rats and monkeys. The animals receiving high doses of the drug either died or suffered organ failure. In monkeys, company scientists found "minor toxic effects" of the drug even at low doses. Company scientists said one of the biggest problems was that L1 had "no . . . safety margin," meaning that the amount of drug needed to treat a patient's disease approximated the amount that would be poisonous.

The company hadn't run human clinical trials, but it had been in touch with doctors doing studies of L1 in patients. Ciba-Geigy had gathered reports of four deaths associated with the drug. The company said four other patients on the drug survived but experienced a serious loss of white blood cells—the same type of life-threatening episode that had landed Hoffbrand's young patient in intensive care. Three and a half years after the *Lancet* declared L1 off-limits for human use, Ciba-Geigy reached the same conclusion. It was throwing away L1.

Within days of receiving the letter from the company, Olivieri flew to Crete for an international meeting on thalassemia. The meeting's "hottest topic" was L1, according to George Dover, who was there from Johns Hopkins. "It was clear there were very strong feelings about whether L1 was the best thing to come down the line or whether it was very dangerous," he said. George Kontoghiorghes argued that L1 was a life-saving alternative for patients who couldn't take Desferal. Speaking in the loud and forceful tones that were normal for him, he declared that the drug's toxicity was limited. Other scientists also debated Ciba-Geigy's conclusions. A key problem, they said, was that the company had tested L1 on animals that weren't overloaded with iron. "It's a drug that must be tested in an iron-loaded animal," Bernadette Modell explained later. Though she wasn't studying L1, she thought Ciba's testing process had major flaws. L1 researchers said the hazards L1 posed were preventable. For example, low white cell counts could be averted by frequent blood tests. If the blood tests showed a problem, the patient was taken off the drug and got better.

The doctors passed figures around among themselves as they sat listening to lectures. A Swiss doctor had heard that Desferal was earning Ciba-Geigy US$500 million annually, up from $100 million a few years earlier. Why give that up for a pill that would be cheaper and could earn less? Maybe the company hadn't really wanted to continue with L1 and was just using the animal data as an excuse. As the discussions grew more heated, Nancy Olivieri took centre stage. "Nancy stood in between these two camps and said she was going to study this," recalls Dover. She hoped that her clinical trials would answer many of the questions being raised about L1. Soon after she got home, Olivieri agreed to participate in an informal protest at Ciba-Geigy headquarters in Basel.

When she and other L1 researchers convened in Basel, they were unanimous in their advice to the company: Don't give up on L1. Olivieri was still hoping that Ciba-Geigy would make her a partner in the drug's development. She was furthest ahead with human trials and had the highest numbers of thalassemia patients enrolled. Her results with patients on L1 were encouraging and her group was about to begin its randomized head-to-head comparison of L1 with Desferal. For the comparison study, she intended to assign patients randomly, half to L1 and half to Desferal. She spoke well, according to another scientist attending the meeting, and she looked terrific, "like an angel, with a halo of golden ringlets around her head." But she did not persuade the men from Ciba-Geigy. They were dropping L1 like a hot potato. In fact, they'd already relinquished their patent agreement.

Back in Toronto, Olivieri had to face her disappointment. With financial and production problems mounting, she called Doug Templeton, who'd been funded steadily by Ciba-Geigy over the past few years, and he offered to speak to an official he'd gotten to know at the company. And she spoke to Gideon Koren, who had been appointed division chief for pharmacology and associate director of the Research Institute at Sick Kids in 1992. The dual administrative responsibilities combined with his many committee appointments meant he was overstretched, but he remained as energetic as ever. And despite his busy schedule, Gidi Koren always had time for Olivieri. As she described her funding crisis, he thought he could help by contacting the officials he'd gotten to know at drug companies. He got a nibble on one of the first calls he placed.

The catch on the other end was Apotex, a Toronto-based firm that had been in business for nearly two decades as a manufacturer of generic drugs. Koren's contact there was Michael Spino, a PhD pharmacologist-pharmacist and a former faculty member at Sick Kids. Spino had been in the hospital's pediatric pharmacology program in the early 1980s when Koren started his fellowship, and was an expert in pharmacokinetics. Doctors treating children with cystic fibrosis used to call Spino for advice when a child had a potentially fatal infection, and he would tell them how to ensure the patient wouldn't excrete the antibiotic medication before it had a chance to work. When a boy with severe asthma was brought in to emergency with an infection that made it hard for him to breathe, Spino told the doctors what antibiotics they could use to avoid triggering a fatal drug interaction between the antibiotics and the child's asthma medications. Spino wrote and lectured on many of the drug problems he solved at Sick Kids, acquiring an international reputation among academic pharmacologists, and Koren thought he had been one of the best teachers at the university.

In the early 1980s, Sick Kids head pharmacologist, Stewart MacLeod, took a call from Apotex CEO Barry Sherman. Sherman said he needed help proving to Health Canada that the generic forms of the drugs his firm produced were the same as the brand-name drugs they replaced. MacLeod referred him to Spino, who began devoting time to Apotex as a consultant, becoming expert in the specialized field of bioequivalence, the match between a generic product and its brand-name original. In 1991 Sherman offered Spino a full-time spot running a totally new venture at the company. Until then, Apotex had only produced generics, but Spino would be heading up a research division aimed at developing novel drugs to be marketed as brand-name products. It was an exciting opportunity and he took the job, but he still came to Sick Kids occasionally to teach and work with his former colleagues. In 1992, when Gidi Koren became head of pharmacology at the hospital, he appointed Michael Spino as a consulting faculty member, a nonsalaried position that gave Spino a line on the pharmacology division's letterhead and a small lab.

At the time, so many academics were developing their own companies or consulting part-time to drug companies that the status of individuals who worked in both spheres was in flux. Spino's arrangement—a job in industry together with a lab at a university hospital—wasn't unheard of. Still, Koren was in good stead when he contacted Spino in the spring of '93 about the L1 trials. Koren said later, "At that time, Dr. Olivieri and myself found an open ear in Apotex, because of the fact that we had people we knew." Michael Spino enjoyed being the open ear. He called it "sourcing out" a new idea, and conceded to a reporter in 1993 that he was vetting hundreds of proposals from scientists in university, hospital and government labs as he searched for products to develop. But the chance that any given product would succeed was exceedingly slim. Each compound had to go through the myriad tests, refinements, animal experiments and clinical trials needed to bring a new drug to market—a process of winnowing that rejects thousands of new agents for every one that becomes a licensed drug. Researchers at the Center for Drug Development at Tufts University in Boston who have tried to quantify it say that thousands of chemicals are run through pre-clinical tests in animals without ever entering human trials, and even when compounds make it to the point of clinical trials, only about one-fourth become marketable products.

When Spino joined Apotex in 1991, the company was producing generic versions of more than one hundred different brand-name drugs. The company's worldwide sales averaged $200 million per year, it had spanking new headquarters, it employed seven hundred people, and Sherman was about to embark on the construction of a facility that the company claimed would be "North America's largest drug packaging plant." As a sign of his commitment to developing new drugs, Sherman had built a state-of-the-art biomedical research facility, equipped with expensive laboratory equipment and a forty-eight-bed research ward for drug trials, which opened in the fall of 1992. Around that time, Spino and his staff had a novel product for AIDS in the pipeline. At a federal hearing on drug patent legislation in January 1993, Spino told people that it could prove fifty times more powerful than AZT, then the most powerful agent available to fight the disease. As Spino raved about his test product, Sherman exulted over Spino's intellect. An Apotex ad in a pharmaceutical publication included a photo of the back of Spino's head under the caption, "One of our laboratories." Hubris aside, though, it wasn't clear how much progress the company was making—and the AIDS drug was never released.

After Koren spoke to him about L1, Spino got in touch with Nancy Olivieri. Olivieri ran through her positive results, offered to provide copies of her many publications and meeting abstracts, and described the comparison study of L1 and Desferal that she was just getting underway. She dropped names and numbers, noting that she ran the largest thalassemia clinic in North America and mentioning her meetings with the FDA's Stephen Fredd. Michael Spino had moved from the university to industry but still thought of himself as an academic. His looks befit his corporate job—he was always well coiffed and immaculately dressed—but his mannerisms were that of the professor, and he would often turn to a blackboard or pull out a notebook to diagram something as he was talking. He asked Olivieri a series of questions, then studied L1 in the medical journals. He read that the drug had been controversial and saw that Ciba-Geigy was dropping it. He thumbed through explicit discussions of its toxic side effects and learned that Koren and Olivieri weren't alone in arguing that it deserved to be studied further, so he arranged to speak with Canadian drug regulators about it. By this point, Health Canada had stopped viewing L1 as a drug that could be allowed only for compassionate use, and was permitting Olivieri to test it directly against Desferal in her comparative study. Spino said later that Health Canada officials told him they thought L1 "would be fantastic."

As a business decision, however, investing in the pill wasn't easy to justify. For one thing, the market for L1 in North America was very small. Spino estimated that, at a maximum, there were perhaps one thousand American patients and two hundred Canadians who would take L1. "Who develops a drug for such a small number of patients?" he asked a reporter later. There were other problems as well. L1 could be made using the formula Kontoghiorghes published, but despite that, a North American company wanting to develop it had to pay royalties to the British Technologies Group. Spino figured that between the royalties and the other problems, an investment in L1 was unlikely to generate a return. Even if Apotex paid the royalties, they had no assurance of being the drug's exclusive manufacturer. Everyone working with L1 knew of the unpatented method for making it. The drug might sell well in Third World countries where thalassemia was common and Desferal was too expensive, but Spino didn't expect Apotex to make a substantial profit on it.

In the spring of 1993, Michael Spino told Nancy Olivieri that he doubted any firm would be willing to take a risk on L1, but he still offered to collaborate with her. He claimed it was an act of generosity. "We took on this project to show that Apotex cares, and that money isn't the only thing that motivates the company," he told a reporter for the *Financial Post* later that year. Apotex agreed to fund the project for three years, providing the drug to all of Olivieri's patients who needed it, including the "compassionate use" patients from the earlier study, some of whom had been taking L1 for four years already.

U of T chemist Bob McLelland breathed a sigh of relief when he heard Apotex would take over production of L1. His lab had reached the point of being barely able to keep up with Olivieri's needs. As for Nancy Olivieri, her excitement was palpable when she spoke to Bob Phillips about the Apotex deal. None of the other doctors working with L1 had an industry sponsor. Though they were all her colleagues and she even counted one or two as friends, they were also scientific competitors. Her agreement with Apotex put her way out ahead of the pack.

On April 23, 1993, Nancy Olivieri and Gideon Koren signed the contract drafted by Apotex. Apotex would make the drug, pay for two research residents and cover other research costs up to $128,000 per year for three years. Olivieri would run the trials; Koren would be her co-principal investigator. Olivieri also brought in an American friend, hematologist Gary Brittenham, as a major collaborator. Brittenham's most unusual claim to fame was an invention called the SQUID. The acronym stood for superconducting quantum interference device—an enormous magnetic apparatus that could be used to "guesstimate" the amount of iron in the liver without a patient having to undergo a biopsy. Brittenham was studying it—in fact it was virtually impossible for anyone to study it without him, since his university owned the apparatus and there were no others in North America. It was part of what made him invaluable to Olivieri.

Olivieri's patients on L1 would have annual liver biopsies, but she also wanted them to have the SQUID test that only Brittenham offered. She convinced Spino that it was cutting-edge technology and wrote the costs of yearly trips to Cleveland for each patient into the budget of her Apotex contract. For Brittenham, it was important to keep the SQUID in use and let other researchers see its value. And he enjoyed working with Olivieri, finding her incredibly industrious. "If you want something done, ask Nancy," he said once. "She'll get it done."

In May, Olivieri and her expanded team applied with Apotex to the Medical Research Council's special granting program—the one that required scientists to have an industry partner. This time, the MRC responded favourably. Beginning that fall, her trial comparing L1 with Desferal would receive federal funds of just over $100,000 per year for three years. The increasing momentum underscored Olivieri's success as a researcher and as an advocate for L1. She'd become a sort of cheerleader, persuading and encouraging patients and their families to take part in her research. In early 1993, a few years after the first British paper alerting scientists to the side effects of L1, she pitched the study to the family of an eleven-year-old patient named Patrizia. Olivieri told her that L1 was a promising new drug that could revolutionize the treatment of thalassemia. If it worked, Patrizia could trade in her nightly injections for a pill. Patrizia had been on Desferal since she was four, and the shots left her upper arms hurting and badly scarred. "When Dr. Olivieri told me about L1, I was happy, oh my God, so happy," Patrizia told a reporter for *Maclean's* a few years later. "No more needles."

Louisa Tonna was a few months shy of her fifteenth birthday and was equally interested in L1. Whenever she injected herself with Desferal, "the site would puff up and be irritated, her whole arm would be red," her mother told me later. When Olivieri put her on the new drug, Louisa's family was "thrilled with relief."

Olivieri made the case for L1 to another patient that year, a girl who was about twelve years old. The girl's mother was present at the time. "Dr. Olivieri described the study and my daughter said, 'Why should I switch from Desferal?' The answer Dr. Olivieri gave was, 'I think we might have finally found something that will work.' She presented it as if she seemed to be extremely confident. She had all these positive reasons for starting on it. There had been other drugs, but this one seemed to be right and seemed to be working. I think she said, 'This time we've hit the nail on the head' or something like that. So we said okay."

Josie, now at university in Hamilton, was taking a course in moral issues. It covered informed consent in research and Josie was surprised to learn that in clinical trials, a patient's own doctor is not supposed to ask the patient to participate. In the thalassemia program at Sick Kids, she explained, "it used to always be the doctor who was doing the inviting."

In order to be valid, a patient's consent has to be given freely. If the patient's doctor extends the invitation to join the research, patients—or their parents—may say yes to avoid jeopardizing their relationship with the doctor. Researchers are encouraged to ensure that someone who has no connection to the patient is the one to describe the study and ask the patient to join. With Olivieri doing the asking herself, Josie said, "you've got the researcher who is also the physician asking permission [to include the patient in the trial]. I thought that was one of the cardinal things that you don't do."

Another strategy to ensure patients don't face external pressure to be in a trial is to make it clear that declining to participate won't change the patient's level of care. Thalassemia patients received care in Toronto whether or not they signed on to a study, but if they joined a clinical trial, they got to see Olivieri. The patients who weren't research subjects saw the program's pediatricians or residents.

As Josie listened to her professor give a textbook description of informed consent, she felt it didn't match what she and her friends had experienced. In the thalassemia program, she said, "it's very much: 'This is what we recommend,' and then the families agree." One staff member of the program said patients and their families were "well informed as to what the studies were all about," but another member of the staff became so worried about Olivieri's interactions with her study subjects that she wrote supervisors about her fears. Patients weren't "having opportunities to have information and to make choices," she wrote, and "weren't getting all the information. They were just being told, 'This is what you need to do.'"

Toward the end of the summer of 1993, Olivieri played research cheerleader with the federal government. This time, the patient was a six-year-old Pakistani girl with thalassemia named Duri-Sadaf Ali. Duri-Sadaf was enrolled in Olivieri's compassionate use trial of L1 and seemed to be doing well. But Canada planned to deport her family back to the U.S., where they'd arrived first from their native Pakistan. At a press conference, Duri-Sadaf showed reporters the space where her two front teeth were missing, and lisped that she wanted to stay in Canada "because I love my doctor and I love my nurse." Olivieri told the reporters that Duri-Sadaf was part of a special clinical trial. "I don't know who is telling you she can receive adequate medical treatment if deported, but that's false," she said. "She'd die in Pakistan, no question, in fact, the L1 treatment she needs isn't even available in the U.S." The girl remained in Canada and on L1.

By sponsoring the L1 trials and producing the drug, Apotex was playing a critical role in the drug's development. Some academics see those sorts of partnerships as necessary evils, though, because funding from industry isn't the same as a grant from the MRC or the NIH and it often comes with strings attached. In Nancy Olivieri's case, she finally had a solid financial base for her research, but unlike federal funding agencies, Apotex wanted something in return. The company planned to use her data to seek approval of L1 in Canada, the U.S. and Europe. Olivieri was a contract researcher now, and her contract included a gag order, noting that her results would be kept confidential for three years; they could not be disclosed to a third party without the company's prior written consent.

"When you do something for someone else as a contractor, they own the data that you collect," neuroscientist Floyd Bloom explained in 1998 in an interview for CBC Radio about the influence of commercial sponsors on academic research. "It's not your choice as to what to do. It's not very appropriate in terms of the scientific thought process, but that, in fact, is what you agreed to do." Bloom works at Scripps Research Institute in La Jolla, California. As editor of *Science* magazine during the 1990s, he dealt repeatedly with the issue of academia-industry collaboration in science. But other scientists see the issue of sponsored research differently. They draw a distinction between "private" research that begins in a company and "public" research that begins in a university but is supported by a company along the way. In the university setting, they say, it's immoral for a company to claim ownership of a research project. But Bloom is correct that when companies foot the bill, they frequently claim rights over the data.

In 1993, NIH director Bernadine Healy testified in Congress against an agreement between Scripps in California and the Swiss drug giant Sandoz that gave the company permission to review papers by Scripps scientists before publication and to dictate who could enter a building in which Sandoz-related research was being done. Healy said the arrangement was "against the spirit of science and possibly against the law." The contract between Scripps and Sandoz was reconfigured. Yet some restrictions are legal. In 2003, Yale researchers reviewing published studies reported in the *Journal of the American Medical Association* (*JAMA*) that scientists conducting industry-sponsored research often face restrictions on publishing and sharing their data. Typically, data from clinical trials belong to the sponsoring company, and making them public is the company's decision, as Thomas Bodenheimer explained in a presentation at the National Institutes of Health in 2000. That year, the portion of biomedical research paid for by the industry on U.S. campuses reached 62 per cent, nearly double what it had been in 1980, when the Bayh-Dole Act came into effect. As academics have extended their collaborations with industry, the question of who owns a researcher's ideas or data has grown into one of the most contentious issues in modern science.

In Canada in 1993, when Nancy Olivieri agreed to work with Apotex, the issue hadn't yet received much attention and the dance steps between academic scientists and private companies weren't very clearly marked out. Olivieri said later that she'd been naive when she had signed the contract the company drew up. But it wasn't just that. Her work on L1 was an enormous effort. She was quarterbacking a diverse research team, encouraging patients to enrol in her studies of the drug, and coping with new adverse effects—all at the same time. She'd presented her data to the FDA and discovered that the agency was interested in L1. But she was rejected in her quest for a federal grant. One of the grant's reviewers told her to find a company to work with. She'd hoped to collaborate with a major international pharmaceutical firm but was turned away by Ciba-Geigy. In a desperate search for funds, she had found a smaller company in Toronto that was interested. Michael Spino later described Olivieri and Koren as "scientists pleading for help." The company had answered her pleas, and she was grateful; she more or less asked them where to sign.

9

UNDOING SUSAN PERRINE

As Olivieri spent time on L1, she also continued to maintain her involvement in collaborations on other drugs for thalassemia or sickle cell disease. One project was going particularly well, involving a new drug called butyrate. The promise of butyrate was that it was almost a cure—it could form a sort of hemoglobin substitute in the body so that patients with defective hemoglobin didn't need blood transfusions. The thought of using butyrate to treat hemoglobin disorders was the brainchild of Susan Perrine, a woman Nancy Olivieri had gotten to know during her years in Boston. As with L1, once Olivieri got involved with butyrate, she devoted so much energy to the project that she began to take it over.

Susan Perrine owed her interest in hematology to her physician father. He was practising internal medicine in Saudi Arabia and became intrigued by a form of sickle cell disease found there that did not cause patients to develop the usual painful episodes associated with the disease: the Saudi patients were protected from the consequences of their anemia because they had high levels of fetal hemoglobin, a form of hemoglobin normally found only in very young babies. Yet these patients had fetal hemoglobin throughout their lives.

From Saudi Arabia, Susan Perrine's father began collaborating with scientists in Oxford and elsewhere to learn more about the puzzle of late-life fetal hemoglobin. Over the next few years, he tested hundreds of people in eastern Saudi Arabia, and his daughter joined his research operation for a summer while she was in medical school. The findings were striking. A sizeable group of Saudi Arabians had sickle cell disease but had never felt its effects—they all had high levels of fetal hemoglobin. Perrine and his collaborators coined the term "benign sickle-cell anaemia" to describe what they were seeing, and their papers triggered a series of similar studies in Jamaica and South Africa, where doctors also described adults who were protected from the disease's consequences because they continued to make fetal hemoglobin instead of "switching" entirely to adult hemoglobin.

Soon, the NIH became interested in the connection between sickle cell disease and fetal hemoglobin, and by the early 1980s "hemoglobin switching"—the switch from fetal to adult hemoglobin during early development—was a hot topic. Around that time, Susan Perrine entered the pediatric hematology-oncology fellowship program at Boston Children's Hospital, intending to focus her research on fetal hemoglobin. But she was entering a crowded playing field. Already, several teams of scientists were looking for a drug that could get patients with severe anemia to start making fetal hemoglobin again.

Nancy Olivieri arrived in Boston toward the end of Perrine's fellowship. Officially, Olivieri was in Stuart Orkin's lab, learning to clone genes. Unofficially, she was spending time at Boston Children's, getting to know the hematologists there. She met most of the hematology residents, including Perrine, one of the few women in the group. Pretty, with a soft smile, Susan Perrine kept to herself and was known for her reserved manner. By contrast, the men in the hematology fellowship were good friends who shared meals and told each other tales about their boss, the thalassemia expert David Nathan. The fellows knew of the so-called Saturday night massacre, when, as Harvard's head pediatrician for hematology and oncology, Nathan fired several faculty members at once—but they also knew him as the befuddled owner of an aging car that was always breaking down. Susan Perrine wasn't the sort to joke about her chief, and she also may have been uncomfortable being the only woman in the crowd.

Perrine's research kept her busy. Working on the labour and delivery suites of another Harvard teaching hospital, she collected blood drawn from the umbilical cords of newborns, analyzing it to see how much fetal hemoglobin it contained. Some of the babies had much higher levels of fetal hemoglobin than others, and when she examined the medical charts for those babies, she discovered that their mothers all had diabetes. Something in diabetic mothers was causing increased production of fetal hemoglobin. It was an intriguing discovery, and in 1985 Perrine published it in the *New England Journal of Medicine.*

On finishing her fellowship, she left Boston and took a job closer to her family, as a staff hematologist at the Children's Hospital in Oakland, California. Once there, she pursued the question of the diabetic mothers, trying to find out what triggered production of fetal hemoglobin in their newborns. She thought she found the answer in a substance called butyrate, a naturally occurring fatty acid found in butter and cod liver oil that also shows up in human sweat. A group at the Medical College of Georgia had experimented with it during the early 1980s and found that when they added it to cord blood, the production of fetal hemoglobin rose significantly. When Perrine tested the cord blood of the infants with diabetic mothers and found butyrate, she thought she might have solved the puzzle.

Butyrate is a natural product used as a flavour enhancer and food additive. It had been tested previously as a therapy for leukemia and though it didn't work, it didn't cause any bad side effects. Perrine was eager to see if she could give it to patients with thalassemia or sickle cell disease and raise their hemoglobin levels. She began by taking samples of blood from patients with thalassemia and using them to grow colonies of red blood cells; then she added butyrate to the resulting cell colonies. It worked: the red cell colonies made fetal hemoglobin and by the late 1980s, Perrine was presenting her results at international conferences.

Sheep were used as a model for hemoglobin switching, so Perrine apprenticed herself to a scientist who taught her how to operate on ewes. Then she began working with the animals when they were pregnant, infusing their lambs with butyrate prior to birth. She discovered that butyrate worked in the lambs just as it had in the red cells: lambs that got butyrate via prenatal infusions were born with higher levels of fetal hemoglobin. Writing up the experiment, Perrine concluded by saying that butyrate might be used to treat sickle cell anemia or thalassemia in the future. She started to put together a clinical trial to test butyrate in patients.

Perrine had been making the butyrate she needed herself, ordering basic ingredients from a chemical warehouse and mixing, filtering and sterilizing them to produce a specific form of the substance. Now she had to develop a form of the drug that patients could take. Unlike Bob McLelland, she had never made experimental compounds for human use. She tried making butyrate according to FDA standards, working completely on her own, and paid for her inexperience: it was two years before she had a product that passed muster with the FDA. Finally, in 1991, she was ready to enrol patients in a clinical trial.

Nancy Olivieri had collaborated with Perrine on a few small projects that involved experimental treatments for sickle cell anemia. When Olivieri heard that Perrine was testing butyrate in a clinical trial, she thought one of the thalassemia patients in Toronto, a woman in her early twenties named Anita, could be a perfect candidate. Anita had an unusual form of thalassemia in which she became resistant to transfusions over time. After age seven, she could

no longer be transfused, so she suffered all the symptoms of thalassemia that had been seen in the 1950s—frequent fractures,
deformed bones, a deformed face, stunted growth and delayed puberty.
She couldn't even exercise. A game of volleyball at age eight had left
her with a broken wrist, and after that doctors had advised that all ath-
letic activities were to be avoided. Listing her medical problems,
Nancy Olivieri noted "gross, progressive skeletal deformities." For
Anita it wasn't a medical observation; it was depressing. She felt terribly unattractive. At sixteen she began asking when she could have
plastic surgery on her face. The surgeons told her that was impossible;
they'd have no way to transfuse her if they ran into a problem of blood
loss. Later, describing herself to a reporter, she said, "My cheekbones
are rather large and the bridge of my nose is rather flat. I'm not fully
grown and I don't look my age. When other people see me, they wonder what happened."

When Anita was twenty, she started having vision problems. She
thought she needed glasses, but it wasn't that simple. Olivieri told a
reporter later, "Bone marrow was forming everywhere, including in
the optic canal, and it was crushing her optic nerves." Olivieri thought
she would go blind. She also had early signs of heart disease—she was
weak and tired all the time. Olivieri saw her as a desperate patient
who could die soon and for whom standard care for thalassemia was
off-limits. A trial of an experimental drug was therefore justified.
Olivieri introduced Perrine to Anita, who says that both doctors were
very positive about butyrate; Anita decided to try it.

Perrine got permission from the FDA to test butyrate as an
investigational new drug, while Olivieri applied to the Health
Protection Branch at Health Canada and the Research Ethics Board
at Sick Kids. All of the monitoring agencies gave the trial a green
light, and Anita started on butyrate in the spring of 1992. Perrine
flew to Toronto and moved in for two weeks with Olivieri. Every
two days, twenty-one-year-old Anita travelled the hour from her

hometown of Guelph to Sick Kids, where a nurse hooked her up to an intravenous line for an infusion of butyrate that lasted eight hours.

After Perrine returned home, Anita continued to come to Sick Kids for butyrate infusions. The drug smelled bad, but it seemed to be working. Her eyesight improved, her fetal hemoglobin levels rose significantly and she had a level of energy she hadn't had for years. It was the sort of result that usually could be achieved only with blood transfusions. Perrine and Olivieri were both excited by how well Anita was doing.

Perrine started more patients on butyrate in California, and Olivieri did the same in Toronto. After a few months, their trial had accumulated six patients—three with sickle cell disease and three with thalassemia. During a few weeks on the drug, all of the patients did well, though the best success story was Anita's. Perrine took the lead on writing up the results, and when the paper was published (in January 1993 in the *New England Journal of Medicine*) hematologists were stunned. "That paper astounded us all," George Dover said. "No one had seen changes like that in any thalassemic patient before . . . This was an astounding response that was seen. The patient was independent of transfusions. That was the cure that every thalassemic patient in the world was looking for."

Susan Perrine had high hopes for the drug and wanted to test it in longer and larger trials, but her grant monies wouldn't cover those costs. Then her *New England Journal of Medicine* article came out. The huge German chemical company BASF was looking to build up its pharmaceutical interests and negotiated a deal with Perrine's hospital in California to make butyrate in an oral form. At first it sounded terrific. The company would make the drug and sponsor the trials. In return, Perrine and her hospital would have data and royalties. But Susan Perrine grew worried. She had never worked with a private company and, like Olivieri, was naive about dealings with industry. She didn't know where to turn for advice on her concerns that Anita wouldn't be able to get the drug once BASF took over the rights to make it. Anxious that her prize patient would be left without the drug she was dependent on, Perrine refused to sign with BASF and the hospital's deal fell apart.

Perrine's bosses at Children's Hospital Oakland had courted BASF assiduously, and they reacted bitterly to the loss. A security guard escorted Perrine off the premises of the hospital; she was even barred from her own lab. When a San Francisco reporter phoned Olivieri for comment, she described Perrine as "a very principled person." In April 1993, Perrine settled her dispute with the hospital, but the experience made it difficult for her to continue working there. She moved back to Boston and took a faculty position at Boston University.

Anita remained on butyrate. It was still working for her and nothing else had. Olivieri wanted to start Anita's ten-year-old brother on the drug too, since he had the same unusual variant of thalassemia. Perrine applied to the FDA for permission to use the "investigational new drug" for longer than originally approved and negotiated with a chemical compounding facility in Texas to make the drug according to her specifications, while Nancy Olivieri obtained grant funding for a longer-term trial.

Over the course of a year, Anita and her brother did well on butyrate and Olivieri signed other patients to the trial, including two kindergartners and a toddler with thalassemia. But the experiment didn't work out the way Olivieri and Perrine had hoped. The youngest patients all experienced anemia after three to four months on butyrate. All ten of the patients Olivieri put on butyrate experienced the significant side effects of lost appetite and lost weight, and most were nauseous to the point that they required anti-nausea drugs. One patient developed intractable vomiting. And then there was a crisis.

One of the patients in the trial, a teenager with sickle cell disease, had a seizure while receiving an intravenous infusion of butyrate at the Hospital for Sick Children. He began to flail uncontrollably, then fell silent; nurses quickly determined that he had seized as a result of a massive overdose. Butyrate was supposed to be given intravenously as a mixture in a 2.5 per cent solution. Instead, a 10 per cent solution of the drug was prepared—four times the dose that had been ordered—and the overdose dripped into the patient's veins for six hours, until he seized. Nurses said afterwards that the drug bottles were poorly labelled.

Olivieri was notified immediately. Worried that her patient could experience permanent neurological damage, she ordered a full battery of tests and everyone was relieved when the tests didn't point to long-term consequences. The patient went off butyrate for two weeks and then was willing to complete the trial, staying on the drug for another few weeks. But seizures hadn't been recorded before in a patient receiving butyrate. It was a new adverse reaction, and the researchers had to alert the drug agencies in Washington and Ottawa.

At Sick Kids there wasn't a clear system for ensuring that adverse reactions to experimental agents got reported promptly, but at the drug agencies, the rules are clear. If researchers testing an experimental drug discover a serious unexpected problem, they have to report it. The basic policy on experimental drugs is "report first and ask questions later." Otherwise, another patient taking the drug at a different research centre may get injured, needlessly. The drug agencies may step in to halt a study if the side effects of a drug are too worrisome, or they can limit the patients who can participate. In this case, they could prohibit patients with a history of seizures from taking part in butyrate experiments.

It was Susan Perrine's responsibility to inform the FDA since she was the one who had obtained official permission to work on an investigational new drug, but she didn't learn about the seizure or the overdose until Olivieri told her about it one month later. When Perrine realized what had happened and how much time had passed, she was shocked. She was afraid they had violated FDA policy because she hadn't contacted the agency. She flew to Toronto for another two-week stint, this time checking into a hotel. She spent her days sifting through the medical charts of patients on butyrate and going to the lab to check their blood tests. She examined the patients herself and met with Olivieri's residents, and she questioned Olivieri about her methods for administering the drug. She and Olivieri implemented a series of safety measures to protect against another overdose and wrote a letter to the FDA and Health Canada describing the overdose and the new safeguards.

Later, one hematologist said, "I don't think anyone had ever questioned Nancy's ability to do a clinical trial." Now Perrine had questioned her about a drug error and a patient's seizure. The relationship between the two women was never the same after that. A few weeks after Perrine left Toronto, Olivieri wrote her about one of the patients she'd seen, a young woman with a cut on her leg. Perrine had told one of Olivieri's residents that they should write about the woman for a scientific journal because her cut had begun healing on butyrate and the healing could be a sign that the drug was working. Olivieri wasn't writing Perrine to discuss the scientific aspects of the issue. Instead, she was worried about who would get credit for the idea. Her letter informed Perrine that if any articles were written about patients on butyrate in Toronto, she would author them. Nancy Olivieri had just moved Susan Perrine from "in" to "out"; she didn't want to collaborate with her any more. That was easier for Olivieri than it would have been for most researchers studying novel drugs because butyrate is a natural product that can't be patented. Olivieri was on familiar ground: she was working with a compound that, like L1, was legally unprotected and she found a way of making it in a form called arginine butyrate.

"One thing to say about Nancy, she's very resourceful," says her hematologist friend and colleague George Dover. "For example,

Nancy made L1, and because Susan had no patent rights to arginine butyrate, Nancy got that made up in Toronto." Once she had a steady local supply of the drug, Olivieri stopped sending data from the butyrate trial to Perrine. At first, Perrine didn't realize what had happened. Then Olivieri gave a presentation about butyrate at a scientific conference and wrote an article about the patient with the cut on her leg but didn't invite Perrine to participate in either venture. The article, co-authored by one of her residents, appeared in *Blood* in the fall of 1994. Perrine felt as if her work as a collaborator had been stolen.

A few months later, Olivieri wrote up her findings on the long-term butyrate trial. Many hematologists were growing skeptical about butyrate as no doctor using a similar substance had been able to reproduce the findings seen with Anita. Olivicri reviewed the data from her patients and decided that she too was unimpressed. Ten patients, five with sickle cell disease and five with thalassemia, had been infused with arginine butyrate on an almost daily basis for about ten weeks. As Olivieri steadily increased the dose, two of the sickle cell patients experienced a significant rise in fetal hemoglobin, then their levels fell back to baseline. Anita and her brother continued to do well on the drug but, in Olivieri's view, their results weren't representative. None of the other thalassemia patients showed any response. She concluded that, overall, butyrate didn't work very well. Susan Perrine saw it differently.

It's not unheard of for a group of scientists to work together and later disagree about their findings. Even scientists who have practised their craft for decades sometimes encounter these situations. To resolve them, the collaborators could write one paper offering two opposing views of the data, or write two separate papers and advise a journal editor of their disagreement. But neither of those things happened. Instead, Olivieri wrote a paper that didn't list Susan Perrine as an author but simply acknowledged her "for arranging the initial supply" of butyrate, and submitted it to the *New England Journal of Medicine* without contacting Perrine. In its first version, the paper was rejected. In Olivieri's second submission, she stated clearly and strongly that butyrate was ineffective. The stark conclusion increased the chance that the paper would be accepted, because the journal has a policy of considering a paper even more seriously if its findings are the reverse of findings the journal has already published. Her paper came out in June 1995.

Perrine's close colleagues published letters in the *New England Journal of Medicine* disputing Olivieri's conclusions, but letters don't have the weight of a published article and Olivieri's evidence against butyrate had swift consequences for the entire field. Proposals to work on the drug got shot down in the next funding round at the NIH. A hematologist who intended to study butyrate in California heard from grant reviewers that it wasn't a promising line of research; a New York–based scientist heard the same thing; and Susan Perrine's federal grants weren't renewed. Perrine's friends thought she'd have to study something else or give up her research career.

The article's impact derived from more than the cachet of the *New England Journal of Medicine*; it was also a sign of the stature Nancy Olivieri had achieved as a scientist by the summer of 1995. Despite her disappointments at the Hospital for Sick Children, she was influential in the international scientific sphere of doctors researching hemoglobin disorders.

Perrine didn't have the same high profile, but she survived her funding hiatus and eventually began studying butyrate again, collaborating with scientists in the U.S. and Europe to figure out why it failed to work for certain patients. It turned out that the drug didn't work properly if patients took it continuously. The solution was to give it intermittently, similar to the way cancer patients take chemotherapy. When patients received butyrate steadily for four weeks and went off it for two weeks—a form of treatment called "pulse therapy"—it was effective enough that some patients no longer needed transfusions. Within a few years, Perrine was involved in a multi-centre study to test butyrate's effectiveness in sickle cell patients and, in 1999, she and her collaborators published their results: pulse therapy with butyrate worked for more than two-thirds of the patients. Meanwhile, Anita and her brother remained on butyrate. Olivieri added hydroxyurea to their regimen and wrote in the *Lancet* in 1997 that their "remarkable response" to the two drugs was probably explained by genetic factors.

Butyrate still has a negative image, and industry funding for large-scale clinical trials has been difficult to come by, but Perrine and other butyrate researchers are encouraged because federal funding agencies have renewed their interest in the drug. The NIH is funding butyrate trials and, in 2004, one of the scientists it funded to do such work was Nancy Olivieri, who planned to treat thirty thalassemia patients with sodium phenyl butyrate and three other drugs in "an attempt to provide definitive therapy" for their disease.

THE TRIPLE THREAT

Olivieri's funding from Apotex started in early 1993. Later that spring, she spoke at the FDA again, after the agency's Stephen Fredd heard about L1 from U.S.-based thalassemia advocacy groups. "The disease advocates were very anxious to get going," Fredd recalled. A group of L1 researchers requested another meeting at the FDA and it was held in October, with Olivieri, Brittenham and others presenting. Olivieri's data showed that L1 was working for patients but the doctors also described its toxic effects. "So all of this was put forth," said Fredd, "and the question was, would we allow clinical trials to go forward." Ciba-Geigy's answer was already on the table: because of the drug's toxicity, the company would not conduct human tests. But Olivieri had Canadian approval to run clinical trials. For the FDA staffers present, Fredd said, the issue was straightforward: "We already knew there was toxicity in humans. The question was, would the benefits outweigh the risks."

Olivieri and others thought the problems with L1 could be managed, and she felt encouraged by her meeting at the FDA. She left believing the agency would probably approve clinical trials of L1. Coming on the heels of her Apotex contract, that was exciting, but it also raised the stakes. FDA approval meant that American scientists interested in working with the drug could begin running their own trials. In New York, doctors at Cornell University's medical school were already experimenting with L1 on a small scale, using it in a few patients every year, and doctors at Harvard and Yale were doing the same thing. The pressure on Olivieri was mounting. To avoid being scooped on L1, she had to compile her results and get them into print as quickly as possible. But it wasn't easy to find time.

By the middle of 1994, Olivieri was at the head of a clinical trial to compare L1 with Desferal, involving her patients from Toronto and thalassemia patients from the Montreal Children's Hospital. She was also continuing her long-term follow-up study of patients on L1, the compassionate use study. She had to send data from both studies to Apotex, since the company now had the responsibility of reporting to the regulatory agencies. There were numerous checklists to keep track of and sheets to fill out on every patient. She was "busier and busier, more involved in the clinical trial, and more stressed," says Doug Templeton.

Olivieri was living the classic catch-22 of the teaching hospital, trying to be a full-time scientist while holding down a clinical post that came with responsibility for scores of patients. She stayed at the hospital until very late at night and spent many of her weekends working. Still, she'd be racing during the day to review manuscript galleys that were due back to a medical journal in forty-eight hours, or to meet a grant deadline that would be up at the end of the week. In the midst of it all, she had to dole out precious moments to her patients and residents. She had become what was known in academic medical circles as a "triple threat": researcher, clinical practitioner and teacher. Though it was the traditional role of academic physicians to be all three, some medical schools in the U.S. and Canada had begun to realize that a single person could no longer master them all. Study after study of medical and surgical outcomes showed that volume mattered. The more patients with a particular disease a doctor treated, the better the patients did. Hospitals—and third-party payers—wanted high-volume clinicians. In earlier decades, physicians could spend the bulk of their time with patients but still do "research with a small R," as some academics called it. But running experiments—including clinical trials—had become much more demanding.

As a result, universities had begun developing different tracks for their medical school faculty. Clinician-teachers, for example, split their time between seeing patients in clinic and teaching residents but didn't do research. On the other side of the coin, scientists at the Hospital for Sick Children's Research Institute taught graduate students in their labs but saw no patients. Yet the idea that a doctor could function simultaneously as a top-notch clinician, an internationally acclaimed scientist and a gifted teacher was still firmly entrenched, and academic physicians were often stuck trying to do it all. For Nancy Olivieri, the time management problem was underscored because she'd won a grant from the Medical Research Council requiring her to devote 80 per cent of her time to science; it was a superhuman feat to meet all of her other demands in only 20 per cent of the workweek.

Officially, she was directing the thalassemia and sickle cell clinics at Sick Kids, scheduled to see patients herself on Wednesday mornings and to supervise their care at other times. But in reality, she'd clamped down on the time she spent in clinic in order to preserve time for her research. Her patients rarely saw her any more, and the residents rotating through the thalassemia and sickle cell clinics didn't see her either.

The patients and families who knew Olivieri felt cut off. In earlier years, she would chat briefly whenever she ran into them on their appointed transfusion day. Now she would walk by a patient without saying a word. She was distracted, and the patients and their families were hurt. Howard would tell those who complained about one of his favourite doctors, "Well, I'm sorry, but she's very busy and can't stop to say hi to everyone." But he knew he was privileged—

he stayed in touch via e-mail and phone. "Sometimes I'd get e-mails from her at two or three in the morning or at five or six in the morning," he said. He'd write back, "Did you actually go home tonight?"

Josie tried telling patients that Olivieri was still keeping an eye on them even if she didn't see them in clinic. But the parents of younger children were frustrated. They would book a child's monthly transfusion session specifically for Wednesday in order to see Dr. Olivieri. Then, for months on end, she wouldn't be there. They had to settle for the pediatricians hired to cover her clinics, or for the nurses and residents.

Over time, parents came to appreciate the pediatricians, who had a fundamental knowledge base about kids and adolescents that Olivieri, who was not a pediatrician, sometimes lacked. But the staff who came closest to filling Olivieri's shoes were the residents, who essentially ran the thalassemia service. In 1993–94, that task fell to Graham Sher, an MD-PhD from South Africa who was taking a year off from his residency at the U of T to be Nancy Olivieri's research fellow. Sher cared for most of the thalassemia patients through his work in their clinic, and he taught the students and residents on the service. A doctor who worked with him said, "You'd like to hate him if he wasn't so nice, because he's just so perfect— a good scientist, a good clinician, an excellent speaker." Many of the patients also became quite fond of Graham Sher that year. They liked the fact they could usually find him "floating around the hospital somewhere."

"Graham had an incredible talent or just knack, and it was his bedside manner," said one patient. "He was just really good at it. There was just something very competent about him. He had an attachment to us."

Whether in his office at the hospital or in an examining room at the clinic, Sher acted as if he were in his own living room. He'd lean his lanky body forward to hear what a person was saying, biting his lips the way a child might to concentrate on the words. Another time he'd sit back in his chair and throw his legs up on the desk, reflecting on the question he'd just been asked. He wasn't in a rush, arrogance wasn't in his nature, and he didn't seem to have a temper to lose.

When Sher left the thalassemia program in the summer of 1994 to complete his residency, neither the patients nor Nancy Olivieri wanted to see him go. For Olivieri, losing Graham Sher had practical and personal implications. She liked him, and she'd become good friends with his wife. Sher was also a vital part of her organization on the ground. She trusted him as a physician. "The whole time I was there, Graham was God," one doctor said. "Nancy would say what a good job he did." The thalassemia patients also knew of Olivieri's high regard for Sher. One patient said of Sher's year in the thalassemia clinic, "He was new to it. And here was Dr. Olivieri putting him up on a pedestal. He could do no wrong. He'd say to us, 'You know, I think we should do this, but I need to ask [Dr. Olivieri's] opinion.' And I'd say to him, 'Oh, come on. You know whatever you say to do, she'll say "Fine."'"

South of the border, the notion of a clinical service being run by a resident was under fire. The U.S. government—through its Medicare and Medicaid programs—was refusing to pay for medical care delivered by students training to become physicians or by physicians training to become specialists. But in Canada, the British model of resident-centred care was still acceptable.

Sher was there to step in when Alex got sick. Alex, Josie's boyfriend, was now in his twenties. Tall and lean, he'd been a leader in the patients' organization, and one of the first thalassemia patients from Toronto to travel to an international meeting and talk with patients from other countries. But, like his friends Howard and Biagio, he often skipped his Desferal shots, explaining to those who asked that it wasn't intentional, it was just that he played hockey. He had to be at practice early in the morning and he didn't think he should have to choose between hockey and his medication.

"Hogwash," said Josie, who didn't accept his excuses, and tried to get him to take his medication regularly. His mother had also tried, but he'd learned to fool her. He'd hook up his pump and put the needle in before saying goodnight to his parents. Then he'd let the drug run out into the bathroom sink.

When Biagio died, Alex approached the clinic nurse who had pleaded with them all to take their Desferal. "You knew this was where we were headed," he said. "You knew it before we knew it." Alex easily won the hearts of the staff, yet despite their efforts, he continued to skip his injections. The nurse spoke to Howard and another patient about it. "[The nurse] pulled us aside—because by that time we were compliant, I was very compliant—and asked us to talk to him," Howard recalled. "We did, and I don't know if it actually worked out or not." A clinic staff member said of Alex, "He just couldn't comply with what seemed to be—for the rest of us— the thing that was going to keep him alive."

In the winter of 1994, soon after he and Josie got engaged, Alex collapsed while playing ball hockey. His heart was overloaded with iron and had gone into a dangerous rhythm. He was rushed to the hospital, where he was treated with cardiac medications and recovered. Olivieri's randomized trial comparing L1 and Desferal was underway and Alex, who had already agreed to be in it, was randomly selected to receive L1. He started on it, but the oral drug didn't help. After only a few months on the pills, the doctors switched him to intravenous Desferal.

It was the same strategy thalassemia specialists were using everywhere for their patients with serious problems. Desferal directly through the veins was their biggest gun. But Alex's heart didn't recover. It went into a dangerous rhythm again and he was moved into intensive care, where Olivieri, who had known him since he was a child, went by to give him encouragement. She believed his only option was a transplant.

Initially, Alex and Josie weren't frightened by the prospect. They knew that their friend Gino had been saved by a transplant. In any given week, Gino might skip his Desferal as many nights as he would take it. Olivieri and other doctors had issued stern warnings of the calamity he faced, but he wouldn't change his ways. By the age of twenty-five his heart was so badly damaged from iron over-load that a transplant was his only option. But the high levels of iron circulating in his system had given him cirrhosis, and his liver wouldn't be able to tolerate the drugs that transplant patients are required to take. In Gino's case, Olivieri had asked the surgeons to consider a novel operation in which the heart and liver were both transplanted simultaneously. Only a handful of "heart-livers" had been done anywhere in the world, and none in Canada. But Gino got his new heart and new liver in May 1991 at age twenty-six. His operation—described by Nancy Olivieri in the *New England Journal of Medicine*—made history in Toronto. And now she wanted Alex to get a new heart and liver, too.

A donor heart became available first. Josie remembers the last words she said to him before the operation: "I'll see you when you wake up." Olivieri was in Europe pursuing her research commit-ments, so the transplant team called Graham Sher, who scrubbed in on the case to help. As a result, Sher was in the operating room when the surgeons ran into trouble with the donor heart. "It was devastating," Sher told Josie afterwards. The heart pumped so sluggishly they assumed the donor had been a drug addict. Still, it was Alex's only hope. Sher and the other doctors began massaging Alex's new heart to try to get it to start. They stayed at the operat-ing table several hours longer, giving Alex different medications to try to get the donated organ to work, but they lost him on the operating room table. Olivieri found out about it only when she got back to Toronto a week later.

Alex was the youngest of four children in a Greek family. He was the only boy and the only one with thalassemia. At a meeting with the doctors that took place after Alex died, his mother blamed his death on the new experimental drug. Given how Alex died, in the middle of a transplant operation, L1 was an extremely unlikely culprit. But he'd taken L1 for a few months before becoming deathly ill, and his mother was convinced the pills had made him sicker.

Olivieri didn't think L1 had harmed Alex, but her worry that she didn't know enough about the drug's side effects grew. L1's most serious toxic effect was the one that had first alarmed Victor Hoffbrand in London: a patient's white cells could be wiped out. But no one knew whether this would occur in 1 out of 1,000 patients taking the drug, or 1 out of 10,000, or at some other rate. Olivieri, believing the FDA could demand an exact figure, began discussing a new study with Gary Brittenham aimed at quantifying all toxic side effects in patients on L1. She also recruited another friend of hers, Dr. Alan Cohen, who headed the thalassemia program at the Children's Hospital of Philadelphia, to work with them, and she talked to several doctors who ran thalassemia clinics in Italy, signing three of them up as collaborators. Research subjects for the toxicity study would be enrolled at the three sites in Italy and in Philadelphia; the plan was to sign up a few hundred patients. It was to be the largest and most expensive of any of Olivieri's L1 studies.

When she approached Michael Spino about it, he accepted her assertion that a toxicity trial was crucial and agreed to fund it. But she and Brittenham had been written into jobs they weren't allowed to hold. The FDA doesn't permit doctors to run a study if they have no patients in it. Olivieri and Brittenham didn't know that and neither did Spino. When they learned of the FDA's rules—in June 1995—Cohen in Philadelphia became the principal investigator and Olivieri became a paid consultant, signing a contract that was retroactive to October 1994 to cover her services to the company.

It was a simple solution to a logistical problem, but it could become an ethical nightmare. Olivieri had intended to evaluate an Apotex product by receiving another research grant from the company; instead, she would now receive consulting fees. It was more than a semantic difference: consulting fees typically went directly to the doctors, while grants for clinical trials—from public or private sources—customarily went to hospitals. In Olivieri's case, her funding from Apotex had always gone into an account in her name at the Sick Kids Research Institute, but there was no requirement for her to deposit private consulting fees into a Sick Kids account.

By 1995, when Olivieri arranged to become a consultant to Apotex, debates over such arrangements were front and centre at U.S. medical schools. Some schools prohibited doctors from entering into consulting arrangements because it was assumed that the consultancy could influence their research. Essentially, the incentive to maintain a lucrative consulting arrangement could get in the way of reporting results without bias. "They're not lying, but they're not as forthright as they would be if they were not receiving these fees," asserts Dr. Steven LaRosa, an infectious disease specialist at Brown Medical School in Rhode Island.

The Cleveland Clinic had enforced a ban on consultancies for doctors studying a company's drug and published it in the *New England Journal of Medicine,* and the NIH had proposed the same sort of ban. Canada, however, had fewer scientists, fewer research dollars to go around and less interaction between scientists and industry. The country also had a different, more open ethic, says Eric Meslin, a Canadian bioethicist who directed the U.S. National

Bioethics Advisory Commission. In Canada, university doctors who consulted to companies and studied their products at the same time weren't under the gun, and Nancy Olivieri's consulting arrangement, which came with a travel budget and an expense account, wasn't unusual.

With the toxicity trial, Apotex was sponsoring three different trials of L1. The results would be crucial to getting the drug approved, and Spino had assigned research monitors to ensure the trials ran smoothly. The monitors—the company's way of meeting the FDA's and Health Canada's rules—were supposed to visit Sick Kids frequently to check the quality of the data. One was there on an almost full-time basis, attending the Monday morning research meetings and scanning the patients' clinic charts for missing data. But the way things worked out, they also wound up monitoring Nancy Olivieri.

Unwittingly, Olivieri had laid herself a trap. Wanting to turn out a top-notch clinical trial, she had designed the L1 trials in a way that maximized the data she could collect. But her research machine was too small to gather it all. Once a year the patients had liver biopsies, then trips to Cleveland to be tested by Brittenham's iron-measuring device, and MRIs of the heart, liver and brain. Every month they had urine tests, blood tests and appointments with other specialists, such as the eye doctors or the endocrinologists. "As they went along, they just kept adding tests," said one of the patients. "There was always something new coming up that [Olivieri] was wanting to do," said a resident. "Some of [the tests] were necessary for patient care but some of them were just for research."

The visits to Brittenham's SQUID facility, which involved an airplane trip, an ultrasound and the SQUID itself, were purely for research, according to the consent forms the patients signed. "We hope to show that the risk and discomfort of biopsy can be avoided by using our instrument to measure heart and liver iron," the form explained. But the test would offer the patients "no direct benefit" because SQUID measurements weren't yet proven to be reliable. Every second week they had blood tests to make sure the L1 wasn't causing their white-cell counts to drop, and those were essential. In 1994–95, a patient in the trial suddenly had no white cells and Olivieri jumped on the case, ordering the patient to be hospitalized and flying back from Europe to manage his care. But they were collecting so much data on the patients Olivieri couldn't keep track of it all.

Years earlier, Howard had been astonished by the number of scans, biopsies and exams he was expected to undergo in the L1 trial. Now it was Nancy Olivieri's turn to be dismayed by how many tests there were. She found documenting the myriad results for all her research subjects in the time frame that Apotex expected unworkable. "We had these huge clinical binders where there were a million things to record," recalled one of Olivieri's residents. The binders were fundamental to the clinical trial process. Ultimately, the intent was to compile them into a collection of materials to be sent to Ottawa and Washington to support Apotex's proposal to register L1.

Drug companies prepare such proposals routinely, using the skills of several different corporate departments. But Olivieri was trying to complete the task on her own, with only her residents, her research nurse and a data manager to help. Discouraged, she decided that the problem lay with the Apotex monitors. In Olivieri's view, they didn't understand the clinical realities she lived with. Later, she described the sorts of interactions she had with them. "The clinical research monitor is at Apotex," she said. "And they come down and they say, 'Do we have so and so's liver function [tests]?' And I say, 'Well, no. It was done in November. It's not in the chart yet.' And they say, 'Okay, well, how about the MRI?' 'He cancelled.' 'Oh, okay, we'll have to rebook.'"

Olivieri tried to explain the problem to them. "You can't tell the patient, 'You have to come in on Christmas Eve, because that's what the protocol says.' People are always late. Many individuals may be late. They may cancel. It's the usual way with protocols."

It was true that lab tests and imaging reports could take a few weeks to get onto a patient's chart. That was typical in clinical trials and in hospitals generally. But the Apotex monitors didn't see what was happening in the L1 trials as typical, and back at company head-quarters they complained to Michael Spino's assistant about it. Patients were having tests such as MRIs done three months later than expected; patients' serum ferritin levels—the blood test for iron—were taking two to three months to get reported; and patients' eye exams weren't being scheduled appropriately. Then the monitors would submit another request to Olivieri. She said, "They'd say, 'Okay, did we get that serum ferritin?' 'Yes, we did.' 'Oh. We don't have the report yet.' 'Well, it's coming back from the laboratory.'"

But the monitors still wanted the information. Spino's assistant would phone Olivieri to pass on the requests and, again, Olivieri would try to explain. "In clinical—in life—the test done on November the 11th does not appear on the chart November 11th," Olivieri said. "It appears—perhaps—January the 11th. So one has to record this when one has the result." The reasons for that sort of delay were unclear and the company kept hounding her for the data.

Spino said in an interview, "You have a protocol—you're supposed to follow that protocol. That's not just a contract. That's a legal requirement from the health minister's point of view. You have an agreement. You filed that protocol with the HPB [Health Canada's Health Protection Branch]."

Olivieri didn't agree. "Any clinical trial person who says my trial had no protocol violations is somebody who doesn't know their clinical trial," she said. "There are always protocol violations." Doctors who participate in clinical trials agree that minor protocol violations aren't uncommon. The issue is not whether violations occur, but what they are and whether they could have a major effect on the analysis.

By the end of 1994, there was almost always friction between Apotex and Olivieri. "Sometimes it was just little things about the protocol," said one observer. "She wanted everything to be her way. I don't think she was used to doing industry trials for licensing, so there were always these arguments about certain things." Said another, "Until 1994, the L1 was Nancy's baby completely, no question. From 1994 on, there started being problems with Apotex." The situation was frustrating for both sides.

"Neither of them—the company or Olivieri—was expert at doing trials," said a resident who worked with Olivieri on the project. "I don't think it was very well budgeted when she started it. Then she kept wanting to add things." Olivieri asked for more clerical assistance to keep track of all the data. The company eventually paid for that, but it turned down many of her other requests.

Apotex had already invested millions to produce the drug and fund the trials, and the company was starting to watch the project's bottom line. If the regulatory agencies weren't requiring it, Apotex didn't want to add it. The company, said one member of the team, "had talked with the FDA, and knew what the FDA wanted." Olivieri's repeated requests for more aid led to "quite a bit of argument back and forth." Spino resented the arguments, and at one point in the spring of 1994, he wrote Olivieri and Brittenham, asking them to "recognize that . . . Apotex is not just supplying the drug and paying the bills."

For Nancy Olivieri, coming up with a substitute for Desferal was still the major crusade of her life. She was putting long hours into testing L1—tabulating the results, analyzing them, discussing them with Brittenham, submitting abstracts to scientific meetings and writing papers for medical journals. To do all that, she was meeting a lot of deadlines already. She may have wanted to meet the

Apotex deadlines, but she didn't see them as more important than others she faced.

As the company's monitors pressed her, Olivieri grew increasingly annoyed with them. Monday morning research meetings occasionally became "bash Apotex" sessions. She "would complain about things they wanted done that weren't reasonable and the things she wanted to do that they were still arguing with her about," said one of her residents. In the late fall of 1994, Olivieri began to withhold certain pieces of data from the company. Explaining to her residents that Apotex monitors had been asking for a particular data point, she'd say, "Don't tell them this," or "Don't give them that," or ask, "Why do they want this?"

When Spino spoke to her about it, she said she didn't have the time to provide the data Apotex needed because she was too busy with the duties spelled out in her research protocol. "You have indicated that there is insufficient time to provide the information needed by Apotex for monitoring the trial," Spino wrote her in 1995. "The result is that data have stopped coming to Apotex since November 1994."

As a collaborator, Olivieri had agreed to certain terms. But when she failed to live up to those terms, there wasn't anyone who could make her. Spino wrote in his March 1995 letter that once she stopped submitting data, the company was in violation of federal rules. "The Government is very clear— they allow us to provide an investigational drug, as long as we continue to monitor progress of the patients," he said in his letter. "Without the data we cannot monitor the patients." If the company couldn't monitor patients, it would be forced "to terminate the supply of the drug or risk the consequences of action by the Health Protection Branch." For Apotex to stop supplying the drug would mean taking all the patients off L1—a drastic proposal that Olivieri didn't take seriously.

Olivieri had attempted to accomplish what was expected of her at the hospital at the same time that she was building her research program, but it was impossible to do so many things at once. Retreating from the effort, she now devoted herself almost entirely to research. Olivieri "would disappear for days," said one physician who worked with her. Sometimes even her secretary didn't know where she was. "She was supposed to be there, meetings were scheduled, and she just didn't show up," said a person on her team. A doctor from Hamilton wanted to share information with her about a mutual patient. He made an appointment through her secretary, but Olivieri wasn't there when he arrived, and though he waited, she never showed. Howard had a similar experience. He wanted to talk to Olivieri about something and twice booked a time with her. Both times she didn't show. She told him she couldn't recall scheduling the appointments.

In earlier years, when personal losses or professional stress had affected Olivieri, her closest colleagues at the hospital had tried to offer support, but now she was more isolated. That was partly by choice, since she'd stopped viewing some of the Sick Kids doctors as friends. But she also saw less of her colleagues—and they of her—because research and travel were eating up her time. Overly taxed and focused on her research, she didn't seem to realize how she appeared to others.

She was still convinced that she was owed more clinical and clerical help, but it wasn't forthcoming. Sick Kids was under tighter constraints now, her bosses told her. The new CEO, an accountant named Michael Strofolino, was intent on reining in spending. Resources for doctors were scarcer than ever before, and Olivieri was forced to lean more heavily on her residents. But as before, her stress took its toll on them. In particular, things weren't working out as she had hoped with one of the female hematology residents, Janet MacKinnon.

MacKinnon was the sort of physician who exuded calm. If a nurse or a patient put a question to her, she would pause to think about her answer. That was reassuring to some of her patients, but it was a marked contrast to the fast-talking, fast-moving Olivieri, who began to berate MacKinnon in public. Said one observer, "Nancy made her life pure hell . . . She treated her like you wouldn't treat a stray cat." At research meetings, Olivieri would complain in front of the others about the way MacKinnon looked after her patients. Sometimes she told her that what she'd done was stupid; other times she would ask why she didn't do a particular test. When MacKinnon responded, Olivieri was dismissive. Yet other hematologists on staff at Sick Kids didn't find MacKinnon lacking in clinical judgment.

Most observers agreed that it was an unpleasant, tense situation. Like Doreen Matsui before her, MacKinnon repeatedly broke down in tears. Her friends say she looked forward to the periods when Olivieri was travelling. At least then she could work without fear of being publicly humiliated. MacKinnon's sister, concerned by how stressful the situation was for her, advised her to leave the program, but MacKinnon wasn't the sort to quit.

During the Monday meetings, Gideon Koren was the only one with the authority to stand up to Olivieri. But direct confrontation wasn't his style. "He was more the mediator type," said one of the residents. He would try to deflect the discussion. "He could gently push it back on track, not really confront her and say, 'You can't call someone "stupid,"' but just try to move it on to something more constructive. He'd say, 'Well, perhaps the way we should do it next time is . . .'" Koren may have felt he had to limit his input. Though he was nominally Olivieri's co-investigator— both their names were listed on the contract with Apotex—his actual involvement in the day-to-day operation of the L1 projects was quite limited. Olivieri's other major collaborator, Gary

Brittenham, lived elsewhere and couldn't be at her team meetings for the project.

Remote from Brittenham and disengaged from Koren, Olivieri slipped, less than two years after signing with Apotex, into a confrontational situation with her residents, and she carried on a complex back-and-forth with the company that resembled guerrilla warfare.

A NEW PROBLEM WITH L1

Clinical trials are designed to reveal all sorts of truths about the drugs they test, and in the course of Olivieri's trials of L1, she and her team of residents discovered an unusual problem with the drug. One of the sisters from London, Ontario, now a teenager, had been doing well on the pills, then suddenly her iron levels began to rise as if L1 had stopped working for her. Olivieri checked to make sure she was taking her pills. Usually that would involve counting the pills that the patient had left in her pill bottle and calculating whether there were more left than there should be, but Olivieri didn't have to rely on pill counts alone, for she and Koren had put a special system in place to track the pills a patient took. The system had a dull medical title: the medication event monitoring system, or MEMS. Essentially, it was a computer chip in the pill bottle caps that recorded every time the cap was removed.

Now, checking the computer readings for the two sisters from London, Olivieri confirmed that their pill bottles were being opened the right number of times. Why would the drug stop working for one sister but keep working for the other? The girls had the same transfusion regimen. Then the team discovered the same phenomenon in a few other patients, and Olivieri decided it could only be the patients not taking the pills as directed. Maybe they were tricking the device in the bottle cap—taking the capsules out but not ingesting them. "She was convinced that they weren't taking their pills," said one person who spoke with her about it at the time. "The MEMS device was showing that they were opening and closing, but she was convinced that they were throwing them down the toilet or something."

While she was trying to understand the phenomenon, she flew to Panang, an island off the coast of Malaysia, for a meeting on thalassemia with many of the doctors working with L1 in attendance. During one of the breaks, Olivieri asked the London hematologist Beatrix Wonke, "Have you noticed that the L1 seems to stop working for some patients?" Wonke hadn't seen that, and she'd been prescribing the drug since 1988. She said that if the drug had "stopped working" in a patient who'd been responding to it previously, Olivieri might be using too low a dose.

Back in Toronto at the Monday morning research meetings, the residents would list the patients' lab values and Olivieri would direct her attention to the patients whose iron levels weren't going down, still certain the problem had to do with the patients discontinuing their medication. Her residents weren't sure she was right.

"Why would you open the drug bottle and take the cap off and put it back on without taking the pills?" one of the residents recalls asking her. Olivieri thought that her patients didn't want to swallow their medication but didn't want to disappoint her by dropping out of the study. "For two years almost, we used to get into this endless debate around compliance," said one of her residents.

The debates were part of the first-pass, informal peer review that's so critical in science. These were Olivieri's lab meetings—a standard tool used by scientists everywhere to validate or reject their ideas at the earliest stage. She was wondering aloud what was going on, and generating a hypothesis. The residents' doubts and questions enabled the meeting to serve as a self-correcting mechanism. The only ones who weren't in on the discussion were the people from Apotex. Olivieri consulted her lab group at that early, uncertain stage of thinking, but not the company. As a sponsored researcher, she was supposed to let Apotex know about any adverse effects of its drug; the company, in turn, had the responsibility for letting the drug agencies know. But since Olivieri had stopped sharing data with Apotex, the company didn't know she thought there could be a new problem with L1.

At that point, Olivieri was worried that L1 might be losing its effectiveness for a few patients. But her data showed that it still worked well for most of them, and that was what she planned to say at ASH. The meeting was in Nashville in December 1994, and Olivieri spoke at its plenary session to an audience of about 8,000 physicians and scientists from around the world. The graphs and scatter plots on her slides demonstrated that patients in the compassionate use trial continued to do well, according to all the various tests they'd been subjected to—serum ferritin, liver iron and cardiac function. Olivieri didn't mention that L1 had stopped working for some of them, believing the problem lay with the patient not taking the drug.

A few months later, U.S. scientists would begin a debate about the data left out of scientific papers. A federal commission assigned to investigate scientific practice—the Commission on Research Integrity—concluded that, in certain cases, a scientist who omitted data was committing misconduct. But the commission's report met with hostility from organized groups of scientists, who argued that omitting important results was simply bad science, not misconduct. In April 1995, John C. Bailar, a long-time statistical consultant to the *New England Journal of Medicine* and head of statistics at McGill University, addressed the issue in an editorial in the *Chronicle of Higher Education*. Bailar thought it was common for scientists to report their data selectively, leaving important findings on the cutting-room floor. He concluded, "While such omissions may not damage the validity of the results reported, the failure to inform seems seriously at variance with standards of good science."

In Olivieri's talk, her failure to recognize or report the anomaly caused her to overstate the value of her study drug. Among researchers sponsored by drug companies, that sort of thing was the norm. Studies published since the 1990s have shown that industry-sponsored scientists are more likely than their publicly funded colleagues to find that a new drug they're testing works, and they're also more likely to editorialize in favour of it. One such study, published in 1996 by California researchers, showed that in 98 per cent of company-sponsored drug studies published during the 1980s, the results favoured the company's drug.

Some of Nancy Olivieri's scientific competitors had worried that she was biased in L1's favour even before Apotex began funding her. At that point, her attachment to the drug was that she was the person who had brought it to North America, and her professional reputation was tied to it. Now she was running two trials as an Apotex-sponsored researcher and was about to embark on a third. Her research funding depended on the company's continuing investment in the drug.

Though Olivieri's paper from the podium at ASH didn't mention that a patient was not responding to L1, Janet MacKinnon had prepared a scientific abstract on it for a poster session, co-authored with Olivieri, Brittenham and the other members of the team. MacKinnon travelled to Nashville with the charts and figures she'd assembled describing the two sisters from London: the younger one who was continuing to do well on L1 and the older one for whom the drug wasn't working. The doctors had calculated the two girls' iron levels from liver biopsies and Brittenham's SQUID measurements, and the poster described the problem. "In the younger girl, initial hepatic iron concentration has declined steadily . . . while in her sister, initial hepatic iron concentration has remained essentially unchanged."The girls had been on L1 for four years and the poster made it clear that the doctors didn't understand why one girl had stopped responding to the pills. In a way, that was the point of presenting the data at an international meeting: maybe some other hematologists working with L1 had encountered the same problem.

Victor Hoffbrand attended the poster session and talked to MacKinnon for a while about the data. Back home, Hoffbrand was in a tug-of-war with George Kontoghiorghes. There continued to be reports from some doctors that Kontoghiorghes was supplying L1 to patients outside the Royal Free Hospital; Kontoghiorghes was denying those allegations and fighting efforts to limit his work. But despite internal strife, the group had managed to continue its clinical trials of L1. Hoffbrand told MacKinnon that he couldn't understand why the sisters were responding differently to L1, but he wondered if they had tried using a higher dose of the drug. At his hospital, they had found that some of their patients didn't do as well on L1 as others. "In some patients it just wasn't strong enough from the beginning," Hoffbrand explained later. By the fall of 1994, his group was finding that "poor responders" to the drug sometimes did better when they raised the dose. Like Beatrix Wonke, he thought that maybe the dose of L1 needed to be higher for the sister who wasn't responding. But the protocol for Olivieri's studies called for all of the patients to receive the same set dose.

One month after the meeting in Nashville, the sisters from London were to be hospitalized on the research ward at the Toronto General. Admitting the girls was another way to study the problem. A research nurse would watch them swallow their capsules, then the amount of iron in their urine would be checked and they would have blood tests, including serum ferritin. But the morning they were scheduled to come in, the hospital shut down. Workers had been using a welding torch to remove asbestos in the basement, and a piece of paper had caught fire. The smoke spread through the hospital's ventilation system, forcing the cancellation of any admissions. The sisters' admission to the research wing was rescheduled.

Meanwhile, the *New England Journal of Medicine* accepted Olivieri's paper describing the L1 trial. It was published in April 1995, a positive study about an experimental drug. Two graphs in the paper showed how L1 removed iron from the body. The graphs had a line corresponding to each patient. Howard, who had taken L1 then gone off it for a while, had his own line. Josie, who had taken the pills for a little over a year before becoming worried about it, also had a line. The text of the paper explained that in ten patients, the drug worked well and their iron levels went down. In the other eleven patients, the iron didn't go down but it stayed at a level that the doctors considered low enough to prevent problems, including early death.

The paper pointed out that the drug wasn't quite as good as Desferal. But L1 was easier to take, and its side effects were rare. The paper described what had happened to Helen—that her liver enzymes had gone up, probably as a result of the drug—and it said that the drug could cause a patient's white blood cell count to drop. But the *New England Journal of Medicine* paper, like Olivieri's talk in Nashville, didn't mention that some patients might have stopped responding to L1.

Olivieri had her reasons for not flagging it. She was still investigating it, for one thing. It seemed as if she wanted more data before concluding that the problem was serious enough to spell out in a journal article. Her paper also didn't mention any deaths in patients who had taken L1. Outside Canada, Ciba-Geigy thought four patients on the drug had died. In Toronto, Paula and Alex had taken L1 before they died. Olivieri might have left the deaths out when she wrote about L1 because she didn't accept that the drug was implicated—there wasn't any evidence that L1 had caused those patients' problems. She also might have decided not to mention them because Paula and Alex were not part of the trial she was writing about—Alex had been in the randomized comparison of L1 and Desferal and Paula might have been classified as a subject of Olivieri's pilot studies. But with a new drug, it's prudent to mention any adverse reactions or deaths among clinical subjects.

When the paper came out, the Hospital for Sick Children held a press conference and Nancy Olivieri spoke to the journalists. The next day, the *Toronto Star* described L1 as "a pill-size reprieve for people with thalassemia." *The Globe and Mail* quoted Olivieri's prediction that the new medication could "alter the treatment of thousands of patients around the world." L1 had proven itself, Olivieri told the Canadian Press. "We can say it's just as good as deferoxamine [Desferal]." But to others, including her mentor, David Nathan, Nancy Olivieri seemed to be overselling L1's promise.

Nathan had been asked to write an editorial about L1 to run in the same issue of the *New England Journal of Medicine* as Olivieri's report on her clinical trial. His skepticism about it, along with his dismay at the work done on it at the Royal Free Hospital, continued to colour his opinions. He warned in his editorial that L1 was "considerably more toxic" than Desferal and that it had to be present in the body "at very high concentrations (close to toxic levels) to be effective." He also cautioned that teenage thalassemia patients might not take enough of the pills for the drug to work.

Later, Stephen Fredd of the FDA spoke in an interview about biases in drug research. In his experience, industry-funded scientists were often biased in favour of the drug they were testing. Apotex had pumped more than $5 million into Nancy Olivieri's various L1 trials when she published on L1 in the *New England Journal of Medicine*. The largest grants she'd received before then paled by comparison.

In the large-scale clinical trials that are the bread and butter of researchers in fields such as cardiology or oncology, trial directors usually take a series of steps to protect themselves from bias in favour of the treatment they're testing. For example, they'll "blind" the doctors and patients to the treatments being tested so that researchers can't be influenced by knowing that a patient is on the study drug. Doctors break the code if they have any worries about a patient, but otherwise, they can't view their results until the study is over. Olivieri's study wasn't blinded, in keeping with the norms of the field. In countries where thalassemia research is conducted, including the U.S. and the United Kingdom, so few patients have the disease that it's hard to take the same sorts of precautions as researchers in larger fields. Blinding is rare in thalassemia research.

Unblinded, Olivieri had discovered that in some cases L1 wasn't working the way she expected. Maybe she was using too low a dose, or maybe the patients weren't taking all of their capsules—it wasn't clear. But while she tried to figure it out, she presented and published her research without discussing the dilemma.

PULLING THE PLUG ON NANCY

Olivieri spent part of the winter and spring of 1995 trying to understand why the response to L1 was "good in some patients and not so good in others," as she put it later. By this point, she'd known about the drug's variable effectiveness for well over a year. She'd spent hours discussing it with her residents. But she still didn't know what was causing the problem. Determined to figure it out, she began to discuss it with Gary Brittenham.

Every few months, her residents took a group of patients to Cleveland, where Brittenham tested them in his SQUID apparatus. He measured the patient's liver iron and got the results back to Olivieri within two to three days. When she asked him about it, he concurred that a few of her patients were no longer responding to L1. The two doctors came up with a name for the problem—"loss of response"—and an acronym, LOR. They developed a plan for how to find a way of predicting which patients would do well on L1 and which ones wouldn't.

Olivieri explained their reasoning later: "There certainly were—we should never forget this—some patients who were doing well on deferiprone [L1], who seemed to have a good response to it." For that group of patients, she thought L1 "was absolutely adequately effective."

Howard was in that group. "I used to do twenty-four-hour

urines," he explained. He'd collect all his urine in a large specimen bottle and bring it in to the clinic. Bev Tyler, the clinic nurse, sent it off for analysis and gave him the results. "I was excreting three times as much iron as a regular, normal, chelated patient," he said. "That's what I was told by Bev." In other words, L1 was taking more iron out of his system than Desferal was for most other patients.

The trick, Olivieri thought, was to sort out the differences between the patients who were responding to L1 and the ones who weren't. "I wrote a new protocol," she said. "There are many factors that affect iron and how iron leaves the body, and all of these we tried to include in the new protocol." Their plan was to follow the patients for five years. She and Brittenham thought they needed that long a period in order to understand what was unusual about the patients who had stopped responding to L1.

At some point that spring, Olivieri finally shared her concerns about the "loss of response" to L1 with Apotex. She thought there were six patients in whom the drug wasn't working well. Until then, Spino hadn't heard anything about a new problem with the drug, and he was stunned. Nancy Olivieri knew thalassemia, but Michael Spino knew drugs. His reaction to the problem with the drug was the same as Olivieri's had been originally. He told her that if L1 was ineffective for a given patient, the individual must have stopped ingesting the pills. He asked to see the raw data; she wanted him to agree to the new protocol.

In June, she contacted the Health Protection Branch in Ottawa and told agency staff about the loss of response to L1. An agency official wrote her about it, recommending that she revise her research protocol so she could study the new problem. In July, she contacted Spino again to discuss the new research protocol she was proposing. In a letter, she explained that she couldn't be sure the drug would continue to have its same effects over the long term, so she wanted to study the patients for another five years. But

Apotex wasn't ready to agree to that. The company worried that she was pushing for five more years because she wanted Apotex to increase her research grant. "It's a great opportunity for any investigator if they can get a confirmed five-year period of time for a whole lot of subjects," Spino said in an interview.

Spino wrote her in August that Apotex had "a legal and moral responsibility" to investigate her concerns about the drug. He said the company needed to "obtain all the raw data" that showed the drug wasn't working. Then Apotex would carry out its own analysis. Olivieri replied that she was revising her research protocol, but Spino wanted the data and was growing increasingly frustrated. The previous spring when she had failed to supply data, he'd intimated that if she didn't send the results, the company would stop supplying the drug, effectively cancelling the study. Now he repeated the threat: he would stop the trial unless she provided the data. She replied by sending him Brittenham's SQUID results showing that in eight of the patients on L1, the iron levels weren't going down— the drug was no longer working.

Spino and his staff reviewed the data and thought there was another explanation. "Was it lost effectiveness?" Spino asked in an interview. "No." Other theories had to do with how quickly the drug was passing through the patients' bodies and whether they were on the correct dose. Spino agreed that L1 wasn't working as well for a few of the patients as it was for others and offered to sponsor a follow-up study of those patients. But Olivieri wasn't asking Spino for research advice; she'd already proposed the study she wanted to do, and she wrote him about it in mid-September. This time, she copied her letter to the head of the hospital's Research Ethics Board, which was no longer Gidi Koren. The new chair was Stanley Zlotkin, a specialist in gastroenterology. Olivieri had known Zlotkin a long time and considered him a friend. Underneath Zlotkin's name she wrote "Head, Human Subjects Review Committee," letting Spino know that his decision on her proposed new research protocol was being watched.

The two continued wrangling with each other throughout the fall of 1995 and into the early winter. Brittenham came up from Cleveland for some of their meetings, and both appreciated his calm presence, but it didn't resolve their dispute. Eventually, Spino decided to consult with other scientists working on L1—Cohen in Philadelphia and the other doctors in Montreal and Italy whom Olivieri had gathered as collaborators. "We forwarded her data that she gave us to all the other investigators that we were working with," Spino said. Apotex was funding their work on the drug along with hers. Individually, each of them got in touch with Spino and told him that when they analyzed the data, it looked as if L1 was working for most of Olivieri's patients.

Olivieri urged him to put together an independent group of experts to resolve his dispute with her and serve as a data safety monitoring board by reviewing the trial data at regular intervals. But she also decided to involve the hospital's Research Ethics Board more directly. Working with Brittenham, she began putting together a formal report to the board on the problem of patients not responding to L1.

Koren argued against making a formal report, suggesting that any new concerns about L1 could go in their annual report to the ethics board, but Olivieri made the final decision. The report—with Koren, Brittenham and Olivieri as authors—went to Apotex and the ethics board in March 1996. It said there were now twelve out of nineteen patients in whom the drug wasn't working or was working poorly. The researchers proposed revising their study consent forms to let the patients know that the drug didn't always work.

Spino and his staff still wondered if Olivieri's proposal for a five-year study was a creative financing manoeuvre. They were correct that she felt that her research was seriously underfunded.

Despite her continued arguments with Spino over the "loss of response" to L1, Olivieri needed Apotex. In the spring of 1996, she wanted the company to fund the new long-term study she'd proposed and to renew her existing contracts. On March 31 she wrote Spino three letters in one day, each a request for further financing. In one, she said that her contract with the company for one of the L1 trials would end on April 23. "I am firmly committed to the successful completion of this trial and hope to hear from you soon," she wrote. In another, she told Spino that she wanted to run a new study of L1 in patients with sickle cell disease. She said she'd already proposed the study to the National Institutes of Health and "would be delighted if Apotex were willing to donate the approximately 50 kilograms of [L1] that will be required."

A hematologist confided later that he thought it was "bizarre" for a doctor to use a drug in sickle cell patients if she thought it wasn't working for some of her thalassemia patients. But despite the setbacks, Olivieri was still an advocate for L1, believing it worked for some thalassemia patients and that it might work in a different way for sickle cell anemia. She thought L1 could benefit sickle cell patients not by removing iron, but by decreasing the destruction of red blood cells, thereby ameliorating their anemia.

However, Spino didn't renew her contracts, nor did he sign a new one to follow patients for five years. He left her in limbo regarding Apotex support. And he wrote the ethics board chair, Zlotkin, whom he knew from his time at Sick Kids, to tell him that the L1 research results were in dispute.

For Zlotkin, the ethical issues of the case seemed fairly straightforward. Human volunteers in a clinical trial are entitled to know about the risks of research they're taking part in, and the responsibility for describing those risks falls to the doctor who is leading the trial. It's the rule of informed consent. Zlotkin contacted the ethics board's legal counsel, and the lawyer agreed with him: having determined that L1's failure in certain patients was more than a statistical anomaly, Olivieri had to warn patients that the experimental drug they were taking might not work. They agreed with her plan to revise the study consent forms, and Zlotkin wrote Spino that the ethics board would not mediate between the company and Olivieri.

In April 1996, the ethics board issued its directions to Olivieri in writing. There it was in black and white: Olivieri had to alter the consent forms for patients taking L1. She faxed the letter from the ethics board to Spino. Taking no chances, she sent it off to him by courier as well. On April 22, she still hadn't heard back from Spino and wrote him to say so. She also let Apotex know that she was holding a group meeting with all her patients to tell them about the new risks associated with the drug. Despite her urgent need for continued financial support, she was not one to kowtow to the company's views. On the contrary, she planned to share her concerns with the patients, a courageous move that was independent of Apotex and against the company's wishes. To help her, she recruited Brittenham and Graham Sher, who had finished his residency and taken over the thalassemia clinic at the Toronto General Hospital in the summer of 1995. Together, the three doctors spent a Wednesday night in early May in a conference room at Sick Kids, talking to patients and answering their questions. In a letter Olivieri wrote Apotex about the meeting, she said it "was prompted by several anxious inquiries from families" after the families learned that some patients were being taken off L1 and put back on Desferal. Olivieri was candid and clear with her patients, telling them it was "extremely important" for those on L1 to keep getting their white blood cell counts checked every two weeks. If the FDA didn't get the data on white cells counts, she warned, L1 couldn't be approved.

Patients asked whether they would have to go back on Desferal once the trial ended and she reassured them that there were protocols in place for them to continue on the drug. But she and Sher let them know L1 was not a panacea. Its effectiveness was extremely variable between individuals, they said, and there were some patients who had experienced a "loss of response." In Olivieri's view, L1 wasn't as good at removing iron as Desferal, but she told the patients she planned to keep studying the drug "to learn how to use it better." She also mentioned that doctors in New York were experimenting with combining L1 and Desferal so that a patient took both drugs. Howard had the impression that Olivieri might want to try that in the future.

Spino was also upset that patients were being switched from one drug to the other. The day after Olivieri's meeting with the patients, he wrote Zlotkin again: "Unfortunately, with the unapproved switching of patients on and off Apotex deferiprone [L1], the data are of even less value to Apotex today than when we started." The company's review of the data had been "most intense," Spino wrote, and Apotex had made a "full and complete response to the situation." In light of that, he thought the ethics board chair would "agree that . . . no further action by Dr. Olivieri at this time is warranted." But, as he already knew, Olivieri was under orders from the board to revise the patient consent forms.

In Boston that spring, David Nathan had new worries about L1. Nathan was now head of Harvard's cancer hospital (the Dana Farber Cancer Institute), a fellow of the National Academy of Science and a winner of the U.S. National Medal of Science, and he had used his predominance in thalassemia to warn against L1 when Olivieri's positive findings appeared in the *New England Journal of Medicine*. But he considered her data seriously, and after it appeared, his centre in Boston obtained a "treatment IND" from the FDA to use L1 experimentally. In July 1995, they began giving the pills to a thirty-three-year-old man with thalassemia. The case gave Nathan a scare.

First the man developed joint pains in both knees and ankles. Then his serum ferritin level began to rise, showing that the iron in his system was increasing. It rose steadily over the course of six months on L1. In February 1996, the man's serum ferritin was more than double what it had been before he started taking L1, and Nathan's team decided to stop the experiment. They told the man to discontinue his pills and go back on nightly Desferal. Over the next few months, the man's ferritin fell back to where it had been origi- nally. Nathan didn't know for sure how to explain what had happened, but he thought the drug could have damaged the man's liver in a new, toxic reaction to L1 that hadn't yet been described. Nathan's staff informed Olivieri, and Nathan also wrote the FDA. He described what had happened to his patient, calling it a "possible toxic effect" of the drug, and sent Olivieri a copy of his letter to the agency.

She phoned him at some point that spring and said that her report about the drug in the *New England Journal of Medicine* no longer matched what she was seeing. "She's a very honest person, and she just said, I've got to tell the world that I was wrong," Nathan recalled in an interview. Finally, she was on his side of the L1 con- troversy. She spent time revising the information and consent forms for her studies, and in May 1996, satisfied with her revisions, she wrote a covering letter. "Dear thalassemia patient or parent of a thal- assemia child," it began. "I am writing to tell you about an un- expected finding in our most recent analysis of studies." The letter said that L1 was working for "only a minority of patients," and that phrase was underlined. The consent forms contained the same wording, with the same phrase underlined. She put all the materi- als in an envelope and sent them to Zlotkin at the Research Ethics Board. She also faxed copies of the revised forms and covering let- ters to Spino at Apotex.

As Michael Spino read his faxes the next week, what registered was Nancy Olivieri's impatience. She knew he disagreed with her about the data. He was putting together an independent panel of experts, which she had asked for, scheduled to meet in Toronto in

July. But Olivieri was no longer waiting for the experts' assessment. Spino said in an interview, "What we had done is, we said, 'There is an independent panel. Please wait . . . Wait until the review of the independent panel.'" But it was clear from the faxes she'd sent him that Olivieri wasn't waiting; she was changing the consent forms.

In Spino's view, he was the coach on a collaborative project and his team captain was acting unilaterally. It was an important project—the company had now spent close to $8 million on L1, and of all the products in the "innovative drugs" pipeline at Apotex, it was the furthest along. He thought Olivieri had misled the Research Ethics Board about the data. He'd tried to rectify the situation by communicating with Zlotkin, but Zlotkin wouldn't allow it. Instead, the board was applying a "report first and ask questions later" policy to L1, advising Olivieri to let her patients know—in writing—what she'd already told them at the evening meeting: that the drug might not work. It was the right thing to do, given Nancy Olivieri's assessment of the drug. But Apotex couldn't accept her assessment.

"At that point, our confidence in her judgment was lost," Spino explained. "We didn't feel that she could be fair and unbiased. We don't know why she was no longer, in our view, unbiased. But for some reason, she had a mission. We didn't know what that mission was and we didn't want to rely on her doing the studies."

In response to the revised consent forms, Spino produced a series of letters. In his letter to Nancy Olivieri, he wrote that her contracts with the company were "terminated, effective immediately." In a letter to Olivieri and Koren, he explained what that meant. "Effective immediately, the deferiprone clinical trials . . . are being discontinued at the Hospital for Sick Children and The Toronto Hospital." He told the doctors to return all study medication in accordance with federal regulations for drug studies that have ended. The last paragraph of the letter was the clincher. All information from the study, "whether written or not, obtained or generated by the Investigators," was to remain "secret and confidential." If there was any breach of confidentiality, Apotex would "vigorously pursue all legal remedies." When all of his letters were ready, he went to Sick Kids to deliver them personally.

It was a Friday at the end of May. At the hospital, Spino managed to meet with Gideon Koren. Spino wrote him afterwards, "Your thoughtful, scientifically sound assessments, and sage advice throughout this period have been most helpful." But Nancy Olivieri was harder to find. He left her a long phone message so that his meaning wouldn't be missed.

"Hi Nancy. I'm sorry we didn't get a chance to meet face to face. It's Mike Spino. I've left you an envelope. I'm sorry but Apotex has decided to terminate the L1 studies at the Hospital for Sick Children." He said that her statement, "the drug is working in only a minority of patients," was "incorrect as verified by other investigators." If she "in any way" attempted to convey her incorrect notions, she would "be subject to legal action." Spino closed on a first-name basis: "Nancy, if you want to reach me this weekend you can, but please read the letters first. Bye."

In one day, with two letters and a voice-mail message, Michael Spino and his company transformed their argument with Olivieri into the biggest scandal ever to hit Canadian science.

FIGHTING BACK

Nancy Olivieri said that as she read Spino's letters and listened to the message he left on her voice mail, her heart was "just racing." She didn't know what she was going to do. Apotex was stopping the trials, creating a clinical emergency for her patients taking L1 as well as a crisis for her entire L1 research program. "I had a sense that I was in this by myself," she told the producer of the British television documentary *Dying for Drugs*. "It was a sick feeling." She was convinced Apotex was trying to hide the fact that there was a problem with the drug. "I wanted to tell the patients there was a problem, but business interests prevented that from happening easily," she said to a reporter for *Business Week* two years later. It wasn't really that simple, but the company's actions smelled bad. Stopping the trials like that—suddenly, without warning the scientists or patients involved—was more than unusual. It bordered on unethical.

The ethics argument goes like this: Once a drug trial is already in progress, sponsors have an ethical obligation to complete it, since patients have exposed themselves to a risk with the idea that the study will be completed and knowledge will be gained. If the drug turns out to be unsafe or ineffective, the trial may have to be stopped. But if the problem is more complicated—say, the study costs a lot more than the sponsor thought it would—stopping the study will prompt a debate. Companies generally argue that it's legitimate to stop a trial for commercial reasons; scientists often argue that it's not. Ethicists advise that the way to stop a trial is to follow "stopping rules" established ahead of time by the sponsor and the scientists.

Apotex is far from the only company to have stopped a drug trial, but the way the company stopped the L1 trials at Sick Kids had the whiff of a reactionary decision. They weren't following stopping rules, and when the studies ended, patients who had been taking the drug—for years, in some cases—had to quickly seek alternative treatment. Though an alternative was available in Desferal, switching treatments abruptly isn't in the best interest of patients.

Stopping the trials was also terribly harmful to Olivieri. Suddenly, she was to be out of the loop on L1 and off the international research juggernaut she'd been on. Her scientific program, already in a precarious financial situation, would become virtually defunct. She was scheduled to fly to Europe the following week, and Gideon Koren would be out of town as well. They had to act quickly.

She phoned Gary Brittenham and spoke to a lawyer, who told her to call the Canadian Medical Protective Association (CMPA), the organization that defends Canadian physicians against claims of medical malpractice. She did and was put in touch with a CMPA lawyer, whom she called at his home on Sunday. After that, she called the dean of the University of Toronto medical school, Arnold Aberman, and told him she had spoken to a lawyer. She also wrote a two-page letter to the hospital's chief of pediatrics, Bob Haslam, describing everything that had happened. She was clear about her biggest problem: she couldn't tell the patients what was going on: "Finally, our patients will . . . under threat of legal action be terminated prematurely on the study without explanation provided to patients and families." She asked for "advice and guidance as to how to proceed."

She got Gideon Koren to sign the letter along with her, copied Spino's letters, highlighted his passages about taking legal action and sent the package off to Haslam and four other high-ranking administrators, including Stan Zlotkin at the Research Ethics Board, Arnie Aberman at the medical school and the new head of the Sick Kids Research Institute, a geneticist named Manuel Buchwald. On Monday, she urged her CMPA lawyer to try to reach Aberman. Then she left for Europe.

Bob Haslam got Olivieri's letter the next day. "I was not aware of the contract that she signed with Apotex," he recalled later. "Then I got a letter from Nancy with two or three weeks to go in my term, sharing her concern about all this." Haslam was preparing to step down as chief of pediatrics, and Hugh O'Brodovich, a Sick Kids lung specialist, was taking over. When Olivieri's letter arrived, Haslam tried to contact her for more information, only to learn from her office that she was away in Italy and wouldn't be back for a few weeks. He didn't try reaching her in Europe, but he met with the Sick Kids CEO, Michael Strofolino, and the hospital vice president, Alan Goldbloom, to discuss her letter. The administrators gave a copy of the letter to O'Brodovich, the incoming chief, who paged Olivieri but got no response.

O'Brodovich had been meeting with Olivieri over the course of the spring to discuss her clinical needs. She felt undersupported, but O'Brodovich had determined that the cash flow to her clinics was already more than for other programs with similar patient loads, and he had turned down her bid for greater resources. Now, after reading her letter about the crisis with Apotex, and getting no response from paging her, he tried Gideon Koren and eventually reached him.

Arnie Aberman also phoned Olivieri when he received her letter, and couldn't reach her either. But he managed to speak to one of the two lawyers who had taken on her case for the CMPA, and through the lawyer, he scheduled a dinner with her. Aberman was an intensive care physician, and crises were familiar territory. He was getting this matter off his desk sooner rather than later, in his usual style.

On Wednesday, May 29, clinic day for the thalassemia patients, patients taking L1 went to get their pill bottles refilled after their monthly transfusions. But there was no L1. Olivieri's residents couldn't tell the patients what to do, and the nurse didn't know either. Nancy Olivieri was away in Europe and hadn't arranged anything before she left. Apparently she didn't realize that the drug could disappear so quickly.

The clinic was discombobulated and the patients were scared. They knew they weren't supposed to get transfusions without any medicine to take the iron out. But were they supposed to go back on Desferal? It wasn't clear. Josie wrote later in an e-mail to me that the clinic staff faced "many pleading, angry, frightened patients." Olivieri heard about the situation when she got back to town and later described it for a television producer: "The people on the front lines with the patients were just saying, 'Well, we'll see what we can do. There's no drug left. You'll just have to continue on the drug you're on right now and keep on until that runs out.'"

Nancy Olivieri arrived home in early June. No one from Sick Kids' administration had reached her yet, but the dean dined with her and her lawyer the night after she returned. She asked Aberman to mediate her dispute with the company. He agreed to do that and more. He said that if the dispute remained unresolved, he would do what he could to obtain the services of the university's lawyers in getting her "proper protection of her intellectual property rights." When it came to protecting a professor's discoveries, the University of Toronto could help.

Like most large universities, the U of T in the 1990s was in the business of doing science. The medical faculty had an annual research budget of close to $200 million, and the campus boasted an active technology transfer office involved in managing multiple contracts between professors and outside commercial concerns, as well as a large legal team that was expert in intellectual property issues. "If a faculty member requested legal support, we would offer it without exception," Aberman said in an interview. But that wasn't what Olivieri was requesting. She wanted the university to tell Apotex to bring the L1 trials back to Sick Kids. Aberman didn't think he could help with that, but he moved immediately on his promise to mediate.

Olivieri saw cancer researcher Bob Phillips the day after her dinner with the dean and told him that the university had shown no signs of supporting her, though Aberman was in fact already putting together a mediation session with the company. That session took place three days later in the dean's conference room. Olivieri met with her lawyers before heading over. They told her, "Be clear about what you want," and she made notes for herself. The thing she wanted most was for her trials to be reinstated. L1 was still her major hope for keeping the next generation's Alexes and Biagios alive. Her work on it represented eight years of her professional life, and she didn't accept that Apotex could simply push her out on Michael Spino's whim. She had high hopes for the mediation session with the dean.

Spino attended the mediation session with two other individuals from Apotex. Gideon Koren and Gary Brittenham were there as well. One of Olivieri's lawyers attended, though he didn't accompany her into the mediation session since the other parties present had no legal counsel. Olivieri said she wanted to continue the L1 trial and gave two reasons: to ensure that her patients on L1 would continue receiving the drug, and to continue studying the pill's effectiveness.

The company was willing to make the drug available to patients. Spino seemed to realize that his company's move to suddenly empty the Sick Kids pharmacy of L1 was clinically unsound, and he agreed to "the Emergency Release of L1 to any patient who was on L1 during the trial." His only stipulation was that the request had to come from Koren; Apotex didn't want to communicate with Olivieri.

Fourteen of the patients in the "compassionate use" study would stay on L1. Others who had started on the pills as part of Olivieri's randomized trial would also stay on it. But the company flatly refused to continue her trial. In a way, she had been so successful in her efforts to collaborate with other centres that Apotex could keep studying the drug without her. The collaborators she'd signed up in Philadelphia, Montreal and, most of all, Italy had sufficient numbers of patients to produce meaningful data.

Meanwhile, the crisis in the thalassemia clinic continued. When the patients turned to Olivieri with questions, her standard reply was that she couldn't say anything because Apotex had threatened to sue her if she did and it was true: Spino's letters warned that if she disclosed her study findings she would breach her confidentiality obligations to the company. Howard decided the patients needed to hear more about what was going on. As head of the Thalassemia Action Group in Toronto—the patients' organization—he arranged for Olivieri to speak to them. But after sharing limited information, she told them she was afraid to say more.

Howard wasn't worried that anyone would try to sue him. The emergency release had been agreed to but it hadn't started yet, and as a result, a number of the thalassemia patients were still scared about what they were supposed to take in the meantime. Howard was on L1 himself and didn't want to go off it. He took the podium. "Whoever wants me to approach Apotex to try and get the pill, let me know at the end of the meeting," he said. Olivieri piped up. "Howard, I don't think you're doing anyone any favours." He thought she was annoyed with him for offering to contact the company. "I think to Nancy, she viewed it as if I was picking Apotex over her," he said. "But I was just picking a pill over a needle."

Spino told Howard that the emergency release program would start soon. Until then, if a hematologist other than Nancy Olivieri prescribed L1, the company would provide it. That was good news to the patients. Several of them headed to Graham Sher's office at the Toronto General, where he met with them, reviewed their charts and answered questions. But he told them he wouldn't pre-scribe L1—he wasn't interested in writing a prescription for a study drug once the study was stopped.

Only one patient found another doctor to prescribe L1. Corrado, who had started on L1 in 1991, couldn't bear the thought of returning to Desferal shots and the outbreaks of hives that, in his case, always followed the injections. He had a close relationship with his pediatrician at St. Joseph's Health Centre in Toronto, and urged the doctor to call Apotex. The pediatrician spoke to Apotex as well as to the hematologists who were testing L1 in Montreal and Philadelphia, and authorities at Health Canada, in order to ensure that Corrado could take L1 and would get the care and monitoring he needed if he was on it.

Those who couldn't finagle a way to get the drug tried to find patients willing to share their supply. "People were taking dribs and drabs of it," Olivieri said. She heard that some patients were taking as little as one pill a day. She told her staff, "A little L1 is worse than none at all," but few of the patients wanted to go back to injecting Desferal.

In some cases they had no choice. About two weeks after Apotex stopped the trial, and just a few days after the mediation session with the dean, Olivieri began telling certain patients that they had to stop taking L1 even if they weren't running out of their pills. They were very surprised. Previously, she had been very positive about L1, and patients and their families had understood that it was the treatment they needed. Apparently, the patients she approached were those she thought had experienced a loss of response to the drug.

Louisa Tonna was now an eighteen-year-old high school student into aerobics. She had been on L1 for nearly three years when Olivieri told her to stop taking it, in mid-June 1996. "It was like, all of a sudden, she was not to take any more L1," her mother, Jan, recalls. The doctor explained that Louisa's liver iron levels had been rising while she was on the pill. But Louisa and Jan hadn't been told that before and they couldn't understand it. Jan Tonna tried talking to the clinic nurse after receiving this shocking news but didn't learn much. "Nobody would tell you anything," she said afterwards. "It was all hush-hush, and if you heard anything, it was behind a closed door." At first, Jan wasn't even sure whether her daughter was supposed to go back on Desferal. Louisa herself couldn't bear the thought of returning to the injections that had left her so sore and puffy. "My daughter really totally resisted the idea of going back to Desferal," said Jan. "She went into an extreme depression." Louisa began crying a lot and having trouble at school, and her teachers told her mother she couldn't concentrate. Off Desferal, her iron levels built up to the point that she had to take the drug intravenously, but that wasn't an easy alternative because the intravenous line frequently clogged up or the site got infected.

The young woman who had developed hives like little balls on Desferal was equally disappointed. She'd logged nearly eight years on L1 and she couldn't figure out why Olivieri was now saying she should return to Desferal.

"I was very upset because I had to go back to Desferal and that was something I didn't want to do," she said. "I was devastated. It took me I don't know how long to get used to the idea that I had to go back on." She, too, was walking around the thalassemia clinic with unanswered questions. "My thing was, like, 'Why? It's [L1's] doing so well for me. Why was I taken off?' That was my question." Eventually, she started on Desferal. Within a few weeks, she noticed she couldn't hear properly. At home, she couldn't hear well enough to follow a TV program; at work, she couldn't hear her customers. She was going deaf in one ear, one of the toxic effects of Desferal that Olivieri and Freedman had reported on.

Around this time—a few weeks after the company stopped the trial—Olivieri also spoke to the girl who had been about twelve when she started taking L1 almost three years earlier, and advised her and her mother that she should stop. She was crushed by the doctor's advice. "For me, it was absolutely incredible to be on the pill," she said. "Because, consider that you don't have to do nightly injections any more. Your whole life is freed up because you're not constantly worrying, 'Am I going to have time to get it all in tonight? Do I have to leave this party early, or do I have to bring medicine to the party?' And the pain factor is gone."

The teenager had seen the nurse or the clinic doctor at the Toronto General regularly when she came for her transfusions and she'd had all the required tests and biopsies. But in June 1996, as she lay in a hospital bed recovering from a scheduled liver biopsy with her mother at her side, Olivieri told her that her iron level was too high. Her mother thought that Olivieri must have made a mistake. "You don't even have the results of the biopsy yet," the mother remembered saying. "How can you know her iron is too high?"

It was a valid question. Olivieri had always told her patients that in order to follow them, she needed them to have annual liver biopsies to assess their iron levels. Her patients dreaded the biopsies, but she had persuaded them that it was the only way she could be certain they were healthy. The teenage girl's biopsy results would be available within a few days, yet Olivieri wasn't waiting for the results before switching her back to Desferal.

It wasn't clear to either mother or daughter when the doctors had first noticed that there was a problem, but Olivieri said that the tests showed L1 wasn't working for the girl and that it was as if she'd been receiving no treatments at all to remove iron.

The mother protested. "We've been coming to clinic every month, and every month they tell us she's doing fine. How come all of a sudden today, you say she's not?"

Olivieri told her, "Please don't ask me any questions because I can't answer them. You have to trust my judgment." Then she wrote a prescription for Desferal and instructed the mother to take it to the hospital pharmacy. She wanted the girl to start back on Desferal injections that night. The mother told Olivieri she needed a chance to talk to her husband and daughter about it first.

The family eventually talked it over with several people. First they met with Mel Freedman. He flipped through the girl's thick medical chart, holding it out so the family could see where the lab had recorded her serum ferritin levels. Based on what was in her chart, Freedman said, she probably needed to go back on Desferal. Her parents asked why it had taken so long for them to find out that L1 wasn't working, but Freedman didn't know. Then the senior hematologist asked the girl how she was feeling about all this. "I don't want to die," she replied. "I'll do whatever I have to do."

The mother took her confusion to Sher. Olivieri and Sher were still close, but he was now more of an equal. One of her colleagues believes that as Sher settled into his new job, he was becoming more popular than Olivieri. To the thalassemia patients, Sher was a clinical doctor with time to spare for them, and even some patients who were officially under Olivieri's care sought him out. The patients still revered Olivieri for her depth of knowledge about the disease and for keeping them so healthy. As one mother put it in an interview for CBC Radio, "I've seen patients from the States and I've seen pictures of them from Europe and none of them look as healthy as our patients do, so Dr. Olivieri must be doing something right and I trust her." Other patients expressed simiar feelings, but when they were in clinic for their transfusions and follow-up appointments, Olivieri was often away or hard to reach. Sher was more accessible.

Olivieri's patient and her family headed to the Toronto General to meet with Sher. But if they were looking for an argument to stay on L1, they didn't find it. Sher told them what he'd heard: L1 was working for some patients but not for everyone. He said he couldn't explain why they hadn't been told sooner that there was a problem. The girl started back on her injections of Desferal with the pump, and marked the date in her school agenda with a Band-Aid taken off a sore injection site. It was a sad day for the family.

Olivieri never spoke to the mother after that. "She sees me coming down a hallway and she'll go in the first door she sees," the mother said. She couldn't understand how she could lose her relationship of more than a decade with her daughter's doctor. Olivieri had treated her daughter from the age of two, and over the years the two women had developed a friendship. Occasionally, the mother would give the doctor a lift home from the hospital. "I would like to have it out with her, because I don't think I've done anything to deserve this," the mother said a few years later. She assumes the doctor stopped speaking to her because she questioned Olivieri's judgment.

In mid-July, six weeks after the study ended, Michael Spino went ahead with his planned advisory meeting on the L1 research. Elias Schwartz, former head of pediatrics at the Children's Hospital of Philadelphia, came as a senior figure in thalassemia research. Schwartz had devoted part of his time during the 1970s and '80s to studies of Desferal. Beatrix Wonke came from the Royal Free Hospital in London, bringing nearly a decade of clinical and research experience with L1. A pediatric clinical pharmacologist came from Case Western Reserve medical school in Ohio, and epidemiologist Mary Corey was there from Sick Kids. Their task was the same as the one usually given to data safety monitoring boards: they were supposed to review all the data from Olivieri's trial and determine whether patients taking the drug were safe.

Each expert received a set of data from the company and a set of sealed envelopes prepared by Olivieri and Brittenham. They spent a day and a half crunching numbers. Said Corey, "I had the Apotex printouts, the Apotex disc and the Nancy data—so I scoured them endlessly for discrepancies." The experts understood that Olivieri wanted to change the consent forms for her studies of L1 and that, as a result, the studies had been halted. According to Corey, the basic message the company gave them was, "Dr. Olivieri had this interpretation; we have a different interpretation. We feel it needs an objective look."

The company was paying them for their time and provided them with coffee and lunch. But company representatives weren't in the room for their discussions or deliberations. Corey described the group as "people who were struggling objectively to come up with an interpretation." As the panel's second day of work drew to a close, Brittenham, Koren and Olivieri came to Apotex headquarters to hear its conclusions. Many of the L1 scientists whom Olivieri had involved as collaborators were also there, including Alan Cohen, the Philadelphia hematologist.

Cohen had published papers together with Olivieri more than once and he considered her a friend. He called her frequently to run a difficult patient case by her and hear her opinion. He'd even asked her to go hear his teenage daughter when she came through Toronto as a singer in a band. For her part, Olivieri had listed Cohen as a suggested outside reviewer for her MRC grant application in 1990. Four years later, when Cohen began working with her on L1, they were both excited about the project. Then, in the spring of 1996,

Spino sent him Olivieri's data—the data that supposedly documented a loss of response in several patients. Cohen reviewed it but
couldn't see a problem with how the drug was working, and he
shared his opinion with Spino. Though it was a scientific question to
Cohen, it was a personal affront to Nancy Olivieri, who now gave
Cohen the cold shoulder.

Soon the expert panellists delivered their opinion. Like
Olivieri, they didn't want the L1 trials stopped in the middle; they
recommended strongly that the trials should continue. But that
was the only point they agreed with Olivieri on. The panellists said
they couldn't corroborate her concerns. She said the drug had lost
its efficacy in most of her patients who took it, while they thought
the drug was working for most of the patients. Olivieri later
spoke with Corey and determined that the panellists hadn't
received all of the material she and Brittenham had sent Apotex.
But it wasn't clear that more data would have changed the panel's
decision. The disagreement seemed to centre on how Olivieri
defined her terms. One panellist explained that the question had to
do with how far a patient's iron level needed to drop for the drug
to be considered successful. Olivieri and Brittenham used one cut-
off point, the panellists another. As a result, patients whom Olivieri
judged to be "treatment failures" were judged by several panellists
to be successes.

Two groups of scientists had looked at the data set and interpreted it differently, which wasn't surprising. This isn't unheard of
in science or medicine. The same set of laboratory results can be
viewed differently, just as the same amount of water in a glass can
be seen as half empty or half full. But the difference between the
expert panel's interpretation and Olivieri's was striking. The panel
had been asked to review the new consent forms that Olivieri had
drafted and was emphatic in its rebuke. They concluded that the
change Olivieri was proposing in the consent forms—her line that

most of the patients were not responding to L1—was unwarranted. She had used the word "unexpected" to describe her discovery that L1 didn't always work, but, like Spino, several panellists thought that individual variations in the response to a drug were normal and to be expected. "The Committee suggests that the words 'unexpectedly' and 'loss of efficacy' be removed from the new consent forms, since the Committee does not find that they are substantiated during the review of the data," they wrote in their report. Mary Corey said afterwards, "There was clearly something that aroused the clinical intuition of someone like Nancy," but she and the other panellists weren't sure what it was.

Toward the end of July, Olivieri finally met with O'Brodovich, who was now officially the chief of pediatrics. She brought the two lawyers who had been assigned to her case back in May when she called the doctors' malpractice association. The hospital vice-president, Alan Goldbloom, was also there, and the meeting was held in his office. Olivieri said she wanted to describe her findings in an abstract for the upcoming ASH meeting; O'Brodovich replied that from a moral and ethical standpoint, he fully supported her right to publish her results. When Olivieri explained that Apotex was threatening to sue her if she published, the chief recommended that she and Apotex resolve their conflict by publishing "dual abstracts" for ASH: Nancy could submit one and Apotex could submit the other, each with the same data but reaching different conclusions. O'Brodovich also asked what Koren thought about the findings. Then he told her that the administration wouldn't weigh in on a debate. "We said Hospital for Sick Children's is not the arbitrator of scientific discrepancies," he wrote in his notes of the meeting. The hospital also didn't want to arbitrate the company's threats to sue her. Her argument with the company over her "contractual obligations" was a legal matter, he told her, and the hospital didn't want to be involved in it.

People left the meeting with different impressions of what had transpired. Nancy Olivieri walked away believing she could no longer turn to the professor of pediatrics or the rest of the hospital administration—they'd abandoned her to the company's machinations. She said later, "The university and Sick Kids haven't supported me. They've presented it as a scientific debate."

In August, Dean Arnie Aberman went alone to a Toronto restaurant to talk to Apotex. He met with Jack Kay, Barry Sherman's second-in-command, and told him: "Irrespective of rights that Apotex may believe it has, Apotex should stop threatening legal action against Nancy and should not proceed with legal action." Kay said that the company wasn't going to sue Olivieri, and apparently, the dean and the hospital accepted those assurances. Administrators at Sick Kids "believed that the position of the company was an empty threat," said Sick Kids research chief Manuel Buchwald, in an attempt to explain why the hospital didn't take concrete action about Apotex.

But Katherine Kay, the lawyer who was handling the company's case for Stikeman Elliott, spoke a different language. Stikeman is one of Canada's largest law firms, and its rosters often included former cabinet ministers and political party leaders. Kay dealt with Nancy Olivieri the way she would with any client's legal opponent. If things ever went to court, she intended to win.

"I have a file full of letters from the company threatening me," Olivieri said later. Kay wrote that Olivieri was bound by her "contractual obligations" to the company and didn't have the right to publish, especially since other scientists, namely "the members of the Expert Advisory Panel," disagreed with her conclusions. In Kay's view, Olivieri's obligations to Apotex were clear, "not overridden by any public interest in the publication of the data," and Olivieri's strong wish to publish wasn't standard scientific discourse; it was evidence of her "desire to see this matter escalate."

If Kay's aim was to intimidate, she succeeded. It's not clear if Olivieri knew about the meeting between Aberman and the president of Apotex, but she was aware of the millions the company had invested in the drug and she thought they stood to lose much more than that if L1 went off the rails. Given what the company had at stake, she was terrified of what they might do to keep her from talking about her concerns. She said that every time her fax machine rang, she jumped. But she didn't tell the patients what had happened and this led to confusion, with many families believing it was Olivieri who had stopped the study. In August, on a conference call with Josie and another member of the patients' organization, Olivieri read aloud from the letter Spino had written her in May, closing out the trials and emphasizing the confidentiality clause in her contract. This proved it wasn't her decision to remove L1 from the hospital pharmacy. Josie and the other patient urged her to speak at their upcoming conference in October and explain the situation, but she said she wasn't sure she could—she'd have to consult with legal counsel first. The patients didn't understand that and Josie asked point-blank if her obligations to the company were more important than her legal obligation as a physician to inform her patients. Once again, Olivieri told them she'd have to consult her lawyers before answering.

The patients were asking excellent questions—a legal expert would argue later that no court in Canada would uphold the company's effort to prevent a doctor from telling patients her concerns. But in August 1996, Olivieri was checking everything with her CMPA legal team, which left patients feeling they couldn't get the information they needed about their care or about the L1 studies that so many of them had enrolled in.

Olivieri was planning to keep studying L1 surreptitiously. She intended to continue collecting her patients' blood tests and biopsy results, since those were available to her clinically. Though she lacked research funds to pay for the tests, they could be billed to the provincial health insurance plan if she ordered them for clinical purposes. Olivieri explained in an interview that after the company "cut the trials off . . . we kept going, so we have follow-up data." But it was unofficial research, and she decided not to collaborate on it with Koren. She simply didn't discuss it with him. It was similar to what she'd done with Perrine and with the Apotex research monitors. And Koren, like Perrine and the Apotex monitors, took a while to notice that things had changed.

Her lawyers worked with her on a plan to share her data with Health Canada. In mid-August, Nancy Olivieri went to Ottawa accompanied by a lawyer and Brittenham. In a meeting with the director of the Bureau of Biologics at the Health Protection Branch, Olivieri and Brittenham both made presentations about why they thought the agency should be concerned about L1; Spino and a company scientist sat in as interested observers. The agency official was noncommittal in her responses, and Olivieri concluded that she was the company's ally.

Olivieri felt under siege. Submissions to ASH were due, and she had prepared an abstract about the patients who weren't responding to L1, but her lawyers had advised her to send the company a copy of the abstract. She thought the company might sue to keep her from submitting it. The hospital seemed obtuse or oblivious to what was going on, and the federal government wasn't coming to her aid either. She began to erect what one person later described as "an invisible fence." She was on one side with a few trusted friends; everyone who couldn't understand how she felt or didn't try to was on the other.

She turned to her colleagues outside Toronto for support. She relied heavily on Brittenham and said she counted him and his wife among her closest friends. He stood by her even at the cost of losing Apotex funding. Early in the summer of 1996, he told Spino that he wouldn't work on L1 without Olivieri, and he began planning with Olivieri how and where they would present their L1 findings—the very findings the company was trying to embargo.

Olivieri later recalled a restaurant dinner she had with Brittenham that summer. "I was saying, 'Do you know that we could be sued for millions? You could lose your house!' And he said, 'I know. Do you want red or white wine?'" When she thanked him for backing her, he replied, "Nancy, I'm not doing this for you. I'm doing this because it's the right thing to do." If it came to it, he told her, he would sell his house.

Olivieri was also in close touch with the British thalassemia expert Sir David Weatherall. Weatherall had been knighted for his contributions to research on thalassemia and was now head of a major research institute at Oxford and a recognized scientific leader in the U.K. He'd been president of both the Association of Physicians of Great Britain and Ireland and the British Association for the Advancement of Science. And he was clearly close to Olivieri.

During the heat of her firestorm with Apotex, she phoned Weatherall often. In the summer of 1996, he spoke to her lawyer to support her need to present her results at scientific meetings. After the expert panel met, she sent him a copy of their report. He agreed with her that the panel's conclusions were invalid. He said it was "impossible to assess the scientific validity" of the panel's approach and that he had "concerns about some of the statistical analysis." Since the differences between Olivieri and the experts hinged on how to define a treatment success or failure, it wasn't clear if Weatherall's concerns simply reflected the fact that he accepted Olivieri's definitions, but because of what he termed "these fundamental flaws," he decided that the panel's assertions were "not supportable." He wrote up his opinion and filed it as a legal affidavit so that if Apotex sued, Olivieri's legal team would have his opinion on file.

Olivieri also kept David Nathan apprised of what was going on. He thought the company's legal threats were outrageous and he was unimpressed by the independent panel. He followed Weatherall's example, filing an affidavit that described the experts' report as "scientifically impenetrable and without any substance." Olivieri loved Nathan's choice of words. The phrase "scientifically impenetrable" made her laugh. But Nathan's affidavit was serious. The company's lawyers said Olivieri couldn't disclose her L1 findings; David Nathan said she had to "inform physicians about her most recent findings to enable them to properly advise their patients." Put that way, disclosure to her colleagues via abstracts at ASH and elsewhere was a moral necessity, and Nathan made similar comments in a conversation with Olivieri's lawyer.

Yet even with strong support from powerful men, Olivieri was losing the battle. She'd tried diplomacy, a mediation session with the dean during which she had hoped to have her studies reinstated. That had helped her patients, who were now able to take L1 if she thought it was in their interests. But it hadn't helped Olivieri as a scientist. The trials she'd founded and designed remained on hold while the company's lawyers sent her intimidating letters and the independent panel poked holes in her analysis. Somehow her bosses at the hospital didn't realize what she was up against and failed to take up her cause. Nathan and Weatherall committed themselves to her fight and explained themselves eloquently, but that didn't seem to influence Apotex.

By the end of the summer, Nancy Olivieri was fighting for her reputation and struggling to assert the validity of her science. Apotex was carrying the flag for L1 without her, and she seemed helpless to stop them. Incensed, she dropped her crusade to replace Desferal with an oral drug. In the fall of 1996, the complicated woman who'd birthed L1 in North America began trying to kill it off—at home and around the world.

ON THE WRONG SIDE OF THE FENCE

Over the next few months, many of Olivieri's former colleagues began to find themselves on the other side of her fence. And then, after all that had happened, L1 itself wound up there. After that summer, when Apotex made it clear that it would develop the pill without her, Olivieri became increasingly concerned about the drug. She said she got worried because of a call from Gary Brittenham. While looking for an explanation of why the patients had stopped responding to L1, he had heard about a British study that Bob Hider collaborated on, involving a drug in the same family as L1—an experimental agent called CP-94. Hider and scientists from Leicester had tested CP-94 in gerbils who were overloaded with iron. The drug initially prevented iron from accumulating in the liver, but subsequently stopped working, and when the animals were sacrificed, the investigators found extensive scarring of the liver and some scarring of the heart. When Brittenham read Olivieri the conclusions of the paper, they wondered if the same thing that had happened to the gerbils on CP-94 had happened to their patients. Olivieri thought that if they'd developed liver scarring from using L1, that could explain why they'd stopped responding to the drug.

The L1 patients had all undergone annual liver biopsies, and a significant liver problem such as scarring should have been detected at the time of biopsy by pathologists, so Olivieri called for the pathology reports. In the case of patients on L1, none of the pathologists who had reviewed the slides had picked up scarring of the liver. Normally, Olivieri would simply rely on the pathologists' interpretation and leave it at that, as most doctors would.

"Most doctors, you order an X-ray and whatever the radiologist says, that's what you go with," explained the liver expert Marshall Kaplan, of Tufts University in Boston, when I asked him about it later. "Same with the pathologist. You order a liver biopsy, and what-ever the pathologist says, that's what you go with." It was a matter of expertise, but Olivieri was about to make an exception.

She requested the old slides, too, and as she peered through the microscope, she was certain she saw scarring. She thought the pathology service had missed the problem because they'd examined the biopsies differently. "You see, what happens is, you send a liver biopsy down," she explained in an interview. "And a liver biopsy has to go to the pathology lab to be read, to be graded on necrosis, inflammation, fibrosis etc. . . . And most of the time the pathologist will examine that and look at the last biopsy and say, 'Looks about the same,' 'Looks a bit different.' But they will not say, 'Well, let's go back. This patient's on an experimental drug. Let's go back and look at the biopsies from 1990, '91, '92, '93, '94.' They don't normally do that. Nor would they say, 'Well, I better look at the other twenty patients who are taking the same drug.'" Her research protocol hadn't called for the pathologists to examine the biopsies in that way, she said. Yet once she organized the slides by patient and by year and re-examined them in order, she saw liver scarring (fibrosis) in some of the patients on L1.

However, she'd neglected to take precautions against bias. In pathology, where everything rides on what a doctor thinks he sees under the microscope, bias can change everything. Marshall Kaplan described how he once studied a drug for hepatitis, knowing that his hopes for it could affect what he saw. "If I looked at all the slides of the biopsies of patients before they took the drug, then I looked at all the slides after they took the drug, I might be able to convince myself that the 'after' looked better," he said. Instead, he took all the slides and numbered them randomly. Then he examined them under the microscope. "I didn't know anything about when the slide was from. I simply looked at each slide and filled out a form with questions: 'How much scarring?' 'How much inflammation?'" Nancy Olivieri had reviewed her patients' biopsies knowing that they were taking L1 and even knowing how long they'd been on the drug. Based on what she saw, she decided L1 had damaged their livers.

In most spheres of academia, professors' personal views on an issue are expected to colour their research. But if scientists are too dedicated to finding a particular result, their reports may be biased. Patricia Huston, a Canadian expert on the ethics of science publishing, believes the problems of bias are widespread. "It's not just pharmaceutical companies that are guilty of this," she said. "People's personal agendas interfere with a kind of dispassionate, objective interpretation of science." Nancy Olivieri had never considered that her personal commitment to L1 or her financial relationship with Apotex threatened her ability to be dispassionate about L1, but it had looked to outsiders as if she was overstating the drug's benefits. Now, locked in battle with Apotex, she didn't question whether her animus toward the company could affect her interpretation of data on L1's risks. Certain she had discovered a new, unreported problem with the drug, she did an abrupt about-face, deciding L1 was potentially so toxic, no one should take it. She began focusing on how to get her new findings out to other doctors.

She and Brittenham had a review article on thalassemia that was coming out in February 1997 in *Blood*, so she contacted the journal editors to see if she could add a few lines about L1 causing liver damage. She got a thumbs-up and wrote a quick addendum. She would be attending ASH in early December and called the meeting organizers to see about arranging a special symposium there. She got an evening slot and set to work organizing the effort. She also started preparing her L1 findings for publication in a medical journal. She got in touch with David Nathan about it, and he said he would write the *New England Journal of Medicine* to let them know some of the background of the L1 controversy. That could smooth the way for her paper when it got there. In the early fall of 1996, she began sharing her findings that L1 could cause liver damage with other physicians, including her colleague at the Toronto General thalassemia clinic, Graham Sher.

Sher and Olivieri chatted regularly and continued to collaborate on research. Over the course of the summer they'd spoken about her conflict with Apotex a few times. When patients asked Sher about L1, he reiterated what she had told him: the pills didn't work for everyone. Then she told him that L1 caused liver scarring— hepatic fibrosis. Her reasoning was straightforward: some patients' biopsies showed fibrosis, and L1 was the most probable cause. But Sher, like Olivieri, knew the patients' clinical histories by heart and wouldn't accept what she was saying.

"You can't claim that there's drug-induced fibrosis in these individuals," he told her. "There are just too many confounding factors." A lot of the patients on L1 had other liver conditions that could lead to scarring. Some had the beginnings of cirrhosis— hardening of the liver tissue. Others, including Howard, had suffered the effects of iron overload on their livers for years before starting Desferal or L1. A few patients were heavy drinkers and that could have damaged their livers. Still others had viral hepatitis—an infection of the liver. A lot of Canadian thalassemia patients had developed hepatitis as a result of receiving tainted blood transfusions, and in some cases patients were infected with more than one hepatitis virus. Sher believed that the patients' pre-existing liver problems made it difficult to ascribe any liver damage they had to a drug reaction.

Sher was thinking of his patients and the complexities of their disease. "These are multiple virally infected, cirrhotic individuals," he told Olivieri. On the question of what was harming the patients' livers, he was voting for multiple phenomena as opposed to a single drug. It was an intellectual argument, not intended to be insensitive or to undermine, but on this issue Olivieri wasn't seeking skepticism. What Sher treated as one more scientific disagreement with his mentor—the sort of academic back-and-forth he might have with a colleague at rounds—she took to heart.

Around the same time, Michael Spino asked Sher to consult to the company on hematology. Sher's wife was pregnant with their first child, and they'd been looking to buy a house. Several of his academic colleagues consulted to drug companies on the side. Spino told Sher he would receive an annual fee of $15,000, and Sher accepted. When Nancy Olivieri learned what he'd done, it was another blow. She couldn't understand how a friend of hers could partner with the company, given how badly they had treated her.

By the middle of October 1996, Sher's once close relationship with Olivieri had dissolved. When they spoke, she cut their talks short. Bev Tyler, the nurse who co-ordinated the thalassemia clinic at the Toronto General, acted as their conduit for information about patients. And Graham Sher got caught up in a conflict that had nothing to do with him.

Sick Kids administrators had decided to move one of Olivieri's clinics—a clinic for the sickle cell patients—to a community hospital. Although she would still be in charge, the clinic would be off-site. Olivieri had opposed the move because she felt it would be too risky for her patients, but in the fall of 1996 the fight was nearing an end. In spite of her protests, Sick Kids' executive committee was going ahead with its plan to transfer her clinic. If she didn't like it, she could step down from the leadership of her clinical program.

Olivieri quickly understood that she was facing an ultimatum. "I received a letter from senior administrators saying that if I did not co-operate with this initiative . . . I would be dismissed as director of the hemoglobinopathy program," she explained. She couldn't imagine co-operating, but she also couldn't risk losing her program directorship, a high-profile position within her field that had been crucial to her research. It was a professional crisis. For help, Olivieri turned to Michael Baker, the hematologist she'd been close to since her days as a resident at the Toronto Western. He was now physician-in-chief at the Toronto General.

Somehow, a plan was developed. Graham Sher would leave the Toronto General's adult thalassemia clinic and move to something else, possibly the transfusion service; Nancy Olivieri would take over the clinic's leadership. In an interview later, Michael Baker explained what happened: "Dr. Olivieri was offered the position of head of the thalassemia clinic at the Toronto Hospital because of her expertise and reputation. And Dr. Sher, having just arrived, felt that his career had to go elsewhere. There was an opportunity opening up in transfusion."

Nancy Olivieri "engineered" her way into the job, said a senior hematologist in Toronto. It all hinged on Baker, according to people who watched the plan unfold. The chief offered Sher a lateral move from director of the thalassemia program to director of the hospital's transfusion service, also known as the blood bank. The Toronto General had the largest blood bank in the country, and transfusion medicine was under-researched, Baker told Sher. It needed someone of his calibre to take it to a higher level.

Sher turned him down, telling Baker that he wasn't interested in leaving the thalassemia and sickle cell clinics; he felt too attached to the patients and to his work there. He had devoted three years of his life to hemoglobin disorders, and he had research projects in progress. Moving to the blood bank meant building his reputation all over again in a different field. In addition, the patients would have to start again with another doctor.

"Graham, if you don't want to go, you don't have to," the hospital chief said. Then Baker talked about Olivieri. "You know, she's difficult," he told Sher. "But all these very bright people are difficult. And she's very important to the division." He was referring to the hematology division at the Toronto General, where Sher, Baker and Olivieri all held appointments and where Olivieri was probably the division's most successful scientist.

Sher felt that if he stayed, his bosses wouldn't support him. He told his colleagues that he had seen thalassemia as his life's work but he felt forced to quit. "I was desperately disappointed in that," said one hematologist. "Graham was the one that we groomed to take over the clinic."

On a Saturday in October, the patients caught wind of the idea. They were holding an educational conference at a Howard Johnson's north of Toronto. Olivieri was scheduled to speak and came with a lawyer in tow. She continued to receive letters from Apotex threatening legal action if she presented or communicated her findings, and was increasingly worried that anything she said about L1 could land her with a lawsuit. Graham Sher was also on the podium but barely said a word.

Later, he took some of the patients aside and told them he would no longer be their doctor. "I'm being relieved," he told them. "I'm moving on." They asked why he was leaving but didn't get a clear answer.

Sher was in charge of more than 120 patients at the Toronto General. Bev Tyler scheduled an appointment for him with every one of them, and he met with each face to face to tell them he was leaving. Subsequently, many patients wrote to the hospital administration protesting his transfer. "They felt close to Graham because they saw him every time they were in clinic, whereas they didn't see Nancy," Howard explained.

Josie and Howard, who were serving respectively as director of the National Thalassemia Foundation and president of the patients' organization, decided to write Baker themselves after hearing from the patients. In their letter, they said the patients were "vehemently opposed" to Olivieri's taking over Sher's position. One thing that worried them was that Olivieri had so many "international commitments." They wrote, "We feel she is taking on too much responsibility and as a result the patients' health care will be compromised." They also feared her effect on the clinic's "stability," given the "high turnover of doctors and nurses working for Dr. Olivieri." They also wrote that patients who "do not agree with her methods feel that their care will be jeopardized."

They scheduled a meeting to address the patients' concerns and urged Michael Baker to attend. The meeting took place in mid-November. Baker showed up, as did Olivieri, Sher and more than fifty patients. Baker told the group that Sher was being promoted into a better position. The leadership of the thalassemia program at the Toronto General would shift to Nancy Olivieri, he said.

"We heard the reasons why Graham was being let go," Howard said, making the hand motions for "shoveling the shit." "This meeting about Graham was all political mumbo-jumbo," said Josie. When it was Sher's turn to speak, he was near tears. "You guys mean a lot to me," he told the patients. "I've dedicated my life to you these past few years. I'm not doing this lightly. But I think this is ultimately better for patient care."

Years later, Howard remembered his own reaction vividly. He remained sympathetic to Olivieri personally, but he objected to what was happening to the clinic. "We were so upset—the patients were," he said. "Patients really liked Graham."

Baker met with the patients once more. Josie remembers him saying, "I know Dr. Olivieri's a little wacky sometimes." Josie had the impression that the chief was trying to woo the patients to a sort of understanding by including them in "all that sort of closed-door stuff." She thought the patients hadn't fallen for the ploy. "Everyone was angry," she said. Corrado described feeling frustrated that their protests hadn't been listened to. The experience left him feeling bitter and cynical toward the city's leading hospitals.

Cynicism seemed like a valid response. The unchecked authority of administrators at Toronto's teaching hospitals and the backroom deals, bullying and intimidation it engendered were well known to doctors but shocking to the patients. They couldn't understand how a qualified physician could be forced from his job though he didn't want to go—and it would have been hard for anyone to explain. Though the drama of Olivieri's replacing Sher at the Toronto General thalassemia program was unfolding at the University of Toronto's largest teaching hospital, there was no input from the university, its faculty union or the patients' organization. The absence of oversight underscored the teaching hospital administrators' lock on power; in Toronto, they routinely make unilateral decisions at their institutions, answering only to their boards, who rarely question them. For patients such as Corrado, sophisticated enough to catch a glimpse of the workings of the hospital at that level, it was a disturbing revelation.

The patients threw a goodbye party for Sher. A few of the doctors and nurses who'd worked in the thalassemia clinic came, and Howard showed up with the requisite gag gift, a game of Operation, presented with a letter that he read aloud. "This came by FedEx today," he announced. "And it says, 'I wish you well. With fond regards, Nancy.'"

Olivieri *was* writing letters, though none of them were to Sher. Many of them went to Michael Spino and his staff at Apotex. That fall, Olivieri wrote someone at the company once every few days. She wrote about the drug, the patients and the data. She faxed her correspondence or had it sent by courier, and she requested prompt replies. In one letter she said Spino's assistant had told her that Apotex no longer wanted to provide the drug for the patients through the emergency release program. Spino wrote back denying that his assistant had ever said that. She faxed another letter asking Spino to send her reports out to all the other investigators working on L1, and another requesting that she be allowed to attend meetings related to the L1 toxicity study in Europe.

Previously, lawyers for Apotex had been the ones sending letters to Olivieri. In August, Spino or the company's lawyers had warned Olivieri or her lawyers about possible legal action in four separate letters; now it was the other way around. Apotex lawyers complained to Olivieri's lawyers about her "letter-writing campaign" in early December and demanded that future correspondence be between the law firms. The lawyers reached an agreement that prohibited Nancy Olivieri from writing to Apotex directly. She could only ask her lawyers to write to the company's lawyers. Around the same time, the company hired auditors to investigate Olivieri's research accounts at the hospital. Olivieri told her lawyers she didn't want to answer the auditors' questions, and she wrote the hospital to ask that staff at the Research Institute and the hospital accounts office not answer them either.

At ASH on the first weekend of December 1996, Olivieri went public with the claim that L1 caused scarring of the liver. Given the continued threats from Apotex lawyers and the company's attempt to prevent her from presenting her results, it was a bold move. ASH was in Orlando, Florida, that year, and she and Brittenham were co-chairing a scientific program on iron. Olivieri's talk was supposed to describe the "optimal management" of a patient with too much iron in his system as a result of frequent blood transfusions.

Essentially, she delivered a clinical argument in favour of Desferal and against L1. At one point she raced through a description of the 1994 study in which the drug CP-94 caused progressive liver scarring in gerbils. Then she described her own patients who had taken L1, asserting that four who had no liver scarring when they started on L1 had progressed to scarring and that four others who had scarring when they started on the drug had progressed to cirrhosis of the liver.

Scientific conferences are typically open meetings where anyone who registers can attend. Olivieri's audience was predominantly hematologists, but there were thalassemia patients in the crowd as well, along with company officials. When she finished speaking, Spino raised his hand, identified himself as being from Apotex and announced that she hadn't presented the data in their entirety. His exchange with Olivieri struck one reporter as "quite sharp" and "really unpleasant." Others objected to her drawing parallels between L1 and CP-94 because the drugs were metabolized differently. "You can't compare them," said one of the doctors from London. Victor Hoffbrand, who was still studying L1 in England, said he thought that if L1 wasn't working for patients, the dosing could be inadequate. He and Wonke were testing the use of higher doses of L1 and had found that some patients didn't respond unless they used a dose significantly higher than Olivieri's patients were on. But Olivieri's friend Elliott Vichinsky, from the thalassemia program in Oakland, California, stood and commended her for her bravery in speaking about the problems she'd discovered with L1.

In addition to the formal meetings, Olivieri was to speak at a special evening symposium she'd organized. "Space is limited; attendance is by invitation only" read the symposium announcement. Fernando Tricta, an Italian thalassemia researcher who had begun working as a medical adviser to Apotex, requested an invitation and got one, though Olivieri told him he would not be able to present his data. Spino didn't attend. The meeting went from nine in the evening until past eleven. Olivieri stressed that for patients on L1, liver scarring was a serious issue, but once again, her audience argued with her about it. An Australian L1 researcher said L1 was very effective, and Beatrix Wonke objected to the report on gerbils, saying that data on CP-94 should not be extrapolated to L1.

Gideon Koren wasn't in Florida for the meeting. As a non-hematologist, he didn't attend ASH. But he still thought he was collaborating with Olivieri, especially since she was now dependent on him to procure L1. Under the emergency release program worked out by the dean, Koren was the go-between. He spoke to Apotex and arranged for the pills to get to the Sick Kids pharmacy, while Olivieri and her staff followed the patients clinically.

When he heard from an Israeli friend what she'd reported about liver scarring, he was hurt that Olivieri hadn't filled him in. "You have done this without me despite my being the toxicologist on the team!" he wrote her. "More shocking, you have used me as a conduit to receive L1 for your patients, but did not tell me of the life-threatening toxicity of the drug!" The last lines of Koren's letter read, "As of today, I will not continue my collaborative work or data interpretation with you." Of course, Nancy Olivieri had ceased collaborating with Gideon Koren many months earlier, without telling him. Later, she said that as "the toxicologist on the team," he should have detected the drug's effect on the liver. "Gidi Koren didn't identify this toxicity, and he was supposed to," she told me.

After she returned from ASH, Olivieri took the time to review the patients' liver biopsies more thoroughly. It was a complicated process. Some of the patients' slides were at Sick Kids; others were at the Toronto General. She wasn't an expert in liver pathology, so she had to work with a pathologist. As she described it later, "You have to get all these seventy-two biopsies from two hospitals and it's not an easy task. But all of those were collected. And on Christmas

Eve of December 1996, I sat with the pathologists and they reviewed these and concluded that there was indeed worsening of hepatic fibrosis, worsening of liver damage in patients on [L1]."

But it wasn't enough to decide what the biopsies showed; she had to prove it to others by showing them pictures. After viewing the slides with a pathologist, she "shot" micrographs of them and developed the film. Then the pathologist looked over the photos and gave her his final opinion; after this, they had to describe the results in graphs and tables. It was hours of work, marred by flaws, for the pathologist she worked with was not blinded to the characteristics of the patients whose biopsies they were viewing and, according to some reports, he didn't use an accepted, standard system for evaluating liver biopsies—two factors that could lead to biased results.

In January 1997, Olivieri worked with Brittenham to incorporate the graphs and tables into a report describing the liver scarring. Brittenham thought that once they sent their report to Apotex, it would be a no-brainer for the company to discontinue its work on L1. But Spino had just come through Olivieri's letter campaign and her accusations about his assistant. He knew that Olivieri had dumped Koren, who disagreed with her about the patients' "loss of response" to L1, and had dumped Sher, who disagreed with her about how to explain the patients' liver biopsies; he'd also sat through her presentation at ASH, where he had become convinced that she was presenting parts of her data set but not others—a tactic that could skew her results. "Scientific integrity requires that you look at all the evidence and you look at it in an unbiased fashion," Spino said later. He hired three consultants to review the report and told his company's lawyers that he wouldn't act on the issue of liver scarring until those reviews were in.

That month, an old friend called up to ask Olivieri how she was doing, and she described her experience fighting Apotex as "very isolating." She discussed her feelings with Brittenham in Cleveland

and with Weatherall in Oxford but not with many of the friends she'd once been close to in Toronto. Her major efforts went toward getting her L1 findings into print. She was preparing abstracts for international meetings on thalassemia that were coming up in the spring, she'd started to write a journal article about her L1 findings, and she was composing a letter to the FDA, letting them know that a new and serious problem had been discovered with L1. She was writing that she didn't think anyone should be taking the drug because the risk of liver scarring was too great.

In her battle with Apotex, the letter to the FDA was a shot over the bow. When researchers are experimenting with an investigational new drug and learn of a serious and unexpected problem, they're supposed to report it. If the study is investigator-driven, as Susan Perrine and Nancy Olivieri's study of butyrate had been, reporting is the responsibility of the researchers. If it's company-driven, as the L1 trials were, the duty lies with the company. Olivieri didn't trust that Spino would inform the drug agencies of her concerns.

Her lawyers had told her they would have to show her FDA letter to Apotex first, given the company's threats. When Spino got it, he called Koren, who said he couldn't understand why Olivieri was writing the FDA that no one should take the pills. He thought she was still prescribing it at Sick Kids and the Toronto General, because as her liaison to Apotex he was still obtaining the pills from the company. Spino realized that he'd just been given crucial information and he phoned Sick Kids' chief of pediatrics.

"Dr. Michael Spino contacted me by phone on Tuesday evening February 18, 1997," Hugh O'Brodovich wrote later in a letter to Olivieri's lawyer. "He asked if I was aware of Dr. Olivieri's opinion that she had observed a 'severe adverse reaction' during her use of L1." The next morning, the chief phoned Olivieri. "I tried to page her, tried to get hold of her," he said in an interview. Instead, he reached Koren and confirmed what Spino had hinted at: despite Olivieri's opinion about the drug, she still had patients on it. O'Brodovich couldn't figure it out. If the drug was so toxic that the FDA needed to be informed, wasn't it too toxic for patients at Sick Kids? Olivieri told her lawyer that when O'Brodovich's secretary reached her, she was given one hour's notice to report to the chief's office. When she arrived, O'Brodovich was there with his administrative assistant and the hematology division head, Mel Freedman.

"How can you be saying this to the FDA, but you're still using the drug?" O'Brodovich asked. "There's absolutely no doubt that I'm right about this," was her reply. O'Brodovich asked how many patients were still on L1 and whether she'd told them how dangerous she now thought it was; Olivieri wasn't forthcoming with the information. "This is an urgent situation," he told her.

He claims he intended the meeting to be supportive. He said in an interview, "We were saying, 'This is a real problem.' We were concerned for Nancy and for her patients." But Olivieri was facing a three-on-one situation as one woman addressing her male adversaries, while the chief's administrative assistant took detailed notes that O'Brodovich would later refer to as "minutes."

Olivieri described what she'd done to confirm her finding of toxicity—how she had reviewed the biopsy specimens with the pathologist, photographed the slides and given the photos to the pathologist for a final opinion. She assured Freedman and O'Brodovich that there was no scientific controversy over her claims, as if the debates she'd been part of at ASH had never occurred. But O'Brodovich wanted to know why she hadn't informed the Research Ethics Board yet. She said she'd been told by her lawyer not to tell anyone else until Apotex was informed, leaving it unclear whether she'd asked her legal team if she could talk to the REB. The chief asked her to please, now, notify the board.

She wrote in her notes that O'Brodovich was extremely agitated. "As I told these idiots today," she began a letter to her lawyer, and detailed for him what she'd said to O'Brodovich and Freedman. "The whole thing was a reversal of the attitude held by the Dept. of Pediatrics in the summer," she wrote her lawyer. "Now it is: 'What have I done? Why haven't I done more, done it faster? Do I know what a risky position I am in?' There is no more: 'What does Dr. Koren think?' All of a sudden *I'm* the expert of the Western world on all this (this was actually stated). I think you get the drift."

It would have been hard for anyone to miss Olivieri's drift. She felt as if her bosses were attacking her when they should have been supporting her. She'd never forgiven O'Brodovich for failing to tell Apotex in the summer of 1996 that she had a right to proceed with her trials and to publish. And in her view, she'd been working all along to protect patients. Yet her own lawyers couldn't understand why her patients were still taking L1 (under the emergency release program worked out by the dean) when she was writing the FDA to say no one should be on it. "I could not stand up from [the pathologist]'s office . . . and cancel everyone's supply of L1 within one hour," she wrote her lawyer.

Olivieri planned to talk to the patients about her new findings at group meetings. She had scheduled a meeting with one group of patients for an evening in the first week of February and was holding a second meeting with another group in March. "Patients see us in clinic every 4–5 weeks," she explained to her lawyers. "That is why I have called the evening meetings, so nobody has to wait more than one month to speak with us about this." Later, the provincial College of Physicians and Surgeons would determine that Nancy Olivieri had acted in the best interests of her patients in informing them of the new risk she'd identified with L1. The College concluded that she'd acted promptly "to co-ordinate a safe and orderly transition to the standard treatment." But at the time, it was confusing—to Olivieri's bosses and to her lawyers.

Unsure what to make of it, O'Brodovich contacted the neo-natologist who was now head of the hospital's Research Ethics Board, a woman named Aideen Moore, who agreed to meet with Olivieri and her lawyer.

After her meeting with Moore, Olivieri spoke to her patients about her liver findings. She wrote in her notes later, "I spoke to all 14 families and instructed them to go off deferiprone after discussion with Aideen Moore who recommended this as a prudent course."

O'Brodovich next wrote Michael Baker to fill him in on the L1 situation and let him know that there were patients at the Toronto General Hospital who were also taking L1 and could, based on Olivieri's claims about the drug, be at significant risk. He copied that letter to Sick Kids CEO Michael Strofolino.

The next week he wrote Olivieri to ask what she was going to do about her patients who were on the drug. He also sent her the "minutes" of their meeting and asked her to sign them. She had already sent him a summary of her plans for the patients but he wanted more details about what she was doing "to ensure the safety of the patients" and about the information she'd shared with them. She replied by quoting the summary she'd given him earlier, adding, "Obviously, there is no information that can further be communicated to these patients, at this time." She didn't sign the minutes. The next day he wrote her again, and this time her lawyer tried to cajole her into writing him back with more details.

"In attempting to discern what exactly is troubling Dr. O'Brodovich, I thought that it would be helpful if I could let you have the benefit of my thoughts," Olivieri's lawyer began his letter to her. "I have the impression that Dr. O'Brodovich would like some assurance from you that your patients have been fully and properly informed about the findings which you and your colleague have reported to Dr. Fredd [Stephen Fredd of the FDA] . . . I suspect that Dr. O'Brodovich is concerned that the issue of 'informed consent' is appropriately dealt with." Tactfully, the lawyer sent Olivieri a copy of a CMPA publication entitled "Consent: A Guide for Canadian Physicians," and asked her to "note in particular the comments . . . relating to disclosure in research and experimentation."

Eventually she did respond to O'Brodovich, in a long memo commenting on the minutes and correcting the points with which she disagreed. At the same time, her lawyer wrote the chief to ask for another meeting, which took place a few days later. "The foundation was laid for the reestablishing of a good professional relationship between you and Drs. O'Brodovich and Freedman," her lawyer wrote Olivieri afterwards, but he warned her that O'Brodovich could limit her hospital privileges and he offered some advice. "Insofar as your ongoing dialogue with the Chief of Pediatrics and the Chief of Division is concerned, I would urge you to speak with them and correspond with them in a manner and in a tone which are at all times in substance and in appearance, professional and courteous." Olivieri took his instructions to heart and, that same day, sent her chiefs a memo reviewing everything she was planning for the patients and describing exactly what she was telling patients about the new risks of L1.

As the chiefs considered the gravity of Olivieri's claim that L1 caused liver scarring, the thalassemia patients contemplated the reality of returning to Desferal. Olivieri told them fibrosis could "be pictured like a series of rubber bands running through the liver or heart," and advised them to stop L1. But not all of them were willing to go off the pill. Olivieri said later, "The patients have not been on my side. To them, it's 'How can you withhold this wonderful drug?'"

Howard may have been one of the patients she was referring to. Nancy Olivieri had shown him the micrographs of his liver slides and had told him he had cirrhosis. But he was skeptical about the dangers of L1. He already knew he had liver damage, and he didn't blame it on the pill. "I think Nancy would like me to believe that L1 was solely responsible for what happened to my liver," he said. "But I have chronic hepatitis C, I drank like a fish in college and I have chronic iron overload." Howard knew, as most of the adult thalassemia patients did, that all three conditions could injure the liver. He continued, "So that's what she would like me to believe, but I'm not blind. I'm not stupid." He also dreaded returning to Desferal injections.

For a few months, he kept taking L1. When he ran out of it, he took nothing. Then, in the fall of 1997, he approached his former pediatrician at Mississauga Hospital, asking for a prescription for L1, and got referred to a hematologist who turned him down. "Unfortunately, I share the concerns about L1," the hematologist wrote to Howard's former doctor. He had heard Olivieri's presentation at ASH in 1996 and it left him concerned about L1's potential toxicity. He advised Howard to stay on Desferal. A few months later Howard vacationed in California and visited a friend who got worried about what she was hearing and also urged him to get back on Desferal. Howard said, "She knows me quite well and she just said, 'You're being a wimp. Give it another shot.'"

"I stewed over this all the way from LAX to Pearson. Then I made my decision and I e-mailed Nancy to let her know." Olivieri was thrilled that he was willing to go back on Desferal.

American patients who'd been at ASH were cynical about what Olivieri had to say. Though they didn't have access to L1, they didn't want to lose the prospect of ever having it approved. Taking their cue from the activists who had pushed successfully for speedy approval of AIDS drugs, the U.S. branch of the Thalassemia Action Group decided to press the FDA on L1. They were gathering letters from across the country to send to the agency. Among the more than 150 notes they would enclose was one from a nine-year-old patient who wrote, "If the pill comes, it will help me not to get bumps on my stomach." A twenty-six-year-old wrote, "I have been on Desferal 17 years and I hate it with a passion. It hurts to stick myself daily but the bumps that are left behind every morning are the worst." The group's leaders also laid out their argument for the FDA: "L1 is not a perfect drug, but it is better than no chelating therapy."

Apotex was also talking to the FDA. Spino had gone to a meeting there, but he thought the agency staffers were hostile to him. Staff at the drug agency had serious doubts about L1. David Nathan had written them that L1 could be toxic to the liver back in May 1996; then Olivieri wrote in 1997 to say she thought it was too dangerous for anyone to be on it. FDA officials were frank in their meeting with Spino. "They told us, 'This drug is a toxic drug and you've got to do a lot more work to bring this to market,'" he said.

It would have been foolish for him to try to explain that he thought Nancy Olivieri was biased against L1. That would suggest that there was something improper about her science, and after all, it was her research on L1 that had gotten the agency to consider the drug in the first place. He didn't go that route. But Nancy Olivieri did, by attacking the credibility of scientists who disagreed with her, accusing one—her former resident, Graham Sher—of scientific misconduct.

UNDOING GRAHAM SHER

Olivieri was planning to say, at an upcoming thalassemia conference in Malta, that L1 was toxic. She wrote an abstract for the meeting describing the liver scarring she'd found, but when her lawyers sent it to Apotex, Spino thought she had intentionally skewed her analysis to present the drug in the worst possible light. Based on the company's response, her lawyers advised her to withdraw the abstract and give a different paper in its place.

Apotex scientist Fernando Tricta was also getting ready for the Malta meeting, preparing a paper by combing through the data Olivieri had filed with the company over the years. Gideon Koren had agreed to collaborate with Tricta on his paper, and Michael Spino was contacting other researchers who had worked with the L1 patients to see if they were willing to get involved. He reached Graham Sher in his new post at the Toronto General Hospital's blood bank, and Sher agreed to look at Tricta's abstract.

The Toronto General is famous for its winding corridors where patients routinely get lost. Graham Sher had a windowless cubicle on one such corridor, and he sat there on a winter evening reading Tricta's description of thalassemia patients on L1. Sher knew them all. He had followed some of them clinically in 1993 and '94, when he was the resident on the thalassemia service at Sick Kids, and he got to know the others during 1995 and '96, when he was medical director for thalassemia at the Toronto General. His clinical impression of the drug was that it worked reasonably well. That fit with Tricta's abstract, which concluded that the pills were effective for most of the patients, and Sher agreed to co-author it.

The difference between Tricta's conclusions and Olivieri's reflected other divisions that had developed in the small community of thalassemia researchers who had experience with L1. David Nathan agreed with Olivieri; so did Gary Brittenham. But in London, Victor Hoffbrand and Beatrix Wonke were saying that L1, while less effective than Desferal, was working well for many patients. They had patients who had been on the pills for several years already. It worked better for some than for others, but they had seen no signs that it suddenly became ineffective or that it was toxic to the liver.

David Weatherall was on the scientific organizing committee for the conference in Malta, and Olivieri soon learned about the company's abstracts and heard that Koren and Sher were listed as co-authors. She thought Tricta, Koren and the other authors of their abstract were publishing her data without her approval. Certain it was against the rules of science for them to do that, she asked her lawyers to request copies of Tricta's abstracts. Its conclusions galled her.

"Dr. Brittenham generated the data," she said later. "But Dr. Koren, together with Dr. Spino from Apotex, took the data, rearranged it, and said, 'See? That makes it look like the drug is favourable and effective.'"

Medical journal editors today publish rules about who can rightfully claim to be the author of a scientific article. Yet even with clear rules, it's such a complicated issue that some journals, including the *British Medical Journal* and the *Journal of the American Medical Association,* ask all authors to specify exactly how they've contributed to a piece of scientific work. Viewed one way, Olivieri was correct: the data belonged to her and Brittenham, and no one else could quote it. Viewed another way, the results of the investigation belonged to all the investigators and they were supposed to work with each other to figure out a way to handle their disagreements. In a conversation at a meeting of journal editors, Frank Davidoff, former editor of the *Annals of Internal Medicine,* compared solving authorship disputes in science to counting angels on the head of a pin.

Olivieri's former collaborators were at least supposed to contact her if they were writing about the L1 trials, but they hadn't. Just as Olivieri had bypassed Susan Perrine in her articles that derived from their collaborative efforts, so too Tricta avoided contacting Nancy Olivieri about his abstract. The difference was that Olivieri knew what was happening and fought back. She wrote the Malta conference chairman and questioned "the propriety" of Tricta presenting at the meeting, given the circumstances. "She tried to stop them from presenting their views," Spino said. Spino saw Koren and Sher as collaborators on the trials with as much right to present the data as Olivieri, and the company's lawyers accepted his perspective. "Dr. Olivieri has repeatedly stated that she wishes the academic community to be made aware of the facts and we anticipate therefore that she will have no difficulty with the presentation of the full data set," they wrote to Olivieri's lawyers when they sent over the abstracts in March 1997. Olivieri disagreed—no one else had the right to present it without asking her permission.

David Weatherall was astounded that the company hadn't told Olivieri about its plans to write up the data and present it in Malta. "They put in an abstract presenting this stuff without showing it to Olivieri and Brittenham," he said in an interview. "I thought that was unbelievable, really . . . I think most universities would take a pretty dim view of it." The scientific committee didn't pull Tricta's abstracts off the program, but it did write a letter to meeting participants "to put on record that [we] do not consider that the authors of these abstracts behaved in a manner that is consistent with the accepted standard of scientific communication."

Olivieri contacted the university's vice-dean, a scientist named Cecil Yip, whose office handled all complaints of scientific misconduct at the U of T. She spoke with Yip long enough to describe what had happened. He said later that he followed the same process with her as he did with every professor who contacted him about potential cases of misconduct: he listened first, then he offered casual advice.

"A faculty member says, 'I have this problem, what do you think?'" Yip said in an interview. "And I say, 'It sounds like it falls within the framework of misconduct.' They say, 'Somebody stole my data or fudged my data.' And I say, 'Yeah, that's misconduct as defined by the framework.'"

After their conversation, Olivieri wrote administrators at the Toronto General, including the hospital's head hematologist, Armand Keating, that Graham Sher had plagiarized her work by publishing her data in an abstract without her permission and without giving her credit: "Dr. Cecil Yip . . . confirmed that, indeed, as was my impression, Graham Sher's actions represent professional research misconduct."

It was a serious charge. If Sher was guilty of stealing her data and calling it his own, then everything he'd ever published could be called into question. Papers he'd written would appear contaminated and his position at the hospital could be jeopardized. But the administrators at the General didn't call Yip or say anything to Sher; they seemed to be hoping that the problem would go away.

In the second week of April, Fernando Tricta flew to Malta to present his two abstracts on L1. Olivieri gave her talk as well. Kosta Papageorgiou was listening in the audience. A board member of the Thalassemia International Federation and father of two girls with thalassemia, Papageorgiou was surprised by what he was hearing from Nancy Olivieri. He couldn't understand her complete and sudden reversal on L1.

"Nancy was presenting beautiful data on L1 for years," he explained. "When she used to be coming to the international conferences, she was a legend . . . This continued until 1997. And in 1997 in Malta was the first time that Nancy Olivieri stood up and she said that L1 has a problem and is creating fibrosis. Everyone was saying, 'Why?'"

One of Papageorgiou's daughters had always taken her Desferal; the other hadn't. When L1 became available in Greece, it was a welcome relief for the family. Now, hearing Olivieri condemn the medication as unsafe, he worried for his daughter. "For us it was a big blow," he said of Olivieri's talk. But afterwards, when Papageorgiou learned that Olivieri's contract with Apotex had been terminated, he became skeptical.

Olivieri knew that Papageorgiou and others were raising questions behind her back, but she blamed it on Michael Spino. In her presence, he told the Malta gathering that her conclusions were misleading and false, and she found his comments hurtful. "I believe that many individuals have been convinced that ours are not solid and dependable views," she wrote her lawyer afterwards.

Back in Toronto, she again contacted Keating, the hospital's head of hematology, about Sher's role in the abstract. She had drafted a two-page letter of apology—a confession of sorts—that she wanted hospital administrators to send to Sher for his signature. She thought Sher should admit to professional research misconduct, say he was very sorry, belittle his own knowledge of iron overload and apologize "for any embarrassment, professional and personal, that this has afforded Dr. Olivieri, who provided me with a year of training in iron overload and iron chelating therapy in the Hemoglobinopathy Program from 1993–1994 during my fellowship." She listed eighteen individuals to whom Sher was to copy the letter if he agreed to sign it. Keating spoke to her and Baker about her letter but didn't call Yip or Sher, and Olivieri began to get impatient. She wrote Keating at the end of April to say she didn't "wish to wait another two weeks on this issue," and after a few days she wrote Sher herself, asking him to justify his participation on the abstract. She added, "Please note that we believe your conduct to be in conflict with guidelines for ethical conduct of research."

It was early May. Sher sat in his office, reading and rereading her letter. He couldn't understand why Nancy Olivieri, whom he thought he knew so well, was accusing him of being unethical. Leaving the hospital, he bumped into a friend and tried to describe his predicament. "I can't believe that this is happening," he said. "I just can't believe it." The friend said later, "He was very upset and very, very sad . . . It was a terrible, terrible time for him."

The next day, Sher wrote a long, heartfelt response to Olivieri. Before sending it, he met with his bosses, including Michael Baker, the physician-in-chief at the Toronto General. Sher didn't know that hospital administrators had discussed the matter with Olivieri several times already, and the men he was meeting with didn't tell him. Instead they asked him not to send his letter. If he gave them time, they said, they could talk to Olivieri. "This will go away," one of the administrators offered.

Sher didn't send his letter. But Olivieri had asked him to reply by a specific deadline, so he wrote to her saying he thought of himself as a collaborator on the L1 "compassionate use" study. He reminded her that she'd often described him in public as her collaborator. And he apologized "for any events which may have caused you to perceive that my conduct was in conflict with the university's guidelines."

"On the contrary, I have not 'perceived' that your conduct is in conflict with these guidelines," Olivieri replied. "I have confirmed that this is indeed the case with Dr. Cecil Yip." Reading her reply, Sher got scared that he could lose his job.

Sher didn't know what to do. He had never been attacked like this before. He phoned Yip's office to ask the vice-dean about his ruling. Yip said he couldn't be guilty because there hadn't been a misconduct investigation yet. Then Yip asked him to read what Olivieri had written. Yip was shocked: "No, I never said that. It's absolutely untrue." Sher asked again if Yip had said he was guilty. "Absolutely not," Yip replied.

Yip said later that his conversation with Sher upset him "no end." At the time, Yip had been on faculty at the University of Toronto for over thirty years. He'd served as president of the faculty union (the U of T Faculty Association) before going over to the other side and joining the ranks of the university administration, and he'd been a vice-dean for several years already. "In all my years, if there's a procedure set up, I follow the procedure," he said. "There's no way that I could come out with a judgment without a thorough investigation."

Sher's clinical records on his patients included much of the data that Tricta had analyzed. After his call to Yip, he went over the numbers in the records and rechecked the statistical calculations in the abstract he'd put his name on. He found no errors. Then he pulled out his hematology journals and found the collection of abstracts that had been presented at ASH that December. When he went through Olivieri's abstract on liver scarring, he thought her calculations seemed wrong. He couldn't reproduce the values she'd published. He wasn't sure what to do about that, and filed it away.

Olivieri wrote him again in mid-May, intent on enforcing her deadlines. "Please indicate if you will be replying to this letter." Two days later, she wrote the hospital administration again, saying that Sher had received money from Apotex for consultation and that she believed he had committed plagiarism and fraud. She italicized the words *plagiarism* and *fraud* and once again attached the apology she wanted Sher to sign.

One of Olivieri's friends at the hospital begged her to fight it out with Sher "in the medical literature." Olivieri was planning to fight "in the literature" by publishing her findings, but she didn't intend to stop accusing Sher of misconduct. Baker decided to try to intervene.

The hospital chief shared a hematology clinic with Sher. Since Baker was often travelling, that meant Sher often covered for the chief and took care of his patients. As a result, they'd gotten to know one another. Baker called Sher into his office and proceeded to explain the ins and outs of a misconduct investigation, as he understood them. "You don't want to go that route," he said. "It'll take months. It'll escalate. It'll cost everything you have emotionally." Instead, Baker advised Sher to simply apologize. He'd drafted an apology already. Baker handed it to Sher. "Sign this," he said, explaining that Nancy Olivieri had said that if he did, she would drop her complaints.

Sher read Baker's apology, but he thought his department head was asking him to apologize for things he'd never done. "Michael, I don't know what to do," he said. "I'm going home. I'll talk to you tomorrow." Then he left the hospital, got in his car and drove up University Avenue. As the avenue heads north from downtown, its name changes to Avenue Road. A few blocks later, it makes a sharp right-hand turn to clear the way for the grassy fields of one of the city's best-known preparatory schools, Upper Canada College. As Sher rounded that bend, he felt as if he could see his choice illuminated before him. He told friends later that it was among the clearest moments of his life.

The next morning he entered Baker's office full of self-righteous indignation and tore the chief's paragraph of apology up in front of him. He said that if he signed that letter, everything he stood for would be wiped away. "I will not suspend my principles," he told his boss. "You want to hold a review process, I'm ready."

But Baker wasn't giving up so fast. He told Sher, "We'll give you a letter." Again, he had it ready and handed it to Sher. "We hold you in the highest regard for your academic and scientific integrity," it read. Baker's plan was for Sher to sign the apology he'd drafted and gotten Nancy Olivieri to approve. Then Michael Baker and other hospital administrators would sign a letter about Sher. "Nancy wanted Graham Sher to . . . put his name to [what Sher considered to be] a falsehood," said a doctor who spoke with Sher at the time. "And Baker and [others] were asking him to do that."

Sher tried to defend his reputation. He wrote Olivieri accusing her of "outrageous and defamatory statements." And he wrote the hospital administration saying that he hadn't committed plagiarism or fraud. He acknowledged that he'd consulted to Apotex for a one-year period, but protested Olivieri's suggestion that the consultancy formed the basis of his disagreement with her about L1. "If Dr. Olivieri wishes to debate a scientific issue, that is in order," he wrote. "To insinuate that my opinions may be 'bought' is not."

Sher had also returned to Olivieri's abstract on the patients in the L1 trials, the one she'd presented at ASH. He'd taken the time to figure out what was bothering him about her calculations, and he outlined one of the problems with the abstract in a letter to Keating. According to Olivieri, six of the patients on L1 had a rise in the level of iron in their livers. But when Sher did the math, it didn't come out that way. He thought she'd presented findings as statistically significant when they weren't. He wrote Keating, "The claim of this statistically significant rise in hepatic iron is erroneous." Then he listed the specific figures that he thought proved Olivieri had made an error in her calculations.

Statistical errors are the sort of thing that can happen if a scientist is rushed or sloppy. They can make a meaningless finding look as if it means something, and they can lead to a published paper—or abstract—being withdrawn. There have been many instances of this. One was at Boston's Children's Hospital in the early 1990s. Cancer researcher Judah Folkman published a paper in the *New England Journal of Medicine*. After it appeared, other scientists at Children's Hospital claimed that it contained faulty statistics and multiple errors. The charges went to the hospital's physician-in-chief, who appointed a committee to investigate. Some of the charges were substantiated, and Folkman submitted corrections to the journal. Children's physician-in-chief at the time was Harvard hematologist David Nathan.

In Toronto, Sher made his charges about Olivieri's abstract in his letter to the hospital's head hematologist and copied the letter to the physician-in-chief, but Baker and Keating didn't appoint a committee to look into the abstract he'd criticized. The university had a system to deal with claims of scientific misconduct, beginning at Cecil Yip's office and ending with a judgment issued by a three-person committee. But it was different at the teaching hospitals, each of which functioned as an autonomous unit with its own policies and procedures. At the Toronto General, Sher's letter claiming that Olivieri had made serious statistical errors didn't produce a response.

Deena Weinstein, a sociologist at De Paul University in Chicago who has studied scientific misconduct, has said that "persons in positions of authority will not consider condemning a researcher who pulls in a lot of grants," preferring instead to "just let him do his own thing and not make any trouble." In the case of Olivieri, Baker and his fellow administrators at the General didn't follow up on Sher's charges against her, and later it was as if Sher had never written to anyone about it in the first place. Sher had other decisions to make, though. He was being recruited to become the medical and scientific head of the Canadian Blood Services, the Ottawa-based organization that oversees all blood donations in Canada. It would mean leaving the university, but it would be a substantial promotion.

Olivieri was determined to pursue her charges against him. She took them higher up the chain of command at the U of T, to the university-wide chair of medicine, and that office initiated a formal investigation by a misconduct committee. Martin Friedland, who had been dean of the law school for most of the 1970s, was the committee's head; the other two members were a psychiatrist who had served as head of a hospital research ethics board for several years and a clinical trials expert based at the medical school. The professors met twice in July 1997 to review the material that Sher and Olivieri provided. They asked Olivieri for more information, such as the original protocols for the L1 trials, the Apotex contract to sponsor the trials and her consulting contracts with Apotex, and they met with Gideon Koren and Michael Baker. Then, in late August, they interviewed Olivieri.

She told the committee that there was no debate about L1, writing Friedland, "There is no substantive argument to support the effectiveness of [L1] . . . Every center investigating [L1] would now support this statement, with the exception of Dr. Sher and his colleagues." Once again, she was ignoring the debates she'd been part of at scientific meetings in 1996 and 1997. But the misconduct committee didn't accept her assertions, and she said later that they made her feel as if she was the one under investigation. She also wrote Yip to complain. She asked that the committee meet with several other experts, including David Nathan, and she said she wanted to meet with them again when they were done with the additional meetings she'd advised.

The misconduct committee didn't accept Olivieri's advice to invite Nathan up. They met with Sher and consulted various articles and guidelines about the authorship of scientific articles. Then, in a long and detailed report, they issued their decision: Sher's work on Tricta's abstract for Malta met the definition of authorship, they said. He should have made sure Olivieri had a copy of his abstract

"to comment on before it was finalized," but he was innocent of plagiarism or any other sort of misconduct.

The committee described Olivieri as a scientist embroiled in "a
long-standing and often hostile scientific dispute." They also mentioned Sher's transfer out of the Toronto General's thalassemia program to the blood bank, writing that leaving thalassemia "was not
initially Dr. Sher's wish." They were especially disturbed by their
discovery that a number of the scientific papers Sher had in preparation were left incomplete as a result of "the conflict with Dr.
Olivieri."

Friedland phoned Arnie Aberman to let him know their decision. It was late at night, but the dean called Graham Sher at home,
where he was looking after his newborn while his wife slept. When
he heard the dean's voice on the other end of the line, he put the
infant down in its crib and went into the next room. Then he listened to Aberman tell him he'd been exonerated. He was so
relieved that he broke down in tears.

Olivieri also got a call that night. The next day she wrote Yip to
ask if she could appeal the committee's decision, but she couldn't.
Only those charged with misconduct could appeal.

By this point, Cecil Yip had figured out why she'd misinterpreted what he'd said and told Sher that he'd been charged with
misconduct before any investigation had taken place. Yip said it
had to do with the passions that drove "this affair, this whole 'Nancy
affair.'" He'd talked to others at the university about it. "The passion
in it is beyond understanding," he said.

Unable to appeal the committee's ruling, Olivieri wrote
Buchwald, the new head of the Research Institute at Sick Kids, to
complain about Sher's actions. She also sought out her occasional
mentor Bob Phillips for advice. After losing his bid for the research
chief's job to Buchwald, Phillips had left Sick Kids and was now
medical director of the National Cancer Institute of Canada. Olivieri

visited him there, and when Phillips promised to do what he could to help, she sent him a copy of the confidential report prepared by Friedland's committee. That was a breach of the university's rules for confidential misconduct proceedings, and the dean of the medical school criticized her for that sort of breach later.

Phillips had never met Graham Sher, but after speaking to Nancy Olivieri and reading the misconduct committee's report, he thought he understood what had happened. In the fall of 1997, he wrote a long letter to Buchwald, O'Brodovich and Strofolino at Sick Kids and Aberman at the medical school, praising Olivieri, castigating them for not supporting her in her fight with Apotex, and listing his complaints about the misconduct investigation. "Sher was not involved in the study; he is a young investigator who is a former fellow of Nancy's and who has yet to establish a research reputation," he wrote in his letter. He suggested that Koren and Sher be required to apologize publicly to Nancy for publishing their abstract without her participation. Sher didn't. Within the next few months he moved to Ottawa and put his arguments with Nancy Olivieri behind him.

THE MAKING OF A WHISTLEBLOWER

After the 1996 ASH meeting in Florida, hemotologists were often confused about what exactly happened in the L1 trials at the Hospital for Sick Children. Here's what we know. Nancy Olivieri had learned that L1 was ineffective for some of her patients by 1994. While she tried to figure it out, she delayed telling Apotex about it. Her relationship with the company was tense at that point. She wanted greater resources, but Apotex wanted to limit its outlay. The company was accusing her of violating her research protocols, and she'd begun to withhold data. The loss of data upped the ante for the company, and its vice-president, Michael Spino, threatened to stop the study.

In 1995, Olivieri started taking some patients off L1. Then she told Apotex the drug wasn't working the way she had expected it to. Spino asked to see the raw data, and when she failed to provide it, he again threatened to stop the study. Eventually the company got the data and reviewed them, but Spino said Apotex disagreed with her interpretation. As the stand-off continued, Olivieri took her concerns to the hospital's Research Ethics Board. In March 1996, she filed a formal report with the company and the ethics board that proposed warning the patients taking L1 that the drug didn't work in most cases.

Her relationship with the company continued to deteriorate. Apotex was her major funding source, and she was asking the company to support a new five-year study because of the new problem she'd identified, but Apotex didn't write her a new research contract. Instead, in April 1996, the company began allowing her existing contracts to expire. That same month, the ethics board responded to her report on L1 by directing her to revise the study consent forms. She sent the revised forms to the ethics board and the company in May. Within a few days, Apotex cancelled her trials, terminated her contracts and her consulting agreement, and threatened to sue her if she spoke about her findings.

Olivieri tried to have the trials reinstated. The dean mediated, and Apotex agreed to provide the drug to patients who needed it, but it wouldn't do more. The company invited an independent panel of experts to review Olivieri's data; the panel found that her data didn't support her claims. But she was tightly linked to powerful figures in the field who disagreed with the panel and took her claims seriously, including David Nathan, who had long been skeptical of L1's value, and David Weatherall, whose opinion was highly regarded among thalassemia researchers. Meanwhile, the company's lawyers frightened Olivieri with threatening letters.

In the fall of 1996, upset by the company's legal threats and professionally hounded by its assessment of her research by independent experts, Olivieri discovered an article showing that a drug in the same family as L1 was ineffective for the treatment of iron overload and toxic to the liver in animal experiments. She hunted for a similar toxic effect in patients, found it, completed her preliminary investigations quickly—in time to present her conclusions in December— and resolved, based on the new toxicity she'd discovered, that the drug was too dangerous for use. She began telling colleagues that L1 was poisonous and could cause liver scarring, voicing her claims at ASH and other meetings and publishing them in *Blood*.

Olivieri was among the most respected figures in her small scientific field of research on drug treatment for thalassemia and sickle cell disease. Her stature in the field gave her influence at home and abroad. When her colleague Graham Sher argued with her that liver scarring in her patients could be due to something other than L1, she said he was biased in the company's favour and stopped speaking to him. She was given his job toward the end of 1996. In 1997 she began telling patients that the drug was dangerous. The company, with its deep pockets and extensive legal resources, objected to Olivieri's presentations and forced her to withdraw an abstract.

Her former collaborators who disagreed with her—Sher and Koren—presented an alternative view of the drug in an abstract, which the company co-authored. No one told Olivieri about the abstract—she heard about it through the grapevine—and since she had gathered the data, she argued that the authors were plagiarizing her work. They presented anyway. Back in Toronto, she accused Sher, but not Koren, of scientific misconduct because of the presentation. When a university committee cleared Sher of the charges, she protested the committee's findings.

That brings us up to the fall of 1997. Olivieri's colleagues abroad generally understood that things were simple: first she discovered that L1 was toxic; next Apotex tried to muzzle her because it didn't want anyone to know. It was how Olivieri told the story. "We found what we believe to be very damning evidence of liver toxicity," she once told reporters. "As soon as those concerns looked like they were going to be official, the company prematurely abruptly stopped the trial and then threatened me with legal action."

Since that's what she said, it's what her colleagues and supporters believed. David Nathan and David Weatherall later wrote in the *New England Journal of Medicine* that Olivieri had discovered L1 was toxic to the liver and that that was what had led the company to cancel her study. They didn't realize that Apotex had stopped Olivieri's trials when she was worried that the drug was ineffective, months before she ever spoke about the drug causing an increase in liver scarring. When I interviewed George Dover, pediatrics chair at Johns Hopkins University, he said the company had cut Olivieri out of its research program because she claimed L1 was toxic. Yale hematologist Howard Pearson was equally certain of it, telling me that Olivieri had stopped studying L1 because she'd discovered the drug was toxic. "No matter what, given what she was seeing, you'd have to stop the study," he said. "She not only stopped it, but announced it at a public meeting and published a paper."

The revised timeline quickly acquired a ring of truth for Olivieri and her fellow hematologists. It wasn't what had happened, but it was less convoluted and more compelling. In the new version of the story, the company's transgressions were even more heinous than they had been in the earlier version, while Olivieri's actions were simple and heroic. She discovered that a drug was dangerous; the company threatened her to keep her quiet, so she became a whistleblower, determined to protect her patients.

As this idea of the Olivieri affair persisted, it gathered the power of myth. Apotex was the greedy Goliath threatening a powerless David who had right—but not might—on her side. She was a whistleblower from academia facing down Big Pharma; she'd had the guts and courage to fight back when a wealthy company kept threatening her.

A reporter for Canada's *Medical Post*—a controlled-circulation newspaper that goes primarily to physicians—had attended ASH that year, and in January 1997 the paper ran a story on the L1 controversy. Olivieri "declined comment" for the article, but her lawyer confirmed the basic facts of the story for the paper. Then a long-time medical journalist picked up the story for the *Toronto Star*. The take-home message in both papers was the same: a physician from the Hospital for Sick Children was blowing the whistle on Apotex, Canada's largest drug firm.

Olivieri began getting calls from TV and radio shows in Toronto. Before she returned the calls, she checked with her lawyers. They'd been advising all along that disclosure of confidential information to other scientists via peer-reviewed presentations and publications was easier for them to justify than talking to the press. As she expected, they advised her not to give interviews. And she had her own reasons to steer clear of reporters: the submission she was preparing for the *New England Journal of Medicine*.

One of the rules at top-ranked medical journals is that if the contents of an article have already appeared in print, even in the lay press, the journal won't publish it. If Olivieri talked to a reporter, it could jeopardize the chances of her L1 data appearing in the *New England Journal of Medicine*. But as a recognized whistleblower, she was going to make it into a major journal a lot sooner than she expected.

After ASH, Nancy Olivieri got a call from Drummond Rennie, a senior editor at the *Journal of the American Medical Association* (*JAMA*) and a U.S. authority on scientific misconduct. She was careful to say that she couldn't tell him anything on the record, but Rennie didn't need to quote her. He listened, and she poured out her story, detailing all that had happened to her since she first told Spino that L1 wasn't working the way she expected it to.

Rennie grew intensely worried for her. She was preoccupied with the intricacies of everything she'd lived through in the past year, yet she seemed naive about the gravity of her situation. He knew that she could lose everything—her office, her lab, her career, her professional reputation, her livelihood—and she didn't seem to realize that.

For Rennie, the tale of the L1 clinical trials bore a striking resemblance to events he was intimately involved with in the United States. As a member of the federal Commission on Research Integrity during 1994 and 1995, he'd heard extensive testimony from scientists across the country who had become whistleblowers. Each had suffered by speaking out about research violations. From their sorry tales of ruined careers, Rennie had determined that the best protection a whistleblower has is the light of day. He planned to spotlight what was happening to Olivieri by writing about her in *JAMA*, but he thought it wouldn't be enough.

A large, tall man with thick white hair, Rennie had trained at Oxford as a physician and scientist before immigrating to the U.S. in the 1970s. His first contact with a whistleblowing scientist was in 1979. The issue caught him then and he never let it go. Nearly two decades later, a 1998 analysis by the U.S. Office of Research Integrity would conclude that scientists who blow the whistle on scientific misconduct are primarily males and nearly half hold senior appointments at their institutions. But that didn't match Rennie's personal experience. "It's very frequently young women who feel that they're stuck in a corner," he told me. "It's unjust, and they've just got to cry out."

When he heard from that first whistleblower, he was an editor at the *New England Journal of Medicine*. She was a researcher at the NIH, and she had sent the journal an article on anorexia. The journal had sent it on to a doctor at Yale University for peer review. At Yale, her article on anorexia was copied, material was added and the authors were changed to two professors at the university. Then it was submitted to the *American Journal of Medicine,* a lower-ranked journal. The woman found out she'd been plagiarized when the *American Journal of Medicine* asked her to act as a peer reviewer for the article from Yale.

In the young woman's case, the most basic rules of scientific peer review had been broken. The reviewers at Yale, like all peer reviewers, were obliged to guard the secrecy of her paper. But they'd violated the system in the worst way, using the anonymity of peer review as a shield to hide them while they stole her work. She sent Rennie all of the documents that proved her case. He was shocked by what had happened but found what followed its revelation even more disturbing.

The anorexia researcher, Helena Wachslicht-Rodbard, complained to Yale and told her superiors at the NIH what had happened, but the paper containing the plagiarized material was published anyway, in a different journal. Finally, the doctors who had plagiarized her work, Vijay Soman and Philip Felig, were investigated. Soman was a junior faculty member still at the beginning of his career. Two outside audits of his work showed that not only had he plagiarized in his work, he had also fabricated data and even invented patients. An immigrant from India who had been in the U.S. for many years, he resigned and returned to India. Felig, Soman's mentor at Yale, had recently left for New York to be chief physician at the major teaching hospital affiliated with Columbia University. When the plagiarism charges surfaced, he left Columbia under pressure but was soon reappointed at Yale; though Soman implied that Felig had pressured him to produce results, university officials said the senior scientist wasn't a party to his junior colleague's conduct. He retracted the papers he'd co-authored with Soman that contained fabricated data, and he testified in Congress about how difficult it was to detect outright fraud in science. A few years later, he became CEO of Sandoz, at that time one of the world's largest drug companies. Wachslicht-Rodbard, on the other hand, became disillusioned with science and gave up doing research.

Close friends of Rennie's say he's a sensitive man who takes other people's losses personally. He hated what had happened to Wachslicht-Rodbard. Over the course of the next decade, as he moved from the *New England Journal of Medicine* to *JAMA* and became active in the leading organizations of medical editors, he dedicated himself to whistleblowers in science, primarily scientists who accused their colleagues of research misconduct. "I've seen scores and scores of these fights," he told me. Too many times, he felt, the essential elements of the 1979 case were repeated. The career of a young scientist who complained was left in tatters while senior figures who committed the wrong—or allowed it to happen—walked away unharmed.

His experience on the Commission on Research Integrity (also known as the Ryan Commission for its chair, Kenneth Ryan) didn't leave him optimistic. Rennie recalled "one quite dreadful afternoon" when he and his colleagues on the commission were holed up in a hotel room with five young women, "all of whom were right, all of whom had been shown to have correct accusations and all of whom had had their lives ruined by this." In *JAMA*, he wrote of whistleblowers who had been "abused for their courage and persistence." The Ryan Commission viewed whistleblowers as the underdogs of science, in vital need of assistance, and its report, issued in November 1995, demanded that universities protect them and grant them a bill of rights. It was a controversial idea.

As a rationale, the commission listed the appalling experiences of retaliation that scientists who became whistleblowers described—threats, censorship, physical isolation, expulsion from their labs or institutions, even physical injury. To those who said whistleblowers sometimes acted out for the wrong reasons, the commission essentially replied that motivations were irrelevant: the scientific community had the responsibility to establish the facts of any given case and protect the whistleblower in the process. Whistleblowers also had responsibilities, the commission said—scientists who blew the whistle were obliged to avoid false statements, to respect the confidentiality of sensitive information, and to act within legitimate institutional channels—but if that was the commission's olive branch to the organized scientific community, it was roundly rejected.

Scientists' professional associations—including the National Academy of Sciences—argued that there was another face to the whistleblower coin. Whistleblowers couldn't always be trusted to get it right. Sometimes the scientists they accused of misconduct had done no wrong, yet whistleblowers would violate a scientist's confidentiality or lie about a scientist. The scientists' organizations didn't even want to label them whistleblowers. They called them "accusers" and "allegators." In Washington, the Federation of American Societies for Experimental Biology, a U.S. coalition of fifty professional societies representing biomedical and bioscience researchers, criticized the Ryan Commission's report, pointing out that it had no provisions directed at unlawful "whistleblower" behaviour. The federation specifically mentioned one form of unlawful behaviour that would be familiar to Graham Sher: violations of confidentiality duties in misconduct proceedings. American medical schools and research universities turned down the idea of a whistleblowers' bill of rights.

The Ryan Commission's critics may have been influenced by the major U.S. science scandal of the 1980s and '90s—the case involving Nobel laureate David Baltimore that was triggered by a whistleblower's accusations. A young woman named Margot O'Toole, who had once worked with an immunologist who happened to collaborate with Baltimore, blew the whistle on the immunologist, believing she had fabricated data in a journal article co-authored with Baltimore. The accused scientist, Thereza Imanishi-Kari of Tufts University, spent nearly a decade fighting the allegations. Tufts University, MIT (where Baltimore had his lab), the U.S. Congress and the NIH all investigated the charges. The Secret Service even got involved in ascertaining whether dates had been altered in Imanishi-Kari's laboratory notebooks. O'Toole was a believable junior scientist, convinced that her former supervisor had committed fraud, but part of the reason her concerns got so much attention was their timing.

A series of reports of flagrant misconduct in science had shocked the American public and left U.S. lawmakers worrying that scientists who made things up and published them were common. Congressional committees held multiple hearings on the issue during the 1980s and early '90s. Meanwhile, the NIH established an office of "scientific integrity" that began receiving reports of misconduct, and, separately, two NIH scientists became self-appointed fraud-busters. The two fraud-busters heard about O'Toole's allegations and persuaded her to take them to Washington, where she was hailed as a courageous martyr. It sounded as if she'd paid a huge price—her position in her lab wasn't renewed, and according to one congressman, she lost her house as a result of blowing the whistle.

In 1994, eight years after the initial charges, Imanishi-Kari was found guilty of fabrication by the NIH and suspended from her university. Baltimore had become president of Rockefeller University in New York City, one of the premiere research institutions in the U.S.; he resigned after the guilty verdict. But the two scientists appealed the decision. In 1996, the findings were overturned and both were exonerated when the appeals board ruled that Imanishi-Kari hadn't lied about her findings. To some observers it looked as if Imanishi-Kari and Baltimore had been falsely accused; to others it seemed that O'Toole was justified in blowing the whistle but that the system for investigating her charges was broken.

Drummond Rennie had already been creating a sort of haven for whistleblowers in his office in downtown San Francisco. (Though *JAMA* is based at the American Medical Association offices in Chicago, Rennie held the title of west coast editor and worked out of the Bay Area.) In the winter of 1995, *JAMA* had received a call from a forty-something pharmacy professor at the University of California in San Francisco named Betty Dong. She didn't intend to blow a whistle; she was calling the journal to withdraw a paper she had submitted. Rennie phoned her back. "It's been accepted," he told her, "and it's already slated for publication." But Dong insisted she had to withdraw it because of her contract with a drug company, Knoll Pharmaceutical of New Jersey. Knoll didn't want her study published, and a confidentiality clause in her contract gave it the right to block publication.

Dong was primarily a clinician and teacher. Her work centred on helping patients untangle complicated drug regimens and on teaching medical residents about drugs. She knew someone at Knoll, and he'd asked her to lead a project comparing Synthroid, the popular thyroid replacement drug made by Knoll and used by millions of North Americans, to its generic counterparts. The company's expectation—and Dong's—was that their product would prove more effective, but it didn't turn out that way. Dong and her collaborators found that the brand-name product and its generic competitors were equivalent. Since all the others were cheaper, doctors—or insurance companies—might use the lower-cost alternatives instead of Synthroid if they heard about her results.

After Dong reported her findings to the company, officials there started complaining to her university that there were problems with her research. The company hired outside consultants, who lobbed further complaints. The University of California responded by investigating—a process that took over two years. Finally, various committees at the university concluded that the company's complaints were trivial. Around that time, the company accused her of giving confidential data away to its competitors and hired a private detective agency to prove it. Detectives parked near Dong's house and began going through her garbage. Lawyers for the company met with her and left her feeling intimidated and scared.

Dong's department chairman at the school of pharmacy, a renowned pharmacist named Les Benet, was outraged. Benet had been asked by the university to review Dong's study, and had determined that the company's criticisms of it were "self-serving." He encouraged Dong to complete her paper, which she did, and she submitted it to *JAMA*. The company threatened to sue if she published, but by this time she had a lot of support from Benet and others at the university and she decided she'd had enough of the company's threats. She didn't care if she was sued; she would take her chances in court. The company's lead scientist made further threats, meeting with one of her co-authors to let him know casually that if they lost their case each author could owe the company for lost revenues. The makers of Synthroid stood to lose market share because of the study, and Dong and the others could be on the hook for millions.

Dong's co-authors included several post-doctoral fellows who barely had faculty appointments. She couldn't bear to jeopardize their careers. They'd done the work; she couldn't take their names off the article, and she couldn't publish without exposing them to the risk of a lawsuit. Benet thought the university would protect her and her co-authors because of their right to publish. But after the university's lawyers reviewed her contract, they concluded that in signing it, she'd given away her right to publish. This was why she was phoning Rennie to withdraw the paper.

Despite Rennie's familiarity with whistleblowers, he was taken aback by her situation. Over the next few months, he teamed up with Benet and they urged the university's legal counsel to reconsider, but the counsel feared the institution would be sued for breach of contract if Dong published. Benet and Rennie then became whistleblowers themselves, contacting a biotechnology reporter at the *Wall Street Journal* and secretly giving him several boxes of papers documenting how the company kept the study covered up. Benet and Rennie both agreed to interviews; Dong herself was too worried to speak more than briefly with a reporter. The report of the company's fight to keep Dong's study out of print appeared on the *Wall Street Journal*'s front page in April 1996 and was soon retold by medical and science journals around the world, but the company still refused to allow the study to be published.

The university chancellor negotiated up front with Knoll's president and with Louis Sullivan, a physician who was a former U.S. Secretary of Health and Human Services and was on the company's board, while Benet went through a back door, contacting former colleagues who were now at the FDA to share details of the results the company was suppressing.

In early 1997, Knoll Pharmaceutical finally capitulated on Betty Dong's paper. The paper would appear in *JAMA* in April with an editorial by Rennie to explain the circumstances of the publication. Rennie wanted to mention Olivieri's situation to illustrate his point that Dong's wasn't an isolated case. He wrote in *JAMA* that Olivieri, too, had signed a confidentiality agreement but had "decided she had to break confidentiality by reporting her results at a meeting." He added, "Because she now feels that she risks litigation for having made her presentation, she would not, on the advice of her attorney, speak with me."

There it was, in one of the world's leading medical journals. Nancy Olivieri, a courageous doctor in Toronto, had followed her conscience as a scientist and a doctor and blown the whistle on an experimental drug. Now she couldn't speak to an editor at *JAMA* because the drug's manufacturer might sue her if she did.

Two months after Rennie's editorial appeared, in June 1997, Nancy Olivieri sat with about one hundred others in a conference room at the Royal Sonesta Hotel in Cambridge, Massachusetts, listening to scientific papers on the latest treatments for thalassemia and waiting for her turn to approach the podium. The occasion was the 1997 symposium of the Cooley's Anemia Foundation, a leading organization for thalassemia research named for the Detroit pediatrician who first described the disease.

Back home in Toronto, Olivieri was arguing with her supervisors at Sick Kids about their plans for her clinics, explaining to her bosses at the Toronto General that Graham Sher had committed misconduct and coping with patients at both hospitals who rejected her advice to go off L1. She was even in a crisis with her lawyers, because the malpractice association felt she was taking advantage of them. An association officer wrote her that her lawyers were "prepared to offer advice and assistance," not "moment-by-moment, day-by-day screening and support." The CMPA was threatening to stop paying her legal bills.

Despite this, Olivieri looked at ease at the Sonesta. She was one of the organizers for the conference and was surrounded by friends. David Nathan was on the organizing committee with her, Gary Brittenham was sitting nearby, and her dear friend David Weatherall had given the keynote address. Olivieri and Weatherall had recently completed their first article together, due out in August in the *Lancet*, and they'd agreed to collaborate on another project, tracking thalassemia patients at a rural Sri Lankan hospital. In his keynote, Weatherall had praised some of her research. Howard Pearson, Yale's senior pediatric hematologist, wanted to know if she would contribute a chapter to a textbook he was editing. When she said she was too wrapped up in "all this L1 business," he became concerned and asked to hear more. George Dover of Johns Hopkins also let her know he was worried. He'd worked with Olivieri on butyrate and other projects; now he pressed her to consider a job in his department in Baltimore. And Elliott Vichinsky, her old friend and collaborator who ran the thalassemia and sickle cell program at Oakland Children's Hospital in California's Bay Area, was urging her to move there and work with him. He offered to create a position that suited her skills and interests, and told her that three other doctors in San Francisco and Berkeley were also interested in recruiting her to the area. Sick Kids scientist John Dick was another familiar face in the room. They'd collaborated once, and she'd talked to him briefly about her dealings with Apotex.

Olivieri kept her distance from some of the other people who were there. The symposium chairman was Alan Cohen, her former friend and collaborator from Philadelphia. He was still working with Apotex, and things between them remained awkward. Michael Spino was at the meeting, along with Fernando Tricta. And three of her patients were there from Toronto, including Josie. Olivieri was officially their doctor now, but in Toronto she rarely spoke to them, and in Cambridge she made no eye contact. Once Josie and the others spotted Olivieri and Brittenham in a corridor. "Basically, inevitably, we were going to cross paths," Josie remembered. "We just said, 'Oh my, there she is,' so the three of us—very clearly— we all looked at them as they walked past us—they were walking, totally not making eye contact with us, and sort of looking more at the ceiling than even ahead of them."

The session was nearly over when Olivieri's name was announced. She walked to the microphone quickly and began going through her slides. Soon she was detailing the problems with L1. The most recent analysis of the eighteen patients in her long-term trial of the drug showed that six of them had iron levels that were too high. As a result, those patients were in danger, at increased risk for heart disease and early death. She said there were other inter-pretations of the data, sounding annoyed as she said it. Listening in the audience, John Dick had the feeling that she'd been told by a lawyer to add that line. Then she described the gerbil study of CP-94, mentioned her findings of liver scarring in patients on L1 and said the pill was toxic to the liver and possibly to the heart as well. She finished and waited for questions.

But before people could raise their hands, another scientist announced, "Well, this research is quite contentious, so we've allowed some people from Apotex to present their side of it." Suddenly, Tricta was up at the podium presenting the company's results, while Spino stood at the overhead projector, flipping hand-drawn transparencies that offered numbers and explanations. "It was sort of like, 'This is hot off the press,'" John Dick said later.

The company's results were from their toxicity study in Philadelphia and Italy, the one Olivieri and Brittenham had pushed Spino to undertake. According to Tricta, nearly two hundred patients in the study took L1 for one year. In general, the patients did well. Tricta concluded that the drug was safe in the short run. When he was through, another man, who was introduced as a pathologist and liver expert from Italy, said the company had asked him to examine the entire series of biopsy specimens from Olivieri's patients on L1 and he had found no evidence of liver toxicity. Next, Elias Schwartz spoke. A former head hematologist at the Children's Hospital of Philadelphia, Schwartz had served on the independent panel that reviewed Olivieri's data for Apotex. Now, as chair of this session of the conference, he offered his audience the independent panel's conclusions: L1 was effective and remained effective over the long term.

It was clear from the look on her face that Olivieri was unprepared for what had happened. Neither Tricta nor the liver expert was listed on the program. Three different people had spoken on behalf of Apotex or L1, and all of them were unscheduled presenters who'd been added at the last minute. Their talks completely undercut everything Nancy Olivieri had said. She had described a small study at a single centre in Canada that involved eighteen patients, while Tricta presented a multi-centre trial in the U.S. and Europe with a sample size more than ten times that. Then the liver pathologist contradicted her claims about scarring and the session chair disputed her findings of ineffectiveness. Her colleagues were as shocked as she was.

Pearson, the Yale hematologist, said that he'd seen cruelty and dishonesty in medicine over the course of his career, but he'd never seen anything like this. The company had bullied Nancy Olivieri in full view of other scientists. "It was what I viewed as essentially the destruction of a young woman," he said.

David Nathan was incensed, and not just because he cared for Olivieri. He thought the company and its hired scientists were spreading false information. He'd always been worried about L1, and in May 1997, amid Olivieri's claims that L1 didn't always work and was toxic to the liver, he wrote the FDA for a second time. "The toxicity is serious," he warned in an e-mail to an acquaintance at the agency.

Now, one month later, Nathan approached the microphone. First he told the audience about Nancy Olivieri's caution and care in her studies of L1. Next he gave them his sense of where things stood. "We don't know who's right or who's wrong here, but just given the concerns that have been raised here, if you asked me should I give this drug to my patients I'd say, 'No way.'"

If they asked, he could say more than that. Nathan was in close contact with Novartis—the pharmaceutical giant that had swallowed Ciba-Geigy—and he knew the company was looking at an oral replacement for Desferal. After testing more than seven hundred compounds, they'd found one called ICL670 that they thought could work. They were testing it in primates, and the initial reports were quite positive. Nathan hoped that it would work out, and that if it didn't, Novartis would go back to the drawing board and find something else that would prove safer and more effective than L1.

Weatherall followed Nathan with a ringing endorsement of Olivieri's research and a casual dismissal of the Italian pathologist's critique. "Look, you know, a single pathologist reading slides can come up with all kinds of different opinions," he remarked to the crowd. He said he'd reviewed the independent panel's report and had found it flawed. Both of thalassemia's leading lights were emphatic in their support for Olivieri, as was Gary Brittenham when he stood to speak. Like Nathan, Brittenham was no longer waiting to see what Apotex turned up on L1. He'd moved on to a different iron-removal drug called HBED and was already collaborating with scientists at the University of Florida to test it in animals.

Afterwards, John Dick hung around, waiting for a chance to talk to Olivieri. In nearly two decades as a scientist, he hadn't seen anything like this play out at a scientific meeting. "It was a very aggressive, very polarized discussion," he said later. Presentations submitted to national and international science symposia are supposed to go through the same sort of competitive peer review process as papers sent to journals. Scientists write abstracts of what they intend to say and send them in for review by a given deadline. Some abstracts are accepted as talks from the podium, others are relegated to poster sessions and still others are rejected. From what Dick was hearing whispered around him, the talks that followed Olivieri's hadn't been submitted as abstracts at all.

He joined a group surrounding Nathan and Weatherall, who were both saying that there were principles at stake. Academic freedom was one: academic scientists were supposed to be free to publish and disseminate their research findings without being harassed. Protection of research subjects was another. According to Nathan and Weatherall, Apotex didn't want Olivieri's patients to know that the experimental drug she was testing had risks. That flew in the face of established codes of research ethics.

Other people were speaking of Nancy Olivieri's hospital. They'd heard that Sick Kids hadn't protected her from the company. John Dick had always thought of himself as one of Sick Kids' "golden boys," because he'd won so many awards and accolades during his time there. He loved his job at the Research Institute. Yet the hematologists who'd convened in Cambridge seemed to view the hospital as an antiquated bastion compared to their own institutions and thought Sick Kids had treated Olivieri badly. Hearing them, Dick felt ashamed. He knew the hospital's leadership was controversial:

the controversy had erupted into a crisis at the Research Institute in the spring of 1995, when the chief scientist, Jim Friesen, suddenly quit. Sick Kids scientists had been angry about losing Friesen and they'd blamed Michael Strofolino, their cost-cutting CEO. Dick was generally ensconced in his lab, though, and was unaware of the degree of dissatisfaction with the CEO on the hospital's wards.

Strofolino, an American from Brooklyn, was a former player in the National Football League who wore a Superbowl ring from his time with the L.A. Rams. He'd come to Canada in his twenties as a linebacker for the Hamilton Tiger-Cats, but after two years and a career-ending ankle injury, he'd gone to school for accounting. Later he moved from a large accounting firm to the hospital supply industry, and in the late 1980s he switched from the supply industry to Sick Kids. Years later he told the *Toronto Star,* "I came to Sick Kids in 1987 as vice-president, finance. I was going to stay for 10 or 11 minutes. What happened is David Martin, my predecessor, allowed me to do more things." Strofolino had a "hearty laugh" about that with the *Star* reporter, but around the hospital it was no laughing matter.

Martin was focused on his legacy to the hospital—the hospital's $230 million expansion, known as the "new Sick Kids," with its brand-new wards and lavish glass-walled atrium. Strofolino was attuned to the bottom line. His promotion to chief operating officer came in 1990. Between 1991 and 1993, the hospital cut 225 jobs. Though the "new" hospital opened in early 1993 to great acclaim, the province was holding the hospital's funding steady. So in addition to the layoffs, there were wage freezes and program cuts. As the cuts continued through 1994, physicians and nurses grew bitter.

"CEOs go and they cut jobs and they fire people and the bottom line looks better," said one pediatrician later. "But you lose the heart of the people who work here. You lose the humanity of the place."

More nurses and technicians were let go, and physicians worried that the tradition of the hospital was going with them. "You get a spiral," explained a pediatrician. "The enthusiastic, capable young nurses leave; the work is overwhelming; it stops being a fun place to work."

The losses were "cataclysmic," said Mary Corey. "The doctors' lives were being altered horribly because programs that they had built up over years and years were pulled out from under them," she said. Doctors were even losing their income. Salaried by the province, Sick Kids pediatricians and surgeons went without a raise for three years. Then they were forced to accept a pay cut.

When Strofolino became president and CEO in 1994, the re-imbursement package he negotiated for himself was higher than that of any other hospital executive in the province. Sick Kids staff read about his pay in the papers (it was public knowledge under the new transparency laws regarding public officials' earnings) and felt like poor cousins. But board members thought he was worth it.

In the same year, Strofolino went from streamlining Sick Kids' clinical services to merging its research laboratories. Until that point, the Sick Kids Research Institute was "quite removed—as far as one could be" from the hospital, said professor of pediatrics Bob Haslam. Yet it was the golden jewel in the Sick Kids crown.

The institute was the wealthiest research institute in the coun-try, and it got its funding from the hospital's foundation, the largest foundation of its kind in Canada. Across the street, the acclaimed research operation at Mount Sinai operated on about $5 million per year; Sick Kids had a research budget of close to $30 million. As research chief from the late 1980s through the early '90s, Jim Friesen put the money toward hiring strong scientists and helping them outfit their labs. When Sick Kids scientists won a series of high-profile races—discovering a gene for Tay-Sachs in 1988, a cystic fibrosis gene in 1989 and a gene for Fanconi's anemia in 1991—Friesen got part of the credit.

Strofolino objected to the institute's independence, however. Research, he said, was only one priority among many. He told his group of administrators, "There's a fine line between being a leader of a discipline and being a member of the executive team. You need to take off your discipline hat." Initially, Friesen went along with that notion. But Strofolino's stance left the research chief feeling that he had "much less freedom," according to one doctor, and Friesen began threatening to resign.

Strofolino and Friesen butted heads for over a year. Their final crisis, in the spring of 1995, involved an American doctor who was a specialist in epilepsy. Strofolino was convinced that epilepsy was an area Sick Kids needed to build up. But when Friesen gave the American doctor's c.v. to his search and selection committee at the Research Institute, the committee recommended against hiring him. Friesen told Strofolino he wouldn't use the research budget for the hire. The pediatrics department could bring the epilepsy doctor in on the clinical side.

Strofolino, who had met the epilepsy specialist and liked him, wasn't willing to leave it there. He urged Friesen to give him a research appointment. "Pressure was put on Jim to say yes," said Haslam. Instead, Friesen quit. John Dick explained, "It's no accident that Jim left two years short of his mandate. Everyone knows that. That was a particular power struggle, and Strofolino won that."

To Strofolino, it was a fight between the old and the new. In the new, reorganized Sick Kids, the research budget was no longer Friesen's to control. Strofolino told a reporter that fall that he was trying to run the hospital "like a business"; to scientists at Sick Kids, the effects were frightening. "

The situation at Sick Kids wasn't unique in Toronto. As the thalassemia patients at Toronto General had learned, managers at the city's teaching hospitals control the dollars assigned to the hospitals by the province. That gives them considerable power, and they function with a high degree of autonomy and secrecy. At Sick Kids, with the institution's independence from the university under-scored by design, doctors who disagree with the administration have few options. When conflicts arise over promotions or programs, they can try to negotiate; if that fails, they can threaten to sue or leave.

"There are healthy cultures and unhealthy cultures, and [the Hospital for Sick Children] was at the edge of unhealthy," said a for-mer member of Strofolino's executive team. "There were aspects of it that one could even call a 'toxic culture.'" The executive described the hospital as "a very unforgiving organization," where "if you . . . tick someone off in senior leadership, you'll pay a price." A scientist described the culture of Sick Kids on Strofolino's watch as a "loyalty" culture: "There's no dissent."

In the weeks that followed the Cambridge meeting, John Dick signed on to Olivieri's cause—her fight with the company, the hospital and the university—and made it his own. He moved from barely knowing her to being consumed by her struggle. He was the first of four senior Sick Kids staff members to do so, none of whom had known Olivieri well to begin with. They hadn't worked under, over or alongside her for any substantial period, and they didn't know the history of L1. Nor were they all close friends with one another. Yet, one by one, as they began to speak with Olivieri and hear her story, they walked into the situation and let it take prece-dence over many other things in their lives.

Together, they became known as the Gang of Four. No one recalls who first used that label, but it stuck. China had its political Gang of Four, Microsoft had used the same label for the company's four major competitors, and Canadians used it to refer to their four leading banks. Now, at Sick Kids, Nancy Olivieri's most dedicated supporters attached it to themselves.

Dick's role was crucial because he was the first. Tall, blond and stocky, with a broad, furrowed forehead and John Lennon–style wire-rimmed glasses, John Dick was a man to whom morals mattered. Colleagues described him as "religious" and "very ethical." Raised in a small town on the prairies of Manitoba, he attended a one-room schoolhouse as a child. At his high school, most of the students never graduated. Dick made it to the local community college and became an X-ray technician before screwing up the courage to apply to the university in Winnipeg. Once there, he fell in love with biology and stayed for his doctorate. He left Manitoba to take a postdoc position in Toronto, and while still in his first few years out of graduate school, he became known in the fields of genetics and molecular biology, publishing in top journals, including *Science* and *Nature,* and winning acclaim for innovative animal models of cancer and leukemia. As his lab expanded, he worked closer to the cutting edge, developing cell lines that opened up new possibilities in immunology, and testing gene therapies in animals.

Dick had beaten the odds but was humble about it. He seemed grateful for the fundamental workings of academic science, where people were rewarded for making discoveries. In his area of molecular biology, benefits also accrued to those who were skilled in collaboration; his papers in the field often included as many as ten or twelve authors. The population-dense environment of his laboratory came naturally to Dick. As the youngest of six children, he told colleagues, he'd learned early to avoid conflict. What appealed to him was the process of building consensus.

The aggressive scene he'd witnessed in Cambridge wasn't part of his normal spectrum. As he listened to the discussion that followed, he began to feel that it was his moral duty to help Nancy Olivieri. He'd seen an injustice and had to speak up. "That's just the kind of responsibility we have as human beings," he told me later. So, as the room cleared out, he sat with Olivieri, listening closely to her description of everything that had been happening in Toronto.

Worried for her, Dick called Manuel Buchwald, the hospital's research chief, as soon as he got back to Toronto. Despite Strofolino's attempt to merge the Research Institute with the clinical hospital for hiring purposes, they were still quite separate domains. As Buchwald explained, "Clinical research was not really seen as the purview of the director of research." Yet he knew of the Olivieri-Apotex affair. In May 1996, when Apotex first stopped Olivieri's studies and she wrote her long letter to Haslam, she sent a copy to Buchwald. At the time, he'd been preparing to go to France on sabbatical. She hadn't come to see him and her line of accountability was through the medical side, so he'd taken no action. But Buchwald was interested in and attentive to what John Dick had to say.

Dick and Buchwald had had labs around the corner from one another for a long time. They admired one another's work and they'd collaborated together. As Dick relayed what he'd heard in Cambridge, Buchwald realized that the situation had festered while he'd been away. Though Olivieri wasn't under his authority, the predicament she was in with Apotex had to do with research. Buchwald said he would meet with her the next morning.

About two hours after their meeting, Dick got a call from Arnie Aberman. He was surprised at first, because he never talked to the dean and didn't really know him. Aberman told Dick he'd heard he was interested in the L1 trials. Then he offered his own position: "This is a scientific dispute, and I don't take sides in a scientific dispute." But Dick knew from what he'd seen in Cambridge that it was more than that. The average scientific dispute doesn't involve underhanded ploys by drug companies to shanghai open scientific meetings. Dick explained why he was worried, but the dean's call made him suspicious. He concluded that by bringing up Olivieri, he "was touching a very sensitive nerve" at the hospital and the university.

Dick spent more time listening to Olivieri and looking over documents she provided, a process he referred to later as "gaining information." Then he relayed what he heard to Buchwald, since the information "would be very difficult for him to gain." Soon, Arnie Aberman phoned him up again. "Whaddya mean you've got problems with the way we've been handling this?" he asked. Dick responded with clear requests. "What I expect," he told the dean during one conversation, "is that you, as a leader in this place, would call up Apotex and say, 'Look, you don't threaten one of my researchers.'"

"Well that's what I did," Aberman replied. "I didn't do it in sky-writing, I didn't put it on paper. But they haven't sued her, have they?"

For Olivieri, it was a relief to have Dick so concerned. With his support, she seemed more ready to talk to others at Sick Kids. Gastroenterologist Peter Durie was increasingly interested in the controversy. An expert on cystic fibrosis, Durie had been at the hospital for nearly a quarter of a century and was known for his sense of humour. It wasn't unusual to find a junior colleague in his office who'd walked in unannounced to complain about a grant proposal that had been rejected or to share the joy of a paper having been accepted. That fall Peter Durie began hearing from Nancy Olivieri. He said later that at first he didn't believe her. But the documents she gave him were convincing. Next, he spoke to John Dick.

Dick had spent the summer asking Aberman and Buchwald to make a statement to Apotex or lead an investigation into what had happened at the hospital. Given Buchwald's evident interest in the situation, Dick expected him to be responsive. Yet it was autumn and nothing had happened. "I was sort of horrified that Manuel hadn't done anything," he said later. Durie wasn't surprised. He had been at the hospital a decade longer than Dick and thought this was Sick Kids' standard operating procedure. He told Dick and Olivieri, "These people need a bit more of a push."

As the chief of gastroenterology during the era of the nursing cuts, Durie had dealt with the hospital administration repeatedly. He found them generally unresponsive. His division—he called them "the GI guys"—had been scheduled to lose nurses from its clinical and research programs. Durie was outspoken in fighting the cuts, arguing that the nurses were the backbone of the hospital.

Durie would invite members of the hospital's management team to his spacious office and motion them to step over a long roll on his floor before ushering them to a seat.

"You know what that is?" he'd ask.

"Carpet?" they'd say.

"Looks okay, doesn't it?" he'd ask.

"Yeah," they'd say, walking into the trap.

He'd explain that it was high-quality carpet that had been removed from the floor of the executive suite when Strofolino took over. There had been a lot of it and "the housekeeping guys" were going to chuck it, but Durie got them to save it for him. He and his wife had used it to carpet two rooms at their home in Toronto, with extra to put in a room at their cottage in the country. And he still had this whole roll left over. Then he began to wonder aloud about the priorities of a hospital that replaced perfectly good carpeting but fired its nurses.

The administration considered him an obstructionist who was attempting to block the new paths they were charting for the hospital. "Peter quite blatantly and beyond any reasonable subterfuge was making enemies," said one observer. "And he was branded as someone who stood in the way."

In 1995, when the professor of pediatrics was stepping down, Durie had been encouraged to run for the position but lost to Hugh O'Brodovich. Once O'Brodovich became the new chief of pediatrics, he hired a U.S. consulting firm to advise him on how to evaluate his staff. Soon the clinical doctors were hearing that their salaries would be tied to new, supposedly objective measures of their performance. Durie got the impression that the new chief was doing Strofolino's bidding and told colleagues he couldn't serve as a leader in O'Brodovich's department. He stepped down as GI division head.

Yet as Durie listened to John Dick describe how he'd been striking out with Buchwald and Aberman, he thought he might be able to turn to some of the other administrators. He set up a meeting and invited Buchwald, O'Brodovich and another hospital administrator, as well as a number of other hospital staff members. Alvin Zipursky, Olivieri's early mentor in hematology, agreed to come, as did Stan Zlotkin, the "GI guy" who'd served as head of the Research Ethics Board, and Brenda Gallie, a cancer researcher who was the Research Institute's newly appointed head of research for heme-onc.

The meeting turned into a small forum. Arnie Aberman showed up uninvited (as far as Durie was concerned) and essentially ran the meeting. The dean spoke for longer than his listeners would have liked, the chiefs responded to questions, and Durie and others argued that the hospital and the university needed to support Olivieri against Apotex. Afterwards, the small group who'd spoken on Olivieri's behalf felt they'd been unsuccessful. The dean hadn't taken them seriously, they said, and the meeting produced no results. However, Brenda Gallie was sufficiently moved by what she heard to become the third member of the Gang. At Dick's urging, she began meeting with Olivieri.

Gallie was an ophthalmologist best known for her pioneering genetic investigations of a rare childhood cancer of the eye called retinoblastoma. In 1997, she'd won a major federal award as a distinguished scientist, and her promotion to division director had followed in 1998. Though she was devoted to her work in the lab and to her surgical efforts for her patients, her new appointment gave her supervisory responsibility over Olivieri's research. "Brenda didn't care about any of this stuff," John Dick said later. "And then she became head of the program and I said to her, 'You're taking this on.'"

A small woman with very short hair and dangling earrings, Brenda Gallie was a risk-taker in her life and in her work. She spent holidays canoeing in the remote backcountry of northern Ontario, and she bicycled every day from her house in Toronto's tony Rosedale neighbourhood through downtown traffic to Sick Kids. She per-formed operations on her patients that surgeons elsewhere said they wouldn't risk. She was also a mother hen, caring for her aging father and a sick dog now that her two children were building their careers. At the hospital, her maternal vision settled on Nancy Olivieri.

Research administration was new to Gallie, and the issue of the L1 trials was the first problem to land on her desk. She spent hours talking to Olivieri and became convinced that the hospital's response—or its lack of response—was "a woman issue." Olivieri was a flamboyant, forthright woman who lacked tact, and Gallie fig-ured that the men at the top at Sick Kids didn't want to deal with her. As a surgeon, Gallie had coped with gender discrimination from the time she was a student. She'd wanted to train in plastic surgery, but at her school (Queen's University in Kingston, Ontario) the residency program in plastics had just accepted a woman one year earlier. Gallie was a competitive candidate—she'd done research as a student and had papers coming out in medical journals—but the plastic surgeons told her they couldn't take a risk on another woman so soon. She knew what they were thinking: what if both decided to opt out and raise children? Unhappily, she looked for another option and chose ophthalmology. After training in eye tumours in New York and molecular biology in Toronto, she put together a position at Sick Kids that allowed her to operate on children with eye disease while simultaneously doing research to transform their treatment.

Now she pulled herself away from her scientific work and began plowing through the sheaf of documents Olivieri had given her. Gallie and her collaborators held a large grant from the Apotex

Foundation, and she'd gotten to know Michael Spino personally, but she still thought that what Apotex had done in the L1 trials was despicable.

Manuel Buchwald was Gallie's boss, and she started meeting with him to fill him in on the L1 issues. She also talked the situation over with pediatric oncologist Helen Chan. Gallie had the feeling that Buchwald didn't understand why she was so concerned, but Chan listened intently. Moved by Gallie's feelings for Olivieri, Chan became the fourth member of the Gang.

Helen Chan was a quiet, solitary woman who was dedicated to her patients. She was a "120 per cent clinician," said one doctor. Another said he thought of her as a saint because she seemed to always be at the hospital, performing the sorts of small miracles required to save a cancer patient's life. Though she often kept to herself and was known as an introvert, Chan felt indebted to her mentor, Brenda Gallie. When Chan first arrived at Sick Kids after medical school in Hong Kong and a residency in the U.S., Gallie suggested they work together. Ever since then, they had managed the young children who suffered from retinoblastoma as a team, with Gallie handling the surgery and Chan serving as the patients' oncologist. Their first case together had shaped their relationship.

Gallie operated on a three-month-old baby, cutting the tiny tumour out of the baby's eye with a laser. Then Chan took over. Chemotherapy was held not to work for retinoblastoma, so radiation was used to stop the cancer from spreading. The three-month-old received radiation therapy on the unaffected eye to prevent the tumour from recurring there. The child recovered and did well. But when he was in first grade, his parents brought him back to Sick Kids because he was having headaches. Chan quickly discovered that he'd developed another cancer—a brain tumour right at the spot where he'd received the radiation. It turned out to be incurable and he died at age seven.

For Chan, the notion that the care she'd rendered had taken a patient's life instead of saving it was horrific. She told Gallie, "You know, I may want to quit working on this." But Gallie had an idea. "Why don't we do a project to see why chemotherapy doesn't work in retinoblastoma?" she asked. If they could get chemotherapy to work, then they wouldn't need to use the radiation that had proven deadly. The question became the subject of Chan's first grant proposal and wound up commanding her energies for the next fifteen years.

Working with Gallie and bench scientist Victor Ling, Chan figured out that a protein on the retinoblastoma tumours made them resistant to cancer drugs, then she found a way to reverse the effects of the protein so that doctors could treat the patients with chemotherapy. The protein was present in children with a number of different tumours, so Chan's discoveries had the potential to make a huge difference in pediatric oncology. Her work on retinoblastoma became her career. Chan "rose from a nothing researcher to someone who was making an international reputation for herself," as one doctor put it.

At one point, though, another scientist at Sick Kids had called her work into question. Chan thought the scientist was just jealous of the attention she was receiving, but his complaints reached the hospital's higher echelons all the same. Research director Jim Friesen conducted an investigation. Gallie stood by Chan the whole time until her name was cleared. Now, with Gallie championing Olivieri's cause, Helen Chan decided to do the same.

The Gang of Four—Dick, Durie, Gallie and Chan—began to work together on Olivieri's behalf. They understood that Nancy was "difficult," and that there was "a character issue," as Durie put it, but that was par for the course at a major teaching hospital. "There are a lot of prima donnas in this place," Durie said. Gallie didn't think the so-called character issue was worth discussing, given the seriousness of the other issues involved. "It's been suggested that this debate is nothing but a personality conflict when it is pretty clear that it is in fact the safety of patients that is the issue," she said.

None of the four had known Olivieri's residents, her nurses, her secretaries or her patients. As a result, they didn't know that her reputation had been affected by the way she treated people, and they weren't aware that her relationships with her chiefs, including Haslam, Freedman and O'Brodovich, had broken down during her persistent battles for greater resources. No one had told them that Arnie Aberman had obtained a sort of backroom promise from the company not to sue Olivieri. The Gang of Four couldn't fathom why hospital and university leaders weren't at Olivieri's side, fighting Apotex.

Olivieri was reinvigorated by all the support. The isolation she'd complained of earlier was gone. Abroad, she had Nathan, Weatherall and Brittenham on active duty—both Nathan and Weatherall had written to Dean Aberman over the summer of 1997, urging support for Olivieri. At home, she had the Gang of Four and her malpractice association, which had decided in the end to continue paying her legal fees. She was becoming known internationally as a whistleblower, and reporters from the U.S. had started to call. Her lawyers told her she couldn't speak on the record—Apotex might sue. But a science journalist with National Public Radio managed to tell her story by interviewing her lawyer, and a producer with CBS told her he was interested in covering her dispute with Apotex before millions of television viewers on *60 Minutes.*

The U.S. recognition was partly due to Drummond Rennie, protector of whistleblowers. "I've tried so very hard to support her," he said afterwards. Rennie called Olivieri frequently and sent funny e-mails that made her laugh. He worried that she was too cut off from support in Toronto and told her that he "loved her to bits." He also made sure Olivieri was an invited guest at meetings he attended on scientific freedom or academic-industry collaborations. She'd gone to one that fall in Washington, D.C., and was scheduled to be at another in the spring in Chicago. At these meetings, she met other scientists who had published or presented data after a private company asked them not to, including Betty Dong, and she frequently met reporters.

Now that they'd pooled their efforts, the members of Olivieri's Gang of Four were disappointed that they weren't making more headway. Dick, especially, couldn't understand why he wasn't getting through to Manuel Buchwald, who was known around the hospital as a scientist with a social conscience. Buchwald held the Order of Canada for his work on the cystic fibrosis gene, and he'd also won awards for working in the inner city to counter illiteracy. Like Dick, he hated it when people broke the rules. Once, in the 1980s, Buchwald had handled a fraud case. A researcher at the hospital claimed he had a doctorate, but it turned out he'd never completed his degree, and he was forced to resign. An official at the U of T called the man's research "superb" and said his resignation was "a modern tragedy," but Buchwald said it was dishonesty and questioned how much "dishonesty at one level spills over into another level."

As the fall of 1997 became the winter of 1998, John Dick and Brenda Gallie were meeting with Buchwald frequently, describing a company that broke the rules. Yet Buchwald wasn't taking any concrete action. Dick, frustrated, felt as if his boss wasn't listening to him. Buchwald may have been listening to Dick, but he was also speaking to Arnie Aberman, Hugh O'Brodovich and Gideon Koren, and their stories contradicted Dick's.

At the hospital and the university, the men in charge viewed Olivieri's supporters as misinformed. Her supposed lack of legal support was a case in point. Gallie and Dick were asking why the hospital hadn't provided legal support—it was one of the things they thought needed to be investigated. Bob Phillips, now at the National Cancer Institute of Canada, even put what he knew in a letter. He wrote the leaders of both institutions that Nancy Olivieri had "hired her own attorney" because "none of her host institutions supported her in this disagreement with Apotex." As he understood it, the CMPA came to her "rescue" several weeks after Apotex stopped her L1 trials.

But her bosses had been there and had seen for themselves the lawyers covered by Olivieri's malpractice insurance who were at her side at their very first meetings with her. Aberman and O'Brodovich hadn't offered legal support because they'd never been asked to, and they thought that this was probably because the CMPA was handling the case almost from the first day. Aberman e-mailed Phillips that his letter was inaccurate. John Dick made similar errors when he described what had happened, and Aberman tried to correct him, too. "You're only getting your information from one source," he told him.

The situation reminded O'Brodovich of other experiences he'd had with Olivieri, when she would say things about her program—for example, that it didn't get the same resources as other programs—but the numbers didn't back her up. He was sure the hospital had never refused to give Olivieri legal support and began to argue with her about what she was telling people. Eventually, Nancy Olivieri wrote her own lawyers to ask whether they remembered the hospital offering legal assistance. They didn't, but they also didn't recall her requesting legal assistance from the hospital or the dean, and they reminded her that Aberman had said, "If the parties were unable to resolve their differences, he would do what he could to obtain the services of the University's lawyers." She also checked with her friend and one-time mentor Alvin Zipursky, who had attended a meeting with Aberman in September 1997. Zipursky sent her his notes of the dean's remarks: "He said that if

Dr. Olivieri had not had legal representation he would have provided it and that even now if she did not have legal representation and required it, he would be prepared to provide it; that was a simple issue in his opinion."

Her lawyers' and colleagues' records didn't change Olivieri's views of what had happened. Convinced that the hospital had been unsupportive and unwilling to help her, she wrote a CMPA official to ask his opinion. The official reviewed Zipursky's notes and advised, "Dr. Zipursky is not saying that the Dean did offer you legal assistance. It is suggested that you feel free to state that at no time did you receive any offer of legal assistance from the Dean."

After this, she wrote O'Brodovich that she had checked with "my legal counsel, as well as advisors of the Canadian Medical Protective Association," and that "these individuals have reviewed their files, in which records of every conversation and any other communication with the Hospital and the Research Institute were impeccably maintained." She said that the records "confirm that no evidence exists . . . that support for legal counsel was offered by a representative of the Administration of the Hospital for Sick Children or its Research Institute at any time." She wasn't dropping the charges; she was adding more.

In October, she accused the hospital of helping Apotex obtain data on her patients who'd taken L1. She wrote Hugh O'Brodovich, "It is inevitable that Apotex Inc. recognizes your . . . potential willingness to assist the company." O'Brodovich wrote back that he didn't know what she was talking about: "I do not know . . . how you believe that I have helped or have a 'potential willingness to assist the company.'"

Olivieri wrote him again two days later. "Please be assured that I anticipate no support from the Hospital for Sick Children or its Research Institute in this matter," she said in one letter. She sent a second letter the same day to say that her lack of support from the hospital had "been recorded with interest" by her "national and international scientific advisors." Bitter that her bosses at Sick Kids hadn't stepped in with concrete assistance in one form or another, she seemed to be repeating the same sort of letter-writing campaign against the hospital that she'd waged against Apotex one year earlier.

One doctor said later that if Nancy Olivieri had been able to devote the same amount of effort to new studies of thalassemia as she was devoting to her fight against Apotex, Sick Kids and L1, she would no doubt have made significant progress. But in Olivieri's view, she *was* making headway. During the spring of 1997, when Rennie described her plight in *JAMA* and the company put its bullying tactics on display before U.S. thalassemia specialists in Boston, Olivieri devoted a portion of her time to re-reviewing her data. She believed it showed that L1 was both ineffective and toxic. By the fall of 1997, she was deeply immersed in preparing the data for publication. A few years earlier she'd nearly wiped butyrate off the NIH map by publishing a negative study on it in the *New England Journal of Medicine*. Now, if she could, she would destroy L1's chances of ever being approved by a regulatory agency.

PREPARING TO PUBLISH

Olivieri was determined to publish her findings about L1, but "the two Davids"—Nathan and Weatherall—thought that peer reviewers might dispute her claim that the drug caused liver scarring. "I don't like little snipped liver biopsies," Nathan said in an interview. "You need big wedge biopsies." Otherwise a pathologist wouldn't know if the biopsy specimen was actually from the liver. It was a judgment call. Liver specialists use a rule of thumb for deciding whether the tissue under a microscope is from the liver: they look for the many spots called the "portal triads," where the liver's vein and artery (the "portal vein" and "portal artery") come together with the bile duct. The more portal triads they see, the more certain they are. "We generally say you need to see eight portal triads," said Tufts' Marshall Kaplan, and he explained why.

"Let's say you were doing a needle biopsy of an apple. You stick a needle in and take a core sample. But you don't go very deep with your needle. Then all you see in your biopsy is the skin of the apple. So your conclusion is that an apple is this thick fibrous thing and you're wondering, why would anyone eat it?

"The capsule of the liver is a thick fibrous tissue. So in order to make sure you're looking at liver and not at liver capsule, you need to see the 'portal triads.'"

Many of the specimens from the patients in Olivieri's L1 trial had fewer than four portal triads, and some of the specimens had only two. That meant the biopsies could include snippets of the liver capsule, making pathologists think they were seeing hardened, fibrotic liver when they were actually looking at the liver's normally thick covering. Knowledgeable specialists might argue that Olivieri and her collaborators couldn't say anything about scarring in the liver because their data were so limited. Weatherall and Nathan thought they needed a number of different liver pathologists to look at the biopsies. Weatherall asked Kenneth Fleming, a liver specialist at Oxford, to look at the slides and arrange for other specialists to view them as well.

Britain had about a dozen liver pathologists who were well known in their field, and Fleming knew all of them. Olivieri prepared seventy-two biopsy slides for transport and sent them to Oxford. Fleming sent them out to two other pathologists and asked them to review them for any signs of "fibrosis" or scarring. But he didn't tell them which patient or which year any of the slides were taken from. That way, their reviews would be blinded, a technical detail that mattered a lot for eliminating bias. The pathologist Olivieri had worked with in Toronto hadn't been blinded.

One of the pathologists who received slides from Fleming was Alastair Burt, an expert on liver scanning from the University of Newcastle; he said in an interview that he saw his task as purely technical. "My role in this was as a sort of independent observer," he explained, "applying a scoring system which is now fairly well accepted." Liver scoring systems are the numbers used by pathologists to grade how much scarring or fibrosis they see on a given biopsy specimen. Part of the problem, as Burt understood it, was that Ross Cameron, the pathologist who had looked at the biopsy slides for Olivieri in Toronto, had used an idiosyncratic system instead of one of the widely accepted scoring systems that liver pathologists live by. On reviewing the slides, Burt discovered that Cameron consistently saw "a higher degree of fibrosis" than he did when examining the same slides.

The other pathologist who received Olivieri's slides from Oxford was Peter Scheuer, head of pathology at University College Hospital in London for many years. Scheuer was a recognized expert on scoring liver slides: he had helped to design one of the most widely used scoring systems himself. When he got the slides from Fleming, he sat down to view them in the lab, and as he peered through the microscope, he rated them on a notepad, giving them a score that ranged from 1 for no scarring to 6 for definite scarring. In a separate column, he made notes about each slide. He wasn't pleased with the overall quality of the set. "Insufficient," he wrote about one slide. "Small specimen," he jotted in his notes about another. "Inadequate," he wrote a few slides later.

He sent his results back to Oxford with a letter saying that many of the biopsies were small and difficult to evaluate. Some were definitely unsuitable for scoring. He asked that any slides he'd marked insufficient or inadequate be omitted from the final tally. That accounted for more than 20 per cent of the slides. He advised that the researchers do their calculations with and without the slides he'd marked as "small," to see if omitting them made a significant difference.

Olivieri phoned later to thank him for his efforts, and he suggested she put together a consensus conference in Toronto. That way, several different pathologists could come to an agreement on which specimens to accept and which to discard. She set up the conference, but Scheuer couldn't make it. Burt, however, was going.

Later, Fleming sent Scheuer the code that revealed which slide went with which patient. It was like being handed the solution to a difficult crossword puzzle, and Scheuer couldn't resist finding out how his own results compared. He pulled out his notepad with the scores he'd given the slides and sat down to check his findings against the code. There were nineteen patients. According to the information Fleming had sent him, scarring in eight had lessened while they were on the study drug. But eight others had developed new scarring or an increase in scarring.

Then Scheuer looked at his own notes. For the eight for whom the scarring was supposed to be worse, four had slides that he'd marked insufficient or inadequate. Of the remaining four, two had the hepatitis C virus. Since hepatitis could scar the liver, Scheuer thought it was hard to ascribe liver scarring in a hepatitis patient to a drug. That left two patients in the category of new or increased scarring. One had odd results: his slides showed scarring at first, then no scarring, then scarring again. The other already had quite serious liver disease with scarring to begin with, and his scarring worsened slightly while on L1. Scheuer thought he was the only patient whose scarring worsened in a way that could possibly be connected to the drug.

Olivieri had been racing to finish a draft of the paper, incorporating the results the pathologists had agreed on in Toronto. She'd decided to exclude nearly one-quarter of the slides, including some of the slides that Scheuer or others had told her were inadequate for evaluation. Then she wrote up an analysis of slides from fourteen of the patients. She said five of them showed progression of scarring while they were on L1. Of the five, four had hepatitis C, but unlike Scheuer—or Sher—she didn't think the presence of the virus raised questions about her findings. She concluded that L1 didn't adequately control thalassemia patients' iron levels and could worsen liver scarring.

She added the three British experts to her list of authors and sent them each a copy of the draft. Peter Scheuer wrote back and asked her to take his name off. The data he'd seen didn't support the paper's discussion. As an author, using the same data, he would have reached different conclusions. Scheuer had no vested interest in whether the drug worked. But Nancy Olivieri, L1's biggest supporter in the early 1990s, had become its biggest detractor after Apotex cut her out. She didn't add Scheuer's alternate explanation of her findings to the paper. She simply took his name off the author list as he'd requested and added a note at the end of the article thanking him "for his independent analysis of the liver-biopsy slides." Fleming and Burt, the other British pathologists, allowed their names to go on the paper, as did Cameron, the Toronto pathologist, and Olivieri sent it off to the *New England Journal of Medicine*. Nathan and Weatherall had already written the journal's editors, explaining the background of the article and the company's bad behaviour.

While Olivieri waited to hear from the journal, the Gang of Four was focusing on principles. Olivieri's supporters were determined to stand up for academic freedom and protection of human research subjects. Dick and Gallie kept talking to Buchwald, while Durie wrote letters to Aberman, urging them to investigate what had happened in Nancy Olivieri's study so that it never happened again. And they waited. "Over the course of months, there were some positive signs that they were going to do this, moving towards establishing some kind of a review," Dick said later. "Unfortunately, that never did occur."

Brenda Gallie was worried about Olivieri, who seemed anxious and under a great deal of stress. She spoke to Durie about it, and he phoned O'Brodovich to make the chief aware that Olivieri's close colleagues were concerned about her. One person said later that the Gang told O'Brodovich that Olivieri would benefit from a medical leave of absence, to reduce her stress level.

In April 1998, Gallie accompanied Olivieri to a meeting with Victor Blanchette, the clinical head of hematology. Olivieri said she was stressed because there wasn't sufficient infrastructure in her clinical programs. She needed more clinical support, more secretarial support and more resources. The administrator offered to hire someone else to run the clinical side of her programs, freeing up her time for research, but Olivieri declined the offer. Giving up the management of a clinical program meant a loss of power in the hospital hierarchy and could make it more difficult to carry out research projects. Adamant that what she needed was more staff for clerical tasks and more cash for her clinical programs, she wrote the administration and said that if the hospital didn't provide the resources she was requesting, she would resign from her position as director of the program for patients with thalassemia and sickle cell disease. She set a deadline of May 31 for the hospital to comply with her requests. She also said she would take "a medical leave of absence"—as if it had already been granted. She planned to leave as of the first of June and to be gone through December.

Blanchette was supportive in his reply and wrote back that he wanted to work with Olivieri to "create an environment in which your clinical and research skills can continue to flourish at their very high level." He added, "I will do everything I can to assist in this regard." But it was up to the department chair, O'Brodovich, to grant a leave, not a lower-level administrator.

O'Brodovich responded to Olivieri in a different tone. He was prepared to grant the leave, but he wasn't interested in being threatened with arbitrary deadlines. "From your letter I understand that in the present circumstances you wish to resign as Director . . . and take a medical leave of absence," he wrote her. "By this letter I accept your resignation as of May 31, 1998 and, at the same time grant you a medical leave of absence."

Olivieri was incensed that O'Brodovich thought she actually intended to resign if he didn't meet her demands. "An attempt to force my 'resignation' . . . when not tendered, and without cause, is of course unjustified," she wrote. "However, for the present, I will consider that your statement is the result of a simple misunderstanding." She said she was neither resigning nor taking a medical leave.

Gallie, who had tried to help, felt as if things had gotten worse. She spoke to Buchwald again and followed that up with requests in writing. Olivieri had to get more resources to do her research, she said. It also would help if the hospital apologized to her and offered her some form of monetary compensation for her stress. And there had to be an inquiry into what had happened in the L1 trials.

Buchwald promised to provide additional secretarial support for Nancy Olivieri. He also said he would ask for an investigation— he called it a review—by a bioethicist. He agreed to talk to Spino about the company's threats and even phoned Gallie on the day he and Spino were scheduled to meet. She said later, "I told him what points he had to bring up." Buchwald's efforts backfired, though, when Spino visited Brenda Gallie uninvited.

Spino knew Gallie as a highly respected researcher, a member of a research team at the U of T that had won a competitive award co-sponsored by Apotex and the Medical Research Council. He thought he could drop by her office as if calling on a colleague. At first, Gallie questioned Spino about the L1 trials. But his story didn't match what Nancy Olivieri had told her. "That's not true," she replied when he described the company's plans for dealing with Olivieri's initial report that L1 had problems, back in the spring of 1996. Spino was surprised. He hadn't expected Gallie, a scientist partly funded by his company's foundation, to doubt his credibility.

For her part, Gallie thought Spino's visit was intended to intimidate her. At one point he accused her of being protective of Nancy. "He made comments like how my mind was closed and I was obviously siding with my scientist, Dr. Olivieri," she said. Gallie saw it as an aggressive interaction and finally said, "I'm sorry, I'd like you to leave." She had never kicked anyone out of her office before and hated being put in that situation. "It made me feel very determined that we would not give up on this and we would not lose Dr. Olivieri for Canada," she said later, aware that Olivieri's friends and colleagues in the U.S. were trying to recruit her to their campuses.

But for all her determination, Gallie felt the hospital administration wasn't taking her seriously, and Durie and Dick agreed. The Gang members had believed that by leveraging their individual clout—which was considerable—they could persuade the hospital to come around. Instead, they had begun to think they were being penalized for their work to support Olivieri.

Peter Durie thought the senior leadership was forcing him to pay a price via the departmental "report card." Salaries in pediatrics were tied to the report cards, and Durie's grades that year weren't high enough to qualify for a pay raise. He blamed O'Brodovich and Strofolino. The report card system, he said, "comes right from the top, it's part of the strategic directions of the hospital." His wife was a schoolteacher and they had two teenagers at home; it was awful to think they'd lost income because he'd stood up for his principles.

Gallie got worried in June when the administration refused to let her talk to the hospital lawyers. In a letter to Buchwald and Strofolino, she listed the things she wanted legal counsel on, including "the aggressive visit by Dr. Spino of Apotex, Inc. to my office." As a division chief in the Research Institute, she figured she deserved the chance to consult with a Sick Kids lawyer.

To Durie's resentment and Gallie's suspicions, John Dick added a lament. In countless meetings with Buchwald and several e-mail exchanges and phone calls with the dean, he'd virtually pleaded with the two men to set the hospital and the university on the right track. "It was a very daunting thing to take this thing on, because you're ending up taking on the dean, your leaders, and that's not my personality," he said. "You don't know exactly what legs you're standing on." Now a year had passed since he'd watched Apotex humiliate Nancy at the conference in Cambridge and no one at the hospital or the university had managed to stand up to the company in a meaningful way. They hadn't even seriously investigated what had happened.

Buchwald had directed an ethicist to conduct a "review," but the ethicist—a junior staff person at the hospital named Mary Rowell—felt that her investigation had no teeth. She'd questioned the various administrators involved, but she felt "so belittled, so used and so lied to" that she had considered resigning from her job. Dick had considered resigning as well. The twelve months from June 1997 to June 1998 amounted to the most troubling year he'd ever had. As he explained, "A scientist by definition has to be optimistic, and I think this situation drained the optimism out of me."

He had his own research on the line—a recent discovery from his lab that he needed to get into print before they got scooped. Dick and his co-workers had unearthed a new class of stem cells, the one-in-a-million blood cells capable of becoming all other types of blood cells. Dick thought it was one of the most important discoveries he had ever been involved in because it made so much other research possible. But for reasons he couldn't understand, two top journals —*Science* and *Cell*—had rejected the work. He was pretty certain the fault lay with the peer review system.

Because the system was anonymous, Dick didn't know who had reviewed his article, but he feared that the two journals had sent it to direct competitors who had an interest in blocking the work from being published. Fearing that his lab had been victimized by jealous scientists, he didn't know whom to complain to. There were supposed to be rules against that sort of misuse of peer review, but the system for enforcing the rules was unclear. Meanwhile, the pressure to publish before someone else produced the same discovery grew more urgent. Discouraged, Dick submitted the work to a second-line journal. Then, one of his kids got sick and had to spend an extended period out of school. Dick had stolen precious time from work and home to get involved in the Olivieri-Apotex crisis. Now he felt as if he'd been spinning his wheels. "This has been a waste in that way," he said. "But more than that, on a personal level, it's been so incredibly emotionally draining and demoralizing."

In June 1998, the Gang of Four began to circulate a petition. Written as a letter to Manuel Buchwald, it spelled out in three pages the principles at stake in the L1 saga: patient protection and academic freedom. It asked for an "independent review of all matters concerning this case" in order to decide whether the hospital had "adequately supported and protected the rights of thalassemia children undergoing a clinical trial of L1 and whether the Hospital for Sick Children supported and protected the role of the principal investigator."

Nancy Olivieri was the investigator who hadn't been supported, but the Strofolino regime had much to do with why people signed the petition. It had been four years since he had taken the reins as CEO. First there were the cuts to the clinical programs and nursing. Then Strofolino centralized power in the executive suite by eroding the power of the traditional fiefdoms of nursing, pediatrics, surgery and research. The push for financial donors to the institution transformed the look of the building. "Sick Kids changed quite a bit," said a surgeon who trained there in the early 1990s. "It became very commercial. All the elevators have a plaque on them [bearing the name of a donor]." On top of that, the directive to fold research into the hospital had led to changes at the Research Institute, including Friesen's departure and twenty-seven demotions. More than a few doctors and scientists "thought they lost out," said Buchwald.

It was true that some of the resentment at Sick Kids stemmed from the losses the doctors and nurses had experienced as programs were discontinued, jobs cut and senior positions reassigned. But it also reflected the growing disconnect between the staff and the head office, with doctors, nurses and scientists feeling that they could not make themselves heard or, worse, that they would be heard and punished for what they were saying. Against that back-drop, Olivieri became more than a woman blowing the whistle on a powerful company: she was a hero standing up to the Strofolino administration. As the Gang of Four shopped their petition around the hospital, many of their colleagues heard the story of the L1 trials as emblematic of what had happened during Strofolino's tenure. Said one physician who signed, "Michael Strofolino handled this like it was a football game: Nancy Olivieri was coming through the line, and he was going to obliterate her." The physician continued, "It requires someone like Nancy to buck the system. Somebody has to have a tremendous determination and a sense of outrage to speak out in this environment."

By adding their names to the Gang's petition, staff agreed to stand with Nancy Olivieri and against Sick Kids. She was their Joan of Arc, crusading against Strofolino's tyrannical regime, and they signed even though they thought it could cost them in the long run. As one doctor put it, "We're all salaried, so merit increases, promotional movement up the ladder could be affected." He thought there could be a special hardship for junior faculty coming up for their three-year or six-year reviews. "These sorts of things can be made a little more difficult, a little less difficult, depending," he said.

As the Gang circulated its petition, David Nathan wrote Strofolino from Boston. Nathan, who had already written to Aberman, had reason to believe he could help guide a medical leader through a crisis. He'd taken the helm of Harvard's cancer hospital, the Dana-Farber Cancer Institute, in 1994, when it was mired in its own scandal after the *Boston Globe*'s health columnist died suddenly from a massive overdose of chemotherapy, administered during routine treatment for breast cancer. The death and the mistake that caused it rocked the Dana-Farber and received national attention. Harvard chose Nathan to lead the hospital through a process of investigations and a makeover. Sick Kids executives, however, weren't interested in what Nathan had to say.

Strofolino acknowledged later that he'd been given advice. "Nathan wrote a letter. It's a letter I can't show anybody that outlines everything he thinks should be done." But Nathan had never worked in Canada, and Strofolino found his tone condescending. He described it this way: "Nathan and Weatherall, they call me up and say, 'Here are the mistakes you're making.' Not 'What are the facts?' They have their opinions formed before even collecting the facts."

With Nathan striking out, Bob Phillips offered to try his hand. Phillips had already written to Aberman, Buchwald and Strofolino, and he felt he'd gotten nowhere. Now his idea was to bypass the executive suite and speak directly to a member of the Sick Kids board. At Sick Kids, it was an unusual route to take. Across the street, at Toronto's Mount Sinai Hospital, researchers occasionally met with board members to defuse conflicts. It was part of the general movement toward greater corporate accountability, with trustees being pressured to exert greater oversight at hospitals, as at private companies. But it wasn't happening at Sick Kids, where trustees were still focused on raising funds. They endowed chairs and created new programs but generally left the running of the institution and the solving of crises to the CEO. Despite the multitude of cuts and "redesigns" that Strofolino had implemented—and the resulting dissatisfaction among staff—the hospital board hadn't gotten involved.

Sick Kids had been warned against this sort of hands-off stewardship back in the 1980s. After the deaths of babies on the cardiac ward, an Ontario provincial commission investigating the hospital slammed its trustees as inactive and unresponsive. The Dubin

Commission had advised the hospital to reconstitute its board with strict term limits and members "drawn less predominantly from the legal, banking and investment communities." But the province's power over the hospital seemed to be as limited as the university's; over fifteen years later, little had changed on the Sick Kids board. Toronto philanthropist James Pitblado chaired a board made up of lawyers, bankers and brokers, some of whom had been trustees for two decades. One man who observed the situation thought the hospital and foundation boards had their roles reversed. At the foundation, trustees worried about what sort of future the massive cutbacks in programs spelled for the hospital, while on the hospital's board, the trustees brought in dollars. Still, Bob Phillips decided to contact Mary Mogford, a trustee he'd gotten to know.

Mogford had overseen the search for a new head of the Research Institute. She wasn't a stranger to politics: she'd been a deputy minister and a treasurer in the provincial cabinet prior to her role as trustee. Now she was vice-chair at Sick Kids. In a phone call, Phillips described what was happening. He asked if he could speak further with her about the situation, and she said she'd call back if she wanted to hear his thoughts, but she never did.

The board was relying on Strofolino for its information. The CEO presented the L1 controversy as a scientific debate: Nancy Olivieri saw things her way; other scientists disagreed with her interpretation, and she wanted the hospital to take her side. Strofolino didn't accept that Phillips or the Gang of Four were motivated by principles; he thought it was sour grapes. At some point during the mid-1990s, Bob Phillips had run for chief of the Research Institute and lost to Manuel Buchwald; Peter Durie had run for professor of pediatrics and lost to Hugh O'Brodovich; Brenda Gallie had run for chief of heme-onc and wound up sharing the post (she was the division's research chief while one of the senior hematologists was its clinical chief). The CEO shared his sour grapes theory with the trustees, and many of them accepted it. "Some of them were bitter," Sick Kids trustee Andrew Baines said later of Olivieri's supporters. "Maybe there are positions they think they should have gotten." Anyone who spent any time in the company of Phillips, Gallie, Durie, Dick and Chan would never doubt that they were the kind of scientists to whom principles mattered deeply.

Phillips, Dick and the others concluded that there was an unseen obstacle preventing those in power from taking action. There were rumours that Barry Sherman of Apotex had promised a substantial donation to the university toward a new building. Olivieri thought the rumours were true, and John Dick decided to look into it.

Barry Sherman didn't spend his money on himself. He drove a 1982 Buick into the late 1990s. He and his wife, Honey, were self-made millionaires, and they'd become one of Toronto's leading philanthropic couples. The University of Toronto—alma mater to both of them—was already a recipient of their largesse, and Sherman wanted to make an even more significant contribution to the school. "Barry and Honey have been involved in discussions over the past five years about possibly making a large commitment to the U of T," said Sue Bloch-Nevitte of the university's public affairs office when I spoke to her about it in the summer of 1998.

John Dick first heard about it that summer when he e-mailed a scientist across campus and asked about a new building that was in the planning stages. His colleague e-mailed back that the building involved a donation in the tens of millions from Apotex CEO Barry Sherman.

The Shermans' discussions with the university centred on a research facility, identified later as the new Centre for Cellular and Biomolecular Research, to which the Shermans would donate more than $20 million. The negotiations with Sherman had included university president Robert Prichard, who had a reputation as a phenomenal fundraiser. Sherman and Prichard later admitted that

Apotex was discussing donations to the university that could eventually total $55 million, a figure larger than any other corporate donation to a university in Canada.

Dick sent a few more e-mails and got more information. In addition to the millions earmarked for the building, it sounded as if Apotex might also offer $10 million to a U of T teaching hospital. If that rumour was true, it was significant. At Sick Kids, as Dick and Durie knew, million-dollar donations represented naming opportunities: $1 million named a professorship, $2 million an endowed chair; conceivably, for $10 million a donor could name the Research Institute itself.

Dianne Lister, head of the Sick Kids Foundation, confirmed in an interview in the summer of 1998 that the U of T teaching hospitals were being asked to submit proposals for $10 million from the Apotex Foundation. As Lister put it, it was a "large naming opportunity" for a donor who "wanted profile and recognition."

In all the time Dick had spent with Buchwald and Aberman discussing L1 and Apotex, neither had ever mentioned Sherman's planned contributions to the U of T or the hospital. Were they purposely keeping the donations hidden? Nancy Olivieri was sure they were, but Dick didn't want to jump to conclusions. He began asking Buchwald and Aberman about the money in an indirect sort of way. "You know, I think there may be a problem here," he told them. "There may be a conflict of interest here. You have to take my concerns seriously." His style was polite and respectful. "I'm not a lawyer," he said. But he was sure they understood what he was asking between the lines. Were they trying to stay on the company's good side because they were expecting a donation? Was that why the university and the hospital wouldn't tell the company to stop threatening Nancy Olivieri? He received no clear response.

There's a well-known rule about financial conflicts of interest in science: they have to be disclosed. In the early 1990s, when the

NIH proposed its rules banning consulting contracts for doctors involved in a drug study, the question of how scientists should deal with their conflicts of interest was still new. But by the late 1990s, the guidelines on disclosing conflicts were clear. Whenever scientists published articles or gave talks, they were supposed to state their financial conflicts upfront. At the U of T and the Hospital for Sick Children, none of the leaders had mentioned Sherman's money to Olivieri, Dick, Gallie, Durie or Phillips, an omission that could have been due to poor management or a lack of explicit policies for disclosing conflicts. But it left open the possible interpretation that Sherman was buying influence with the institutions, especially since neither the university nor the hospital was seriously investigating the Olivieri-Apotex standoff.

What he'd discovered about the money made John Dick more depressed. The Gang of Four had made concerted efforts over the course of a year to persuade the hospital and the university to take up Nancy Olivieri's cause because of the principles involved, but in the end they'd failed. It was upsetting and difficult to understand. If Sherman's money was blocking Buchwald, Aberman, O'Brodovich and the rest from taking action against the company, then Sick Kids was a money-grubbing institution with no backbone and the U of T was equally spineless.

In the end, the hospital turned down the chance for the $10 million from Apotex. Buchwald said later, "Given the circumstances of the L1 trial, we thought it was not in the best interests of this institution to enter into some kind of new venture with them." But they'd been offered it. Nancy Olivieri was certain that Sherman's proposed gifts explained everything. "Apotex supplies the university with a shitload of money," she said during an interview for CBC Radio that summer. "They said, 'Apotex gave us a lot of money; we'll take a risk on the kids.'"

UNDOING MANUEL CARCAO

In the spring of 1998, while John Dick was tracing Sherman's dollars, Nancy Olivieri heard from the *New England Journal of Medicine*. They'd accepted her paper on L1 and scheduled it to come out some time that summer. Now, finally, she could tell journalists her story, as long as they promised to honour the journal's embargo rules and not write anything about her before her article appeared.

Toward the end of May she flew to Chicago for an invitation-only conference that Drummond Rennie had helped organize. Some of the U.S. whistleblowers she'd been getting to know were there, along with journalists from the *Wall Street Journal, Nightline* and National Public Radio. I was there as well, representing CBC Radio. As we all sat together during the meeting's first session, Olivieri was invited to tell us what had happened in her trials.

She said she'd been studying the drug on her own. Then the FDA had urged her to get a drug company involved, so she'd signed with a drug firm, "equally as naively as Betty Dong." When she and her U.S. collaborator discovered that the drug was no longer working adequately, the company suppressed their data. "They said if we published . . . we would be sued for every dime we owned," she explained. "We did publish it in abstract form. They continued to threaten." The story got worse. "There was no university or hospital support given." And worse. "The drug has proven to be toxic. These are children, who could die."

Olivieri was clear and easy to follow. It sounded as if she'd done everything she could to protect her patients but was fighting an uphill battle against powerful forces. Answering questions, she was articulate, poised and passionate—a wonderful speaker. Later, in an interview, she described her current situation. She remained a highly successful researcher, publishing in the top journals. She was waiting to learn when the L1 study would appear, but in the meantime she was working on another article for the *New England Journal of Medicine,* an invited review on thalassemia. It would be one more badge marking her as an expert on the disease. And she continued to study thalassemia and sickle cell disease with collaborators around the world. She had been funded continuously to study thalassemia and sickle cell disease from the late 1980s on, and her operating grants from agencies in Canada, the U.S. and the U.K. totalled $1 million to $1.5 million, a sum that dwarfed the funding many of her colleagues had for their research.

In contrast to the respect she commanded outside Toronto, Olivieri said she felt unsupported at home except by a few close friends. She described feeling so frightened by the actions of Apotex that she lived in terror of what would happen next. Barry Goldwater, the conservative American senator, had died that spring, and Olivieri had seen an obituary that described him as "never terrified." "I read that when he died, and I thought, never afraid!" she told me. "I mean, we must have traded lives, you know what I mean? I got all his fear. How can he never be afraid of anything?" She said she was coping with her fear by phoning her lawyer about six times a day for advice and reassurance.

Olivieri described herself as a busy clinician, with responsibility for all the thalassemia and sickle cell disease patients at Sick Kids and the Toronto General. She said there were more than five hundred patients. Much later, I learned from her patients and her staff that she was so busy coping with her multiple commitments that her patients saw little of her. Her sickle cell patients mostly saw the new staff doctor she'd hired, a young man named Manuel Carcao who had trained at Sick Kids in pediatrics and hematology-oncology. Carcao's work for Olivieri was part of a job he'd patched together—four clinics per week, including two with the sickle cell patients, combined with multiple research projects. He was doing a sort of research fellowship, supporting himself with his clinical earnings.

With Olivieri, he was studying the patients with Diamond Blackfan anemia and performing a genetic analysis of a family with an unusual hemoglobin disorder. She had also put him in touch with her collaborators at the provincial genetics lab in Hamilton, and he was working with them on investigations of a rare form of thalassemia. Then Olivieri asked him to supervise a visiting resident from McMaster, so he'd arranged for the resident to work on the Diamond Blackfan anemia research. And Carcao had begun a project with another hematologist at the hospital to develop guidelines for the care of hospitalized sickle cell patients. He knew why the guidelines mattered: a sickle cell patient had died at the hospital the year before and some doctors thought the death might have been prevented. In two meetings, Sick Kids hematologists, emergency room doctors, intensive care specialists and ward pediatricians had discussed the troubling case, and brainstormed about how to improve the care of children with sickle cell anemia who got admitted to the hospital. A hematologist who attended both meetings wrote the head of hematology in January 1998 that Sick Kids emergency room and intensive care unit doctors were seeking "expertise and leadership in the care of sickle cell disease patients." Olivieri was head of the hospital's sickle cell program, but it wasn't clear if the doctors at the meeting had turned to her. In February, Carcao was assigned to put together the guidelines.

If anyone had asked Manny Carcao what he thought of Nancy Olivieri, he would have said she was brilliant. She always seemed to have an idea of something they could study further. And she knew everyone. Occasionally she'd say, "Manny, I'm just going to make a call," and she would dial David Weatherall's number in Oxford. "David, I have Manny Carcao here, and we were just talking," she'd say, then hand the phone to Carcao. "Here, Manny, say hi to him," she'd command, and Carcao, in his first year out of training, trying to become a researcher in the field of hemoglobin disorders, would find himself speaking to one of the leading figures in the field. It was a thrill.

In their clinical meetings, Olivieri generally praised his work and his clinical intuition. Their research collaborations were also going well. Carcao was scheduled to present on one of their projects at the pediatric hematology meetings in September, and he and the resident from McMaster hoped to present their findings on Diamond Blackfan anemia at ASH. They'd reviewed the medical charts of eleven patients and found that six had occasionally developed low white blood cell counts or low platelet counts. Carcao had already drafted an abstract about their findings and had discussed it with Olivieri. She'd suggested adding more cases and he thought he could do that in time for submission to ASH. He knew she didn't trust her fellow hematologists at the hospital, but he didn't know about her conflict with Apotex. He didn't know her as a whistle-blower on a crusade or as a fighter with an invisible fence to guard her from those she perceived as her enemies. Then he took a wrong turn and was caught in the crossfire.

It happened in May, in a conference room at Sick Kids where Carcao was giving a talk on the guidelines he'd prepared for how to treat the fevers, infections and intensely painful crises that children with sickle cell disease suffer. He'd contacted experts at children's hospitals in the U.S., and they'd sent him volumes of materials on the guidelines and standards they used at their own hospitals. By the end of March, he'd produced a cookbook for how to deal with all the various problems that could land a sickle cell patient in the hospital, and had begun discussing it with other physicians at Sick Kids. One of the doctors asked him to add a section dealing with the needs of "sicklers" who were going for surgery, and he'd done that. A physician from the intensive care unit wrote him that there were still other issues to address, such as which doctors were "primarily responsible for these patients when they enter our institution"— Olivieri ran the outpatient clinics for children with sickle cell disease but it wasn't clear who had primary responsibility for them if they were hospitalized. The head of the Sick Kids emergency room also wrote Carcao with comments on his draft, and she asked the other emergency doctors to do the same. After more than one hundred hours of research and preparation, he was presenting a final draft of the guidelines to representatives from all the different specialties before putting the finishing touches on the project.

As head of the sickle cell program and one of Carcao's supervisors, Nancy Olivieri was scheduled to be there. Carcao had given her drafts of the report as he was writing it, but she'd been too busy to get back to him about it. She arrived twenty minutes after his presentation began and took the only seat available, right next to him. Carcao had already covered most of his material and was at the point of asking for comments and expressing his thanks for the help he'd had from various doctors at the hospital. He noticed that Olivieri seemed angry about his presentation in some way.

After the comment period ended, she told him to come see her "right away" and left the room. A senior hematologist noticed Carcao's expression. "Are you okay?" he asked. Carcao explained that he was about to receive a talking-to from Olivieri. "She's up there right now waiting in her office so I can go in there, and she'll rail at me," he said. His senior colleague told him that Olivieri might simply need a cooling-off period and advised him to wait and not go to her office right away. Carcao had no clue what he'd done wrong, and he decided not to go.

The following week, he expected to see his boss, but she was out of town, attending the meeting Rennie had invited her to in Chicago. Before leaving, she had received the missives from her bosses—the one from a mid-level administrator offering to create an environment where she could flourish, and the other from O'Brodovich asserting that he would accept her resignation and grant her a leave. The hematologists heard that the department heads had cobbled together a plan: Olivieri could take a leave or resign from her clinical post to concentrate on her research, because Manuel Carcao could take over for her on the clinical side. A doctor and a nurse who knew of this idea approached Carcao in the corridor. "Did you hear?" the doctor asked him. "Hear what?" he replied. "Nancy's out. You're probably going to take over the program." Carcao didn't think that was a good idea for his career. He told colleagues he was afraid that if he replaced Nancy Olivieri, she would see him as part of a plot to oust her. But he thought it didn't matter anyway, since no one offered him the job.

Carcao next saw Olivieri a week later, at their usual Thursday-afternoon clinic rounds. She sounded cross with him as she questioned him about everything he'd done with the patients, and she was critical of his answers, saying she couldn't understand why he hadn't talked to one patient about fertility and why he hadn't seen another patient. He tried to explain, but Olivieri didn't accept his explanations and responded with sarcasm.

Carcao felt stupid and ashamed. He tried to arrange a meeting with Olivieri through her secretary, but each time, on the morning they were scheduled to meet, her secretary would phone: "Nancy can't make it." After more than a month, he still hadn't managed to speak to her. In June he sent Olivieri a long letter. "It saddens me the fact that I'm writing this letter as I would much rather speak to you in person. . . . Our relationship for me pretty much deteriorated with that final meeting on the sickle cell protocols," he wrote. "I felt like a child being scolded and a fool for trying to do my best . . . You stopped talking to me and have made me feel very unwelcome in the program in research meetings, clinic meetings, etc. Every day I go home upset by the whole thing . . ." He concluded by asking whether she wanted him to continue working in the clinic. "No response I guess is a response in itself," he closed.

When he heard nothing from her after a few weeks, he tried again to schedule an appointment through her secretary, but the appointment was postponed so he wrote her again: ". . . it gives me great sorrow to write this letter, as I would prefer meeting with you in person . . ." He said he felt "attached to the patients and families," adding, "I could potentially see myself developing a career in this field." But he sounded frustrated by her lack of response to his earlier letter. "All that I was asking was to hear from you that you valued my work, respected me and would want to have me continue working with you." Instead, he wrote, she appeared "suspicious" of him and "totally unapproachable." He then submitted his resignation from the sickle cell program, saying he would work until the end of July. He closed, "Once again I'm available to talk at any time. P.S. I'm usually a good listener, so try me."

This time, she wrote back that she recognized there had been a misunderstanding, and set up a meeting with him in her office.

"Would you be willing to take on a clinician role?" she asked when they finally spoke. He told her he liked the sickle cell patients, but he also liked research. He already had presentations and publications to his credit. He expected to present on their collaborative projects at ASH, but the abstracts were in limbo because he'd been unable to discuss them with Olivieri and get her to sign off on them. First, she wouldn't meet with him. Now they'd met, but she was suggesting he give up doing research and focus solely on the patients.

Carcao couldn't understand it. If she didn't think he was cut out to do research, why had she encouraged him and praised his work before? It was disheartening and depressing, but he didn't think it was because he lacked talent. He was proud of the nearly complete guidelines about how to care for hospitalized sickle cell patients. The head of anesthesia had phoned Carcao asking for a copy of them because he wanted to make his staff aware of the special requirements of that group of patients. The office of one of the surgeons had also called. "The doctor would like to know, would you have a copy of those guidelines?" But Olivieri seemed to ignore his work on the guidelines.

Afterwards, Carcao met with his mentor in hematology. His message was simple: "Take me out of the sickle cell clinic or I'll resign." People in the division who didn't know the whole story heard the rumblings. "Whatever happened [to Manuel Carcao] was very, very unpleasant," said one of the hospital's oncologists. Carcao wrote Olivieri that she should find someone to replace him, and he left the program that summer. The sickle cell guidelines were nearly ready for implementation, and he asked a few people at the hospital how he could continue his work on them. He was told that the guidelines were the property of the hemoglobinopathy program—Nancy Olivieri's program. The guidelines project was left for Olivieri and her staff to finish up; Carcao felt he'd been directed to walk away from it.

Meanwhile, Olivieri began contacting the hematology chief to let him know she needed another clinical doctor to work with the sickle cell patients. As her lawyer put it later, she was seeking the hospital's assistance to deal with the crisis in clinical coverage of her sickle cell patients. She wrote her chief three times in August and four times in the fall to say she needed to hire someone. But in December 1998, the crisis that had resulted from Carcao's departure was still unresolved. Her lawyer couldn't understand why the hospital didn't simply do as she asked.

In July 1998, a new resident had started working with Nancy Olivieri. Soon the resident approached Carcao about one of his research projects and said Nancy Olivieri had discussed the project with her. It seemed as if Olivieri had suggested that Carcao might be willing to provide her with the data he'd gathered. "Can you give it to me?" she asked. Carcao said no. A few weeks later, he was working on one of the computers that the fellows all shared. A file on the computer looked familiar. It was an abstract on the patients at Sick Kids with Diamond Blackfan anemia, similar to the abstract he'd prepared. But Carcao's name wasn't on this new version of the abstract, and neither was the name of the McMaster resident who had worked with him. The name of the new research fellow was listed, along with the name of one of the summer students. The only thing that stayed the same on the list of authors was Nancy Olivieri; she had been listed as senior author when Carcao had prepared the abstract, and she was still listed as senior author on the new version. It was as if he and the McMaster resident had never done the work in the first place.

Carcao didn't think Olivieri was stealing his work; after all, it was her work too. But she was taking a collaborative project that he'd worked on and cutting him out. He didn't think there was anything he could do about it, but he did think it was a lousy way to treat people.

Carcao's mentor in hematology was disturbed by what had happened and conducted an investigation, contacting the McMaster resident, who confirmed his and Carcao's involvement in the research on the patients with Diamond Blackfan anemia. His mentor also got copies of both abstracts—the first one, which Carcao had prepared but not submitted, with the McMaster resident's name listed first, Carcao's second and Olivieri's last, and the second, which had been submitted to ASH and accepted as a poster presentation, with Olivieri's student's name first and her resident's name second, and Carcao and the McMaster resident not listed at all. The first abstract included data on eleven patients; the second had data on seventeen, but the conclusions were nearly the same: a low white cell count and a low platelet count might be "more common than previously reported in Diamond Blackfan anemia." Carcao's mentor wrote Olivieri about it and she wrote back with an explanation. "Because Dr. Carcao has chosen not to discuss the analysis of this work with me despite repeated opportunities to do so, because Dr. Carcao's analysis of the data was preliminary and because of Dr. Carcao's repeated declarations that he would not continue to work within [the sickle cell and thalassemia] program," her summer student had done "a completely new analysis of these data." Olivieri attached guidelines on scientific authorship for Carcao's information.

The division scheduled a meeting to discuss it. Olivieri came carrying a tape recorder and accompanied by Brenda Gallie, but she didn't acknowledge doing anything wrong. "Fuck this," she said at one point. Gallie attempted to mediate. Other hematologists at Sick Kids thought Gallie probably couldn't believe that anyone would undercut a junior doctor's efforts the way Olivieri had undercut Carcao's, since Gallie would never have done it herself. Gallie's junior colleagues felt about her as Helen Chan did—that she'd been one of their best mentors.

Carcao left the sickle cell program as planned but felt bad whenever he saw his former patients. They'd say "Hi, Manny," or "Hi, Dr. Carcao," and he'd say, "I'm sorry, I had to make a decision about where to go." He didn't want to tell them the truth—that he couldn't work with Nancy Olivieri.

THE MAKING OF A MEDIA STAR

Olivieri was getting ready for a moment she'd been anticipating for two years. She knew when her article was coming out in the *New England Journal of Medicine;* the editors had given her a date: August 13, 1998. It was the perfect antidote to the depressed and anxious times she'd had earlier in the spring. Now she would say what she thought of L1—that it was ineffective because it didn't work for a substantial proportion of her patients, and harmful because it could cause liver scarring—where everyone would see it and where Spino and his hired experts couldn't shout her down.

She was scheduled to be in Australia for one of her research projects the last two weeks of July, but she spent some time before that preparing for the media coverage she expected. By June, she was already meeting with reporters, armed with advice on what to say and how to say it. The advice came from Michael Langlois, a man who made his living teaching executives how to speak to the media. He'd offered to help Olivieri on a pro bono basis after hearing from a friend about her situation. "This has to do with integrity," he said, explaining why he'd donated his time. "Here is someone who obviously was facing an unbelievable circumstance, and I wondered, 'Is there any way I can help her deal with what's going on?' . . . There was suppression, defamation, call it what you want to call it . . . I'm working with somebody and trying to help somebody who's trying to do the right thing."

He said that he taught Olivieri to keep her focus on "the real issues" in her interviews and that he helped her and the Gang of Four strategize about which journalists to contact. "I've encouraged them to think about it as, 'This is someone you should be talking to,'" he said later. He also told them to stay in touch with journalists who had already covered her story and to line up experts willing to speak to the press on her behalf. That would give her story more credibility, while keeping Nancy herself from getting too burnt out.

The Gang made lists of people to call. One was pediatrician Michèle Brill-Edwards, who had worked for Health Canada's Health Protection Branch as its top drug reviewer. In 1995, Brill-Edwards had gone on national television in Canada to expose practices she thought led to unsafe drugs staying on the market. Subsequently she became known nationally as an advocate for safer drugs. She was passionate about her issue and had already been in touch with Olivieri, offering to help in any way she could. She told the Gang that she'd be happy to speak to reporters about why it was so crucial for the media to cover what had happened to Olivieri at the hands of Apotex and Sick Kids.

Brill-Edwards had the appearance of a kindly grandmother: she dressed plainly and carried a simple black purse. She was a drug regulator, not a scientist who ran clinical trials, but she and Olivieri had several things in common: both had felt unsupported by their employers, and both were whistleblowers over drugs. Brill-Edwards had blown the whistle on the federal drug agency after more than a decade of reviewing drugs, out of concern that "drugs were being whipped through the system without checks and balances," as she put it in an interview. She'd tried protesting from within. After a while, she felt she wasn't getting anywhere and began sharing confidential information with a reporter for the Montreal *Gazette*.

In 1992, Brill-Edwards was an unnamed source in a story in *The Gazette* about a drug for migraine headaches called Imitrex. Health Canada had approved it, but Brill-Edwards thought that was a mistake, since the drug had dangerous side effects. A few years later, Brill-Edwards spoke out again. This time her concern was a class of widely used blood pressure drugs called calcium channel blockers that had become controversial because of new evidence that they could cause heart problems. The debate was playing out in medical journals, with numerous editorials advocating or criticizing use of the drugs. Brill-Edwards came down heavily against them and thought they should be pulled from the market. Health Canada considered the evidence but kept the drugs on the market. Brill-Edwards decided the system was corrupt because some of the doctors advising the agency on the issue were also advising the manufacturers of the drugs. Fearing that Canadians taking calcium channel blockers were at risk, she resigned from her agency in order to blow the whistle on the CBC's investigative news show, *the fifth estate*. But her decision that calcium channel blockers should not be available to anyone put her at the far end of the spectrum of doctors who were writing about them. Pharmacologist Stewart MacLeod of McMaster thought Brill-Edwards overstated the case against the products. "If they insisted on the kind of drug regulation Michèle is calling for, no drug would ever get approved," he said. The FDA concurred with Health Canada that the drugs were safe, and they continue to be widely prescribed in both countries. Believing the drug agencies set their thresholds too low, Brill-Edwards became a full-time activist for drug safety.

The sea change Stephen Fredd had lived through at the FDA— the "consumer rights" argument that people suffering from very serious diseases deserve to decide for themselves about their willingness to accept greater risks—didn't affect her. She still believed in the idea of "better safe than sorry" and spoke frequently of the "precautionary principle" of public health: the notion that protecting the public requires acting to reduce potential risks even if the evidence is inconclusive. By the end of the 1990s, the precautionary principle was controversial. The drug industry and its supporters in Washington were pushing the FDA for faster drug approvals, and the agency was also under pressure from patient advocacy groups. In 1999, the head of Britain's Royal Society rebuked the precautionary principle as "no way to deal with uncertainty." But for Brill-Edwards it remained an ironclad rule. Nancy Olivieri identified with her struggles, and the two women began to talk frequently.

Olivieri's supporters were also looking for a philosopher to help them out. They found a strong ally in Arthur Schafer, head of the ethics centre at the University of Manitoba in Winnipeg. Schafer had no difficulty distilling the issues. "The Olivieri affair is about corporate values vs. civic values, it's about human well-being vs. profit, it's about institutional corruption," he explained in an interview. He read over at least one of the contracts Olivieri had signed with Apotex and was unimpressed. Though parts of the contract were standard, the confidentiality clause was unusual, and that was the clause that had formed the basis of the company's threats against Olivieri. Typically, a company would protect its intellectual property rights by requesting that results be kept secret for two to six months, but Apotex had specified three years. "To me it was, from the outset, inconceivable that any court in Canada would have upheld such a contract," said Schafer. Like Brill-Edwards, he was happy to help and offered to talk through the issues with any journalist referred to him.

Olivieri, with coaching from Langlois, was spending hours in conversation with the *Globe and Mail*'s medical reporter, Paul Taylor. She also spent several hours with me, taping a lengthy interview for CBC Radio. She was working on obtaining national television coverage in Canada via friends who had contacts at CTV and

Newsworld, and she was hoping for international coverage as well, since she was still in touch with the producer for *60 Minutes*. She made sure that all the journalists she spoke to were aware of the *New England Journal of Medicine*'s embargo policy. They couldn't run a story about her before her article appeared or it would violate the embargo. But if they gave those assurances, she was willing to talk at length, and her story was compelling.

CTV producer Andrew Mitrovica (later with the *Globe and Mail*) wrote later that Olivieri struck him that summer as someone who was "transparently motivated simply by the courage of her convictions to do the right thing." In his earliest meetings with Olivieri, he didn't think she craved attention. "She is a very shy and fastidious woman who was uncomfortable before the glare of lights and the gaggle of reporters, producers and technicians who descended on her modest home," he wrote.

I also had the impression that she wasn't media savvy. She was direct and off the cuff and seemed unconcerned with how she might be quoted. But she was a terrific speaker who was naturally prone to be funny and shocking. "The University of Toronto and the Hospital for Sick Children have tried to present this as some crazy Italian who cannot keep her facts straight," she told me. She said she thought she knew why her university and hospital hadn't supported her. For one thing, she said, "It's not a white disease." Thalassemia was Mediterranean, Middle Eastern and Asian, not North American. For another thing, she explained, Apotex was a wealthy benefactor willing to donate to both institutions.

Olivieri got paged in the middle of one of our conversations and handed me an article from the *Washington Post* as she returned the call. "This is amazing, eh?" she said. The headline was about the FDA's most famous woman: Frances Kelsey, the Canadian-born drug reviewer who kept thalidomide off the market in the U.S. in the early 1960s. The article gave new details about how Kelsey had been pressured by the company that manufactured the drug. "I didn't know she was threatened by a lawyer," Olivieri said, as she waited for the phone to be picked up on the other end. "I wonder what she's like. Have you ever met her? I'd love to meet her, actually. I really, really want to meet her."

Then she continued to describe her own experience standing up to a powerful company and the authorities at her hospital in order to protect children from a drug that could harm them. "What bothers me about this is that there are parents, people, the public who support . . . public institutions such as the Hospital for Sick Children, who have, I believe, always had the understanding and assurance that their children who enter research studies will be protected and informed regardless of any other interest," she explained. "It's the mandate of 'First do no harm.' And in these two particular trials, which were my trials, without the support of my lawyers my patients could not have received that kind of information to make a fully informed choice that might have affected their health."

As she spoke, she made frequent asides, such as "Do you think you can get that in?" or "I'd really like to get that in." She had an axe to grind about how unhelpful the hospital had been, saying that they'd attempted to fire her. "In the last two years, there have been two unsuccessful attempts to dismiss me as director of the hemoglobinopathy program at the Hospital for Sick Children," she explained. "There were two attempts. One was in October 1996 and the other was in May 1998." Her explanations implied a connection between her near-firings and her stance against Apotex.

She explained the second near-firing this way: "In 1998 I submitted a letter to my division chief suggesting that I needed more resources for this program . . . And I did state that I would like a medical leave of absence . . . I received a letter from the Department of Pediatrics Chairman saying that he accepted my resignation as director of the program. The letter accepted my resignation.

I clarified that I had never tendered my resignation and I did not wish to resign as director of the program. And of course, without cause to resign, the hospital accepted that I would maintain my status as director of the program." As an aside to me, she added, "I'd love to use that part of it."

Listening to these stories, I understood that the hospital had been attempting to get rid of Olivieri because she was a whistleblower. I didn't know that her threatened dismissal in 1996 was connected to the hospital's plan to move her clinic and to her attempt to block the move. I didn't realize that her chief accepted her resignation in 1998 after she wrote a letter saying she would resign by a certain date unless she received greater resources. Olivieri herself may have forgotten the exact circumstances of the hospital's threats to dismiss her. She was convinced that Sick Kids administrators were intentionally harassing her, and used the term "constructive dismissal" to describe what her bosses had tried to do.

But if she was angry at her employer, she also came across as a deeply committed doctor. "I've looked after this group of patients since I was a fellow in 1982," she said at one point. "And I know these patients very well . . . I've looked over these charts every month for the lives of these patients." It was clear that Apotex had treated her very badly. She described how scared she'd been. "I was afraid that I couldn't afford the lawyer, I was afraid I was going to lose my job, several times, I was afraid that I was going to be ridiculed in public," she said. Her experience was so stressful that she feared it was making her sick. "I got worried that I was hyperthyroid the other day," she told me. "I think it's ridiculous now. But I'm thinking, 'Why do I have this tremor?'" Knowing that I was a physician, she added, "You don't want to hear this. Besides, I already asked someone. You can't get it from stress. There's no way."

She was a master of the sixty-second soundbite. "I think that there's no real reason to expose patients to a risk, even if there's a chance it might work," she said. "I guess I don't think that chancing it with patients' lives is acceptable." After this zinger, she asked, "Is that too dramatic?" She knew what her message was, and she kept returning to it. "I think a drug that's toxic is something that shouldn't be prescribed to patients," she said. "I don't think patients should take a toxic drug." She urged me to talk to Dick, Gallie, Phillips, Durie, Brittenham or Nathan, and gave me their phone numbers and e-mail addresses.

The Gang's thoughtful, reflective demeanour offset Nancy Olivieri's impassioned tone, as did the documents she provided. She understood that a media outlet such as the CBC would need a way to verify what she was saying, and a few weeks before her article was scheduled to appear she told me I could come by the hospital to collect a carton of papers. She'd carefully organized her materials into three-ring binders and had labelled each one in capital letters. "1995 to June 1996" read the label on one; it contained all the letters Spino had delivered to her on that fateful Friday in May 1996 when he cancelled the L1 trials at Sick Kids. She labelled another "Lay Press and Other Useful Documents"; it included the *Toronto Star* and *Medical Post* articles that had appeared in the winter of 1996–97, as well as Drummond Rennie's 1997 *JAMA* editorial. Another had the suggestive title "Graham Sher Misconduct File" and contained the confidential report from Friedland's committee.

There were ten binders in total. Later, when lawyers for the CBC said they needed certain documents that weren't in the binders, Olivieri obliged, and faxed me a copy of her contract with Apotex.

To Olivieri's voluminous materials, scientists confirming her story added their own. Brenda Gallie offered copies of her letters to the authorities; Bob Phillips gave me a copy of the lengthy treatise he'd sent to the hospital and university leadership; Peter Durie gave me the petition the Gang was still circulating at the hospital.

But Sick Kids wouldn't agree to an interview. After repeated requests, a public affairs officer said, "We're not going to speak on this issue at the moment." Initially, Arnie Aberman couldn't speak about the Apotex-Olivieri dispute either. Later he agreed to an interview but spoke as if the documents I had in my possession didn't exist. "Fundamentally," he told me, "the U of T does not do secret research." He wasn't aware "of a single situation where a faculty member was told not to publish something." When I told him what I knew about Apotex and Olivieri, he said he couldn't comment "on this individual case, because it involves individual faculty members."

At Apotex, Spino spoke to me, but his explanation for why the company had threatened Olivieri was confusing and self-serving. "If you've got something that you have invested in, and you've done everything you think is right to do, to make sure it's brought to fruition," he said, "you do not want someone who's got a vested interest in maligning the drug for whatever reason to lead the charge." He stressed that Apotex had threatened suit but hadn't actually brought one, as if that took the company off the hook. Then he made it clear that the Apotex threats were still in place. "We have not taken action; that doesn't mean we will never take action," he said. "I think she's building a nice case, actually."

The first week in August, the Gang of Four delivered their petition to Manuel Buchwald, making it clear that Nancy Olivieri wasn't an isolated whistleblower, shunned by her co-workers. One hundred and forty doctors and researchers had signed the petition calling for an independent investigation of what had happened in the L1 trials. Toward the end of the week, the hospital announced an "open forum" for all staff, to be chaired by a senior statesman at the hospital: internationally renowned pediatric orthopedic surgeon Robert Salter. Olivieri and the Gang thought it would be a chance to let their colleagues know—in public—exactly where things stood in the conflict. They decided Brenda Gallie should speak for them, and she prepared her remarks in advance.

The forum was held the day before Olivieri's article was scheduled to come out in the *New England Journal of Medicine*. Buchwald went first. He said he would introduce the issues, but his speech was long and drawn out. "You could see he was kind of tortured," said one of the scientists attending. Next, Gallie started to talk. After a few minutes, Salter used his position as chair to interrupt her. "We haven't got time," he announced. Peter Durie shouted from the back, "Let her speak! For God's sake, let her speak." A number of people responded. Soon the serious forum turned into a fracas.

"People were asking all sorts of simple questions," said one observer. "Like, 'I don't understand how a drug company could come in and stop a trial.' 'How could the ethics committee say to change the forms and then the company doesn't have to go along with it?' These were simple questions. And they were saying, 'Hey, if this can happen to her, it can happen to anyone of us.'" Another person at the forum said doctors and scientists were shouting out, "You know, this smacks of money being involved," as Michael Strofolino tried to answer questions. After weeks of Olivieri and the Gang carrying their petition around and describing their frustration with the hospital, the conflict had spilled out onto the administration's front porch. Sick Kids was a battleground.

The next day, Olivieri's paper came out in the *New England Journal of Medicine*. Its conclusions were stated clearly at the end of the abstract that ran on the title page of the article: "Deferiprone [L1] does not adequately control body iron burden in patients with thalassemia major and may worsen hepatic fibrosis." In the same issue, Marshall Kaplan wrote an editorial with Kris Kowdley, a doctor from the University of Washington in Seattle, saying Olivieri's conclusions were weak for several reasons, including the small size of the study and the small size of the liver biopsies. They pointed out that some researchers had "found that deferiprone is an effective iron-chelating agent." But Olivieri herself didn't accept that her study's limitations meant she couldn't be sure of her results. She was certain L1 was dangerous for patients. That spring, Corrado's doctor had written her clinic about his plans to manage Corrado on L1 and she then wrote to Health Canada and the College of Physicians and Surgeons, impugning his clinical judgment and letting the authorities know that in her view, L1 "should not be used in the treatment of iron overload, even in patients such as [Corrado] who presently decline to use standard deferoxamine therapy." Better to take nothing than to take L1 in her view, and it was a view that reporters accepted.

The story that broke on the airwaves that evening didn't comment on whether Olivieri's research findings were strong or weak. It said that Canada's largest drug company had threatened her because she had reached negative conclusions about its drug, which patients were taking. She was trying to protect those patients so she blew the whistle. Torontonians heard it first on CBC Radio's drive-home news show. Those who watched the nightly television news on CTV saw it as the lead item. The next morning, the talk show on CBC Radio included interviews with Olivieri and Spino, and the headline in the *Globe and Mail* filled three lines: "A doctor takes on a drug company. When Nancy Olivieri faced legal action, her hospital wouldn't help. Her colleagues are up in arms." As Michael Langlois had told his clients, it was "the summer news doldrums"—there weren't a lot of other news stories competing for airtime or page space. Soon, Olivieri's blond curls graced the screens of all the television networks, and she was in the headlines day after day.

Long-time Sick Kids board member John McNeil was in Ontario's cottage country, sailing and picking up a paper every time he pulled into a port. He read all the front-page stories and the letters to the editors calling on the hospital to launch an investigation. Then he called the board's chair, Jim Pitblado. Pitblado had been speaking to Strofolino, who was still calling it a scientific dispute. A Sick Kids scientist with personal ties to Pitblado spoke to him later that summer. She said, "He hadn't a clue how the scientists were seeing it—it was all what he'd been fed by the administration."

Andrew Baines, the sole scientist on the Sick Kids board, was at his farm for the month of August but began phoning his scientific colleagues to get the story behind the headlines. Baines had worked closely with Doug Templeton. Both were biochemists, and for years their labs were next door to one another. Templeton gave his old friend an insider's perspective: the dispute wasn't over the science and it wasn't about Olivieri's personality. Apotex really had threatened to sue her. Baines said that after talking to Templeton he argued "strenuously but unsuccessfully" with Pitblado and his fellow trustees that this was more than a scientific disagreement and larger than "a local issue."

Five days after the story broke, Brenda Gallie met with Strofolino alone. She said it was "the stupidest thing" she'd ever done. "He got aggressive, talking about Nancy, and I stood up to leave and said, 'Fine. If that's your point of view, I'm leaving.'" Strofolino called her back and tried to be conciliatory, but wouldn't agree to her requests for an investigation. Strofolino also met with Durie and Chan. The CEO stood occasionally and banged his fist on the table for emphasis. He was such a big man, and Chan was so petite, that he towered over her when he was standing. Durie said he felt as if they were with a bully.

Reporters who had copies of the Gang's petition described it in the press, and that deepened the divisions at the hospital. Apparently some of the signers hadn't known that individuals outside of Sick Kids would see their signatures. Strofolino described the incident afterwards: "Physicians at the hospital were asked to sign a letter addressed to Dr. Buchwald in support of research integrity. Then it was leaked to the press and many people felt absolutely betrayed." He added, "It would have taken courage for them to say, 'Please sign this and this is going to the press,' but they didn't say that."

Now the other side began to solicit signatures on its own petitions. A week after Olivieri's article came out, a dozen heads of research programs at the hospital signed a letter to Pitblado expressing confidence in Buchwald and Strofolino. A few days later, thirteen men and women who were the chiefs of the hospital's clinical divisions signed a similar vote of confidence in the hospital's leadership that also went to Pitblado as chair of the board.

The Gang asked to meet with Pitblado and other board members; the board declined their requests. Journalists accepted their invitations, however. Olivieri and her team scheduled frequent press conferences at the Delta Chelsea Inn, the hotel closest to the hospital. From the podium they announced that board members were refusing to meet with them, that the hospital was refusing to order an independent investigation of what had happened and that Olivieri was being harassed. They gave out copies of press clippings and lists of individuals the media could contact, complete with short biographical sketches and phone numbers. Often the individuals on their lists were on hand to meet with journalists. "Experts from other Canadian cities flew in to demand an independent inquiry," the *Globe and Mail* reported after one news conference.

Arthur Schafer was one of those who had flown in. He told reporters the case was being watched closely. "If this can happen to Nancy Olivieri, it can happen to any physician or researcher in Canada," he said. He'd written an op-ed for the *Globe and Mail* describing the harassment Olivieri had experienced, and was particularly incensed that she was offered a medical leave of absence. "Was that not harassment?" he asked in his article. Apparently he didn't know that Olivieri had written to O'Brodovich saying she was taking "a medical leave of absence." Schafer also didn't understand that it was the Gang of Four who had originally suggested the medical leave, out of concern for Olivieri's mental health.

Brill-Edwards also knew the importance of standing up publicly for a whistleblower. She later told me, "When you're being threatened—and I know this through long experience—the worst thing you can do is complain privately. Because then, they really come after you . . . The advice in the inner circles is 'Seek centre stage.' In other words, once the spotlight is on you, they're not likely to try and break your legs." It was the same lesson that Drummond Rennie had learned, and now the spotlight was on Olivieri. Her supporters helped keep it there by writing about her for the op-ed and correspondence pages of the country's newspapers. Brill-Edwards wrote a letter to the editor of the *Globe and Mail* soon after the story broke, calling for a change in leadership at Sick Kids.

Olivieri kept her focus on patient safety. "If I can't protect patients at the Hospital for Sick Children, I don't see how any one of us can continue with assurance," she said at one news conference. But others signed on to her cause because it involved academic freedom. They included a Nobel Prize winner, University of Toronto chemistry professor John Polanyi, and another senior scientist at the university, geneticist Margaret Thompson.

At one press conference, Brenda Gallie threatened to leave Sick Kids. She announced that she and Helen Chan had been funded by the NIH to carry out a $1.5 million clinical trial of treatments for retinoblastoma but would take the study to a different hospital if Sick Kids didn't hold an independent investigation of the Olivieri-Apotex affair. Chan chimed in, "If we are going to be leading the world in this trial, we want it to be in a place where there is openness and trust."

Nearly a week after the media started calling, the administration finally began a lame attempt to respond. Hospital vice-president Dr.

Alan Goldbloom rebutted Olivieri's charges by saying she and her supporters didn't go through proper channels. For example, they hadn't filed complaints with the Research Ethics Board or the Patient Care Committee. "When you have all those processes in place and nobody accesses them, that's a concern to us," Goldbloom told the *Medical Post*. The hospital announced its intention to conduct an external review of its "policies and procedures surrounding clinical trials and third party funding." But the review wasn't going to deal specifically with the Olivieri-Apotex case. Neither explanation calmed the furor.

At the end of August, with press coverage intensifying, the hospital relented and announced that it was appointing Arnold Naimark, former dean of medicine and former president of the University of Manitoba, to conduct an independent investigation of the Apotex-Olivieri dispute. "One doesn't react in a knee-jerk fashion," Pitblado told the *Globe and Mail* in an attempt to explain the hospital's delay. The *Globe*'s respected columnist and reporter Michael Valpy reported that U of T president Rob Prichard and a former president of the university, John Evans, allied with members of the Hospital for Sick Children Foundation board, had pressured Pitblado to overrule Strofolino and call for an investigation. But the call for a review didn't dampen the intense interest in the story.

In early September, the Olivieri affair was a staple item in Toronto newscasts and was also attracting international attention. *Business Week*'s Joseph Weber came to Toronto to report on the case. "Between Olivieri and Apotex, the vitriol is flowing both ways," he wrote. At the science journal *Nature Medicine,* the story got coverage both in the science news pages and in editorials supporting Olivieri. *New York Times* medical reporter Gina Kolata also flew to town. She and *New York Times* business reporter Kurt Eichenwald were completing a series of articles on conflicts of interest in drug research and wanted to include the Olivieri-Apotex controversy.

But when their series ran in May 1999, the information Kolata gathered on the L1 research didn't appear. In the end, Kolata said she and her editors decided "the issues were clearer" in some of the other stories she was following.

For journalists in Toronto, though, the issues were impossible to ignore, even if they were unclear. Pitblado's announcement of an investigation had provided further fuel for the conflict. Olivieri and her supporters told the press that Naimark was the wrong choice to head up the investigation since Apotex and its financial subsidiaries had been donors to his university: at some point during his fifteen years as president there, the company had given the university $120,000. In any case, she didn't think it should be up to the hospital board to choose the person to lead the investigation. She and the Gang wanted to have a say.

Naimark wrote Olivieri the second week in September to say that his "first priority" was to meet with her, but he received no response. A week later he wrote her again to say that he remained eager to meet and that he would be "particularly grateful for any material you can provide regarding threats or intimidation." Again he didn't hear back. Finally, he met with the Gang of Four in a session he later described as a "group meeting to discuss structure of the Review," but Olivieri didn't attend. According to Naimark, he told the Gang that he was "particularly interested in learning about issues of harassment, threats, or what have you—sometimes they can be quite subtle or implied." But the meeting "to discuss structure" would be the only one they would attend. They didn't share information with him because they thought he would be biased.

Instead, they wanted reviewers "with relevant expertise" whom they would help to select. They submitted a short list of acceptable reviewers, led by a woman Olivieri thought she could trust: Patricia Baird, the pediatrician who chaired medical genetics at the University of British Columbia. Well known to many Canadian doctors for her extensive record of public service, including heading a royal commission, Baird had been outspoken about the need for universities to ensure that research done on campus was in the public interest. Naimark offered her the chance to assist him, but she turned him down, saying she needed to be assured of being able to add her own separate section to the report if she disagreed with its conclusions. When Pitblado objected to her conditions, Naimark offered her the chance to annotate the report instead, but she objected that annotations "would not provide her with appropriate independence."

At that point, the head of the Medical Research Council came to Toronto for a weekend to try to mediate between Olivieri's side and the hospital administration, but he too accomplished little. Brenda Gallie was on a family holiday in the Himalayas and said later that things had fallen apart because she wasn't there. Peter Durie said the hospital administration had resorted to intimidation to try to prevent the Gang's supporters from arguing in favour of including individuals chosen "by consultation between the parties," as the Gang and Olivieri had asked. For Naimark, the result was that neither the whistleblower nor any of her closest supporters agreed to be interviewed.

The Sick Kids press office was on overload, coping with the Olivieri crisis as well as with the hospital's daily events. Public affairs chief Cyndy De Giusti began looking for an outside consultant. The hospital eventually brought in Patrick Gossage, who had once been Pierre Trudeau's press secretary, but Olivieri continued to win the battle for the public's hearts and minds.

Every act against her or for her became news. She tried to attend a meeting Strofolino was holding, and let journalists know she'd been "told—and forced—by Mr. Strofolino to leave the meeting." In early October, Nathan and Weatherall wrote the hospital's board of trustees to say that the hospital's investigation was inadequate; Valpy, who was now covering the story for the women's magazine *Elm Street* as well as for the *Globe,* got an inside scoop about the letter and revealed it in the paper. Toronto journalists saw a whistleblower threatened by a corporation for trying to protect her patients, and they couldn't understand why hospital or university leaders wouldn't agree to at least some of Olivieri's demands. In late October, the *Toronto Star* said in an editorial that the hospital's reputation was "being savaged" and called on hospital leaders to "reassure the most skeptical audience of all—the parents."

Olivieri's patients—and their parents—had lived through the story and had mixed opinions as they watched it go public. Some were willing to vouch for Olivieri—and for Sick Kids. "I have faith in them there. They do everything," the mother of a nine-year-old thalassemia patient told me when I contacted her for CBC Radio. Her daughter had never been offered L1, but she explained that she trusted Olivieri. "She says Desferal, I go with Desferal." Another mother felt similarly toward the doctor and the hospital. She wrote the *Toronto Star,* "We had faith that Dr. Olivieri and the Hospital for Sick Children would always act in the best interests of the patients."

Howard wasn't sure what to make of it. He knew Olivieri was enjoying the attention. "I think the media stuff is an incredible rush for her," he said of his favourite doctor. "She wants her name out there. She likes the fame. She likes her name in the paper, her picture on TV, her voice on the radio."

The Thalassemia Foundation of Canada voted on "whether to take a stance in support of Nancy or no stance and stay neutral," as Howard put it. They took no stance, and Olivieri responded by severing her ties with the organization. Its leaders continued to call to invite her to their meetings, but the only replies they received were messages from Olivieri's secretary to say she wouldn't be attending.

Josie had completed her master's degree in biochemistry and was working in a lab at the University of Ottawa when the story broke. She was disturbed that what she heard on the radio didn't match what she knew, and she sent Howard a quick e-mail. "It seems that the press is picking up the story. . . . Does the Foundation want to have a 'patient' opinion on it? . . . I don't want the patient voice to be lost." They agreed that she would contact CBC Radio.

Olivieri "avoided her patients while she fought this battle," Josie wrote in her e-mail to the CBC. "Her own patients (myself included) openly spoke to others in the worldwide thalassemia community and to physicians about the lack of communication and poor treatment we were receiving. . . ." When I replied, Josie explained what she thought she'd seen happen with L1. "There was this clash, this personality clash," she said.

Colleagues who had worked alongside Olivieri for years seethed over the growing gap between the person they felt they knew and the woman they were reading about in the papers. They especially bristled at the unfamiliar descriptions of familiar events—events they had lived through. Each time an episode was described in the media differently from how it had actually played out, the division between Olivieri's supporters and her detractors grew wider.

In hematology, several doctors had heard that O'Brodovich had offered Olivieri a medical leave because Gallie and Durie had asked him to, yet now the press was reporting that his offer of a leave was the hospital's attempt to ease her out of a job. One doctor was infuriated by it. "I cannot begin to explain to you what it felt like to see this stuff in the papers day after day, and see her on TV as this angel of mercy with patients, and then to see the distortions that appeared," said the doctor. "It was terrible." Referring to Olivieri's personnel file and the complaints from her co-workers that had accumulated there, the doctor added, "Every day you said to yourself, 'The hospital will do something about this. They'll put it in a context of the twelve years of letters.' But it never happened." The doctor was incensed that neither the

Gang nor Olivieri was doing anything to correct the media's mis-interpretation of events.

In an interview, Olivieri described the coverage she was getting in the Toronto papers and on the city's airwaves as "this whole media trip and hype." But most of the "hype" was favourable, and in November 1998 she made the cover of two Toronto-based maga-zines: *Elm Street* and the newsweekly *Maclean's*. The headline in *Maclean's* was simply, "Whistleblower." The hospital administration knew the piece was coming, and several of Olivieri's critics had spo-ken "off the record" to *Maclean's* writer Jane O'Hara, but O'Hara thought their confidences were slander.

"In a display of the lengths Olivieri's critics will go to blacken her name, three people telephoned *Maclean's* last week to complain about her character," she wrote. "One man from within the hospital accused her of stealing money from her research grant, treating her patients unethically, and sleeping with some of the scientists who looked favourably on her research findings."

Olivieri told me later, "Jane O'Hara says you'd have to be braindead not to figure out who's telling the truth here." But when the *Maclean's* article appeared in November, there were several different versions of "the truth" circulating. According to *Maclean's,* Olivieri had been testing L1 as a "promising new drug" until 1995, when she looked at liver biopsies from her patients and "became alarmed" because the iron in some samples was so high. "Disappointed, Olivieri tried to call off the trials," O'Hara wrote. But that wasn't what had happened—Olivieri hadn't wanted to stop her trials. The report in *Maclean's* was similar to the story circulating among U.S. hematologists.

Elm Street had asked Valpy to profile Olivieri, and in his article he described her as "eccentric and wickedly funny." He'd spoken to a close colleague of hers who said she had "spells" where she exploded in anger and "intemperate language," but he hadn't seen that behaviour.

For *Elm Street*'s cover shot, Olivieri posed as a beauty queen in a hospital room. In a tight-fitting black turtleneck with bauble earrings, bright red lipstick, dark eyeliner and her stethoscope strewn around her neck, she looked less a scientist than a film star on the set of a hospital drama. Inside the magazine were further photos, with Helen Chan and Brenda Gallie looking like the attractive middle-aged doctors and scientists they were and Nancy Olivieri looking like a glamour queen with sex appeal.

Later, Valpy and Olivieri admitted to seeing each other on a romantic basis. Olivieri said that their relationship began after Valpy had stopped reporting on her, but some people he interviewed that fall were convinced he'd already had feelings for her when they spoke to him. Said a senior source for his story, "He shouldn't have been writing on it. He was so emotionally involved in it." Gwen Smith, the editor who oversaw the *Elm Street* profile, stood by what she called "Michael Valpy's superb article about this controversy," but Olivieri's supporters worried that she'd gone too far.

"The cover on *Elm Street*," one woman spat out in disgust when we met a few weeks after the magazine appeared on Toronto newsstands. She'd spoken on behalf of Olivieri at Sick Kids and now felt betrayed. "Because of the manner in which the media has covered this, people have lost sight of the principles," she said. Olivieri had become a *cause célèbre,* with the main point in the media being that she was a beauty and a heroine who worked for an institution that treated people terribly. Academic freedom and protecting patients—the principles that had motivated a groundswell of support for her at the hospital and the university—didn't make for photo opportunities.

And just as her supporters were wondering what had happened to the fight for principles, reporters discovered that Olivieri had a media manager. Up until that point, Langlois's existence and extensive advice had eluded the media, or they'd been kind enough not

to mention it. But now there was a brand-new paper in town looking for different angles on the story. Launched in Toronto at the end
of October 1998, the *National Post* intended to be a national paper.
Its founder, Conrad Black, was a major donor to the Hospital for
Sick Children, and the paper's reporters seemed determined to
present another side to the Olivieri controversy. The paper published a series of e-mail notes that had gone back and forth between
Olivieri and Langlois, including his specific coaching about which
reporters she should stay in touch with.

Olivieri was shocked to see her personal e-mails in the paper.
Forced to defend herself, she told her supporters that the basic elements of her story were unchanged. The company had threatened
her, she'd blown the whistle and the hospital hadn't come to her aid.
She couldn't fight them unless she knew how to be effective in the
media. Still, a woman running a media campaign was a different
concept from a woman blowing a whistle and being harassed for it.

All of the Gang's focus was on fighting the hospital, but that was
proving expensive. Olivieri was now paying for legal advice, and she
also had to cover the costs of the public relations effort, with its
rented hotel conference rooms, its multiple mailings, its phone, fax
and transportation bills. That fall, Gallie and Chan mortgaged their
homes to help pay the bills. John Dick, who still had young children
at home, told them he couldn't be involved at that level because he
didn't have the money to do it, and Olivieri began looking for extra
help. In November she found it at the University of Toronto Faculty
Association—the faculty members' union.

The union was housed in three rooms on Spadina Avenue, the
boulevard that marks the university's western border. Its annual
budget was about $1 million, derived from mandatory dues paid by
faculty members and librarians. The funds paid for three staff
lawyers as well as a high-priced Toronto firm that was kept on
retainer. Medical school professors weren't officially union members,

but in this case union leaders made an exception and quickly voted to give Olivieri and the Gang membership status. The Olivieri dispute involved corporate influence, an issue that mattered deeply to William Graham, the philosophy professor who was serving as union president.

Graham had turned the issue into a touchstone for his organization several years earlier. In 1996, the union objected to a $15 million corporate donation to the university's business school, arguing that it would give business leaders unprecedented control. The following year, Graham was equally critical of donations from industry to a U of T centre for international studies ($6 million) and to its centre for telecommunications ($8 million). In the winter of 1998, in a lengthy treatise in the union's newsletter, he urged faculty to remain vigilant about corporate contributions because of the potential for a corporation to "steer" the university's budget priorities. Then came the smoking gun: Nancy Olivieri's fight with Apotex.

Graham believed that Olivieri's case showed that a promised donation from a major Canadian corporation had influenced the university and a university-affiliated hospital with the worst possible results: patients' lives in jeopardy and a scientist harassed. The administrators Olivieri had dealt with hadn't protected her right to academic freedom. "Not only did they not protect it," said Rhonda Love, a social work professor who was the first union official to speak with Olivieri, "they were directly involved in violating it."

Love, an ardent feminist, kept a framed quote in her office from suffragette Nellie McClung, who fought for voting rights for Canadian women at the turn of the century: "Never retreat, never explain, never apologize," read her words on Love's wall. "Get the thing done and let them howl." The union soon threw its counsel and its dollars behind Olivieri and the Gang. "We knew from the beginning that this would be a huge case," Love said.

One of the union's lawyers was assigned to Olivieri's case full-time and began preparing grievances against the university to protest the harassment she and the Gang had suffered. The union also brought in the national organization of faculty associations—the Canadian Association of University Teachers (CAUT)—to help in the battle, since the association represented faculty at sixty universities and the U of T's William Graham was its new president. At its annual meeting in the late fall, the CAUT issued a statement supporting Olivieri and opposing the Naimark Review. "That report should . . . be put on ice immediately," Graham told reporters.

With the union on board, Olivieri shed all the trappings of "a little guy." She had a skilful media coach—the union had hired John Piper, a well-regarded public relations manager, to advise her. She also had widespread public support and legal backing with deep pockets. Her low mood, which had so worried Brenda Gallie in the spring, was gone, and the anxiety and fears she'd complained of over the summer seemed to have dissipated. Olivieri was back in her energetic mode. She hired two prominent Toronto litigators—Clayton Ruby and Beth Symes—to advise her about whether to sue the hospital or Hugh O'Brodovich personally. Ruby was among Toronto's best-known criminal lawyers, famous for his brash style, his many legal successes and his willingness to champion the underdog, while Symes had battled the Hospital for Sick Children successfully many years earlier. As they began to figure out the legal options, Olivieri started another letter-writing campaign. This time her target was the hospital administration.

Buchwald and O'Brodovich had written the editor of *Nature Medicine* after the journal published an editorial supporting Olivieri. Now Olivieri wrote the hospital board demanding that the two men withdraw their letter. She also wanted Strofolino to draft an apology "for wrongly excluding Dr. Gallie and myself" from the meeting they'd tried to attend. In a move that evoked her earlier letter to

O'Brodovich, she gave the CEO a deadline. She told Strofolino his apology was to "be hand-delivered to the offices of Dr. Gallie et al. (Drs. Durie, Chan, Gallie and Olivieri) by 17:00 hours, Oct. 30, 1998."

Though Olivieri remained firmly on the offensive against her institutions and against L1, the drug was rapidly becoming an established part of thalassemia treatment in Europe at the hospitals where clinical trials were in progress. "The drug is not at all controversial in England, Italy or India," Beatrix Wonke told the *National Post* in early December. Instead, among thalassemia researchers worldwide, there was a controversy over Nancy Olivieri's research that became public in December 1998 when the *New England Journal of Medicine* published a series of letters criticizing her study.

The most serious charge came from doctors at Cornell University Medical Center in New York who had been experimenting with L1 since the early 1990s. They objected to Olivieri's analysis being based on figures calculated by averaging all her patients together, instead of analyzing the experience of each patient over time. When they analyzed each patient separately, they got a different result: L1 appeared to be effective. "Olivieri et al. collected a lot of data during their seven-year study but included only selected values in their analyses," the Cornell doctors wrote in their letter to the editor. The implication was that the results could have been skewed.

It was the same thing Peter Scheuer had been afraid of when he compared the original data set Olivieri sent him to the results in her final draft. He thought she had selected data points that bolstered her case and omitted others. "This happens all the time, it's not something terrible," Scheuer said, but the Cornell doctors saw it differently. "All available data should have been presented," they wrote, "so that the effect of any deviations could be assessed." Olivieri's response to her critics, written with Brittenham,

Templeton and Fleming, warned about "the long-term lack of effi
cacy of the drug in many or most patients," but they didn't address
the charge that they had only reported selected values.

Alan Cohen, who was still testing L1 at the Children's Hospital
of Philadelphia, wrote to the journal that, according to his results,
L1 was useful as a second-line treatment. "In instances in which
strong and repeated efforts by staff members to improve patients'
compliance with deferoxamine [Desferal] therapy fail, it seems reasonable to be able to offer these patients the chance to stabilize or
to reduce iron stores with [L1]"—if they couldn't inject Desferal,
L1 was worth trying.

But Olivieri disagreed. Her battle with Apotex had wholly
transformed her views of the difficulties patients faced on the
injection-only drug. "To our knowledge, the total number of children who are unable to use the standard iron-chelating agent,
[Desferal], in North America and Italy combined is less than a
dozen," she wrote with Brittenham, Fleming and Templeton in her
response to the correspondence in the *New England Journal of
Medicine*. She was no longer pleading for children such as Duri-Sadaf
Ali, the six-year-old who would lose access to L1 if she returned to
the U.S. She was no longer pleading for young people whose failure
to take Desferal caused them to get sicker or even die, such as
Howard, Biagio and Alex.

Michael Spino also argued with Olivieri in the *New England
Journal of Medicine,* but North America and its medical journals
weren't his primary focus any more. Apotex was concentrating
most of its L1 efforts on Europe. In Italy, more than six hundred
patients were taking the pills as part of a "controlled use program."
"The Ministry of Health in Italy monitors it," Spino explained when
we spoke. "It's a government-run protocol, and they want to extend
it." There was more good news for Apotex: none of the European
L1 researchers had found the problem of progressive liver scarring

that Olivieri had described, despite their extensive experience with the drug. Petrin Töndury, a hematologist in Switzerland, had patients who'd been on L1 for eight years. "There's been excellent progress in his patients," Spino said, and Töndury later confirmed it. He said in an interview that after hearing about Olivieri's findings, he quickly referred all of his thalassemia patients for biopsies; the liver pathologist at his hospital found no evidence of scarring.

Given the positive reports, Apotex had submitted its L1 files to the European Union's drug agency. If approved, L1 would become available as an option to thalassemia patients across Europe. Olivieri was working to prevent that from happening, crusading against the drug by collecting reports of its toxicity from around the world. When I interviewed her in November 1998, she said an Australian colleague had seen liver scarring in an L1 patient. She was also tracking a case of lung scarring in St. Louis, Missouri, where, she'd heard, "a kid who went on L1 . . . developed progressive and severe pulmonary fibrosis," and she was keeping tabs on one of the Toronto L1 patients, who had developed serious heart disease.

Her patient with heart disease was Michael, a young man in his early twenties who had taken L1 for four years as part of the randomized trial comparing L1 with Desferal. In the winter of 1998, he came into the clinic complaining of severe fatigue and turned out to be in serious heart failure. Heart disease was still the big killer for young thalassemia patients; usually it was caused by a buildup of iron in their hearts. But in this case, Olivieri thought the culprit was L1. To prove it, she wanted Michael to have a procedure rarely done on a thalassemia patient: a biopsy of the heart. It was a risky, invasive test, but the doctors needed it to determine whether his symptoms were due to iron overload or drug toxicity.

Once she had the heart biopsy slides, Olivieri asked a pathologist at the Toronto General to take them to Boston, and she paid for the plane ticket herself; she wanted to have the slides specially analyzed by pathologists at the Brigham and Women's Hospital. At the Brigham, she said they found widespread fibrosis—stiff, scarred areas that would make it difficult for the heart to pump blood effectively to the rest of the body.

To Olivieri, the case proved that L1 could scar the heart, just as she believed it could scar the liver. "We don't usually do cardiac biopsies, but we were concerned about the results that had . . . shown up in animals in a compound directly related to L1," she explained in an interview for CBC Radio's *Quirks and Quarks*. "So we did a biopsy and there were sheets of fibrosis everywhere— this heart was very fibrotic." In November, she told *Maclean's* that the young man's severe heart problems were "a direct result" of L1. It wasn't clear how long he would survive. Olivieri planned to present his case—and his biopsy results—at the American Society of Hematology meeting in December, where she would argue that L1 trials in humans should be stopped and replaced by further testing in animals.

As she flew to Orlando for ASH, Arnold Naimark was completing his review. He'd interviewed more than forty people at Sick Kids, the Toronto General, the university and Apotex. Along with two professors of ethics who were helping him, he'd read through nearly five hundred pieces of correspondence, including many of the letters that Olivieri had sent in her various letter-writing campaigns, and he'd received other documents as well. Sick Kids administrators had written or called Olivieri's former residents, asking them to describe their recollections of the time they'd spent with her. If the former residents provided the information to the hospital, Sick Kids got it to Naimark.

Olivieri knew about these efforts. She'd heard about them from one of her former clinical assistants, who got a letter requesting information. When I interviewed Olivieri that fall, she described it as a "letter requesting the negative things about me." She assumed that at least some of those whom the hospital approached would respond. In addition, Naimark was speaking to staff doctors at Sick Kids who knew some of "the negative things," including her former division heads, Mel Freedman and Mark Greenberg, and her former chair, Bob Haslam.

Olivieri objected loudly and continually to Naimark. "There is no formal way of minuting or recording this inquiry," she said when we spoke in November. "Dr. Naimark has chosen to speak to who he's chosen to speak to . . . so this is a unilateral review, and we know exactly what that will show." One of the things it could show was that Nancy Olivieri had a long-standing reputation as a hot-tempered doctor whose residents, nurses and secretaries complained about her. That wouldn't excuse Apotex for stopping her studies, harassing her with legal threats and prohibiting her from telling patients about her findings, but Olivieri may not have wanted to take that chance.

At ASH she described the case of Michael, the young man in heart failure. It was a poster presentation, and its conclusion was stark: Michael had taken L1 and developed severe heart failure, leading to a biopsy the showed scarring of the heart. The poster implied that L1 could be toxic to the heart in a way that was fatal, and the published abstract concluded, "Deaths from cardiac causes have been reported in patients treated with [L1] for up to 2 years."

To scientists and journalists who read the poster, it was clear why Olivieri was on the warpath against L1: the drug was killing patients. But to a Toronto thalassemia patient who was good friends with the twenty-three-year-old Michael and had visited him every day when he was in the hospital, Olivieri's poster came as a surprise. The patient called Michael as soon as he got home from Florida. "You won't believe what I read about you at the meeting," he began when Michael came to the phone. A reporter who'd attended ASH for the *Medical Post* wrote of "the patient's death," and

Michael Valpy, who was continuing to follow the story for the *Globe and Mail*, had also assumed there was an actual death. He had written in an article in November that L1 "may have been involved in the recent death of an adult patient at the Toronto Hospital"; a week later, the *Globe* had to retract the claim.

Some of Nancy Olivieri's colleagues and supporters knew that her concerns about L1 caused her to cast it in the worst possible light. "She was treated so shabbily that she's convinced it's all shabby and the public's being bamboozled," David Nathan explained in the fall of 1998. He wanted her to go back to research full-time, but he didn't expect it to happen. "I'd love her to drop this," he said. "But when you beat up on a child, you shouldn't be surprised if they turn into gangsters." Others also saw it as Nathan did: Olivieri had been abused. In the face of that, anyone who criticized her could be seen as having joined her abusers.

South of the border, the Ryan Commission had argued in 1995 that whistleblowing scientists had rights but also duties. He or she "must respect the confidentiality of sensitive information . . . give legitimate institutional structures an opportunity to function . . . raise . . . concerns honorably and with foundation." If the institution had provided fair and objective procedures, whistleblowers must "participate honorably in such procedures by respecting the serious consequences for those they accuse of misconduct." Organized science groups in the U.S. had shot back that some so-called whistleblowers were no more than accusers of their colleagues. But in Canada, that sort of discussion and debate hadn't happened yet.

THE WAR OF WORDS

In early October 1998, Nancy Olivieri and the Gang of Four planned to attend a meeting of the hospital's staff association in order to get more help from their Sick Kids colleagues. Peter Durie asked the other members of the Gang of Four to all be at the meeting because the association was scheduled to vote on a motion backing their request to help choose the reviewers who would assist Arnold Naimark. Before leaving home that day, John Dick went to close the skylight at his house but couldn't manoeuvre the window. He tried to tell his wife what was happening, but what came out was gibberish. She soon discovered that he couldn't move his right hand. He was rushed to the hospital—a man in his early forties in the midst of his first stroke.

After recovering from the stroke, Dick developed heartburn that he ascribed to stress. He told his colleagues he was depressed. His work lagged behind his expectations. Later, ethicist Françoise Baylis wrote in a journal article that Dick was reluctant to hire new staff because he considered his lab a suboptimal work environment. "Without new staff, the research team could not move its initial discovery forward, and others have since filled the vacuum," Baylis wrote in the *Journal of Medical Ethics* in 2003.

Helen Chan said of Dick, "He feels things more than us." A scientist who worked with him thought Dick had trouble assimilating his initial take on the Olivieri-Apotex dispute with everything he began hearing once the scandal became public. "John Dick . . . just doesn't believe the world's that complicated, that people have multiple motives," said the scientist. A physician who knew him from the hospital put it more simply: "John Dick—what a swell guy, just the nicest guy—he just got chewed up by this."

Brenda Gallie was getting chewed up too, but in a different way. Her professional reputation was suffering. She'd claimed Olivieri's battle as her own for months. She feared that if she didn't, things might go wrong. Yet as she gave hours to the Gang, she was giving short shrift to her other responsibilities as a division head. Her boss, Manuel Buchwald, had begun complaining about it. Buchwald and Gallie were both molecular biologists, and they'd known each other for twenty years. They didn't collaborate, but they attended the same meetings and understood the importance of one another's work. As research chief, Buchwald promoted Gallie early on. Now, under the weight of the Olivieri affair, their relationship began to crumble.

In August 1998, Buchwald told Gallie that the choices she'd been making were "not in keeping with the leadership position" she held. Then, in November, the *Maclean's* article appeared, with Gallie quoted as saying that the hospital's leadership had "all gone corporate" and that there was no academic voice left "except for the rebels who finally get annoyed enough to do something about it." It was against unwritten rules for a division head to criticize her chief in public—at any hospital or university that was a sin that could not be forgiven—and Buchwald felt personally attacked. He wrote Gallie, "If by some psychological sleight of hand you can exclude yourself from the leadership and believe that it is only the others who lack integrity, then how can we continue to work with you?"

Gallie was caught off guard. It was as if she hadn't thought of how her words in the magazine would sound to her close colleagues. "I am proud to be part of the leadership team at The Hospital for Sick Children and . . . have sought to treat my colleagues, staff and patients with respect and dignity," she replied. "I very much regret if others have misinterpreted my actions."

A few weeks later, Buchwald told her she wasn't performing her job to the level expected, and he put his criticisms in writing. Since she felt compelled "to denigrate this institution and its leadership," he wrote to her, she couldn't be part of its leadership. She didn't proffer her resignation. Instead, she told him she wouldn't discuss her performance without her lawyer present. She'd begun to see his letters as one more form of harassment. When I spoke to her that month, she said she was facing "tremendous persecution" from her peers. Olivieri felt the same way; she was convinced that she was under surveillance, even in her own office. Receiving calls there in November and December, she would answer routinely, "Can't talk, bad phone, call you later, they're bugged."

At this juncture, Sick Kids announced that Arnold Naimark had completed his investigation. His report, titled *A Review of Facts and Circumstances*, was over 150 pages long. The hospital unveiled it at a news conference and planned to post it on its website.

Naimark had gone through all the correspondence and other documents he'd been given. He'd concluded that Sick Kids had weak policies that had allowed Koren and Olivieri to sign an overly restrictive contract with Apotex, and he found that hospital leaders failed to give Olivieri the moral support she deserved. He didn't accuse them of failing to give her legal support—"The question of whether she asked for and was refused legal assistance is still open," he said—and he didn't view the hospital as having a potential conflict of interest because of the monies Sherman had offered the U of T.

He saved his worst condemnations for Olivieri. In his research, Naimark had unearthed the debates that revolved around so many of her claims. Olivieri had alleged that the hospital and the company had done things that placed the thalassemia patients at risk; Naimark described things Olivieri had done that could have harmed the patients. The report states that she had continued to treat patients with L1 for months after saying at ASH that it was a dangerous drug. Naimark also found that she'd waited before telling the Research Ethics Board that it was dangerous. To Naimark, these were serious failings on Olivieri's part.

His report compared the ethics board to a security system, designed to detect problems that arise in research, such as toxic drugs. "There appeared to have been a lapse in the security," he said of Olivieri's waiting to tell the ethics board. "It's like leaving home and forgetting to turn on the alarm."

Naimark didn't know about the early years of Olivieri's research on L1, when she waited before writing the ethics board to say that L1 researchers elsewhere had discovered new risks of the drug. Now, nearly eight years later, Naimark essentially charged her with failing to report to the ethics board that she'd discovered a "serious adverse reaction" involving L1—the reaction of liver scarring. As Michael Valpy wrote in his column in the *Globe* the next day, it was "the most damning statement in the 153-page report."

Though Naimark told reporters that he was "not exonerating the hospital of anything," executives at Sick Kids saw it differently. In the wake of the report, the hospital issued a statement admitting it had made mistakes and apologizing for not supporting Olivieri in her struggle with the company. Strofolino said it was "time to heal" and "to move on." But he didn't really mean it; even as he spoke, the hospital was assigning a staff committee, including doctors, ethicists and nurses, to investigate Olivieri's actions—as detailed by Naimark—and to consider disciplinary measures against her if required.

Sick Kids public affairs staff weren't ready to move on either. They planned to point out the many discrepancies between what

Naimark found and what Olivieri had been telling people, and they'd gone so far as to prepare a three-page document titled "Media Myths Compared with Review Findings," which they handed out to reporters. Under quotations from Olivieri, Durie and Gallie, they listed the review's findings. There was the disputed charge about the hospital's refusal to give her legal assistance: "Dr. Olivieri said she asked the administration to hire a lawyer on her behalf, but her request was refused" was how it had been reported in the *Globe and Mail*. Sick Kids paired it with Naimark's finding: "That legal counsel had been engaged and 'was on the case' was evident as early as June 4, 1996 when Dean Aberman met with Dr. Olivieri and her lawyer."

In response to Naimark's claims, the Gang called three back-to-back press conferences at a downtown hotel. "A defiant Dr. Nancy Olivieri has delivered a scathing indictment of an investigation into her conflict with a drug company and vowed to dig in her heels in the ongoing battle," the *Toronto Star* reported. Olivieri said the review was "fundamentally flawed" and "openly . . . biased." She said she'd notified patients within a week of discovering that L1 had dangerous side effects. "Naimark knew exactly what to say," she told me. "He presented the hospital with a great big Christmas present of exactly what they wanted, and the board took it, opened it and were very happy."

Arthur Schafer told reporters that the Olivieri affair was "without doubt the greatest academic scandal of our time," and criticized the Naimark report for leaving questions unanswered. "Were our children put at risk?" Schafer asked. "Can this happen again? Is this hospital a safe place for our kids?"

Olivieri's close supporters thought Naimark's allegations about Olivieri were based on misinformation or worse. Peter Durie thought hospital leaders had predetermined Naimark's findings by "sort of saying, 'You have to find evidence of X, Y and Z,' and instructing Naimark to find Nancy guilty of it." Though Olivieri and the Gang had refused to talk to Naimark, Durie had a long list of people he thought the reviewers should have contacted to get the full story. Gallie said of Naimark, "He intended a whitewash." Helen Chan described herself as "disillusioned."

Chan said she'd watched the hospital administration persecute Olivieri and that had opened her eyes. Now came the Naimark Review, with its claims that Olivieri was the one who had made mistakes. Chan, who was so obsessive about her own research, began to think that Naimark had been given fraudulent data that made it look as if Olivieri was guilty of wrongdoing when she wasn't. To Olivieri and the Gang, the hospital's decision to refer her for possible disciplinary action was one more episode of harassment. It was retaliation against a whistleblower, and they were determined to fight back. The result for Sick Kids staff was that an independent review intended to settle the controversy had "caused more divisiveness in this institution and made it an even more unpleasant place to be," according to one Olivieri supporter, Dr. Jeff Smallwood.

Olivieri's lawyers—Ruby and Symes—held a press conference and announced that her patients were in jeopardy because her bosses at Sick Kids had cut back on the hours of her clinical assistants. It was the old sawhorse issue of clinical resources, the debate Olivieri had been having with Hugh O'Brodovich for two years. But Clayton Ruby took it a step further, suggesting that the hospital's unwillingness to hire more staff for Olivieri's clinics was a racist move. He let reporters know that the "children at risk" included 350 sickle cell patients, "most of whom are black with sole-support mothers," and 100 thalassemia patients, "none of northern European ancestry." It reminded me of my earliest interviews with Nancy Olivieri, when she hinted that one reason the hospital didn't support her was that thalassemia was "not a white disease."

The words cut like sharp knives for Sick Kids doctors. There were many valid criticisms one could make of Sick Kids, but at Canada's busiest children's hospital in the country's most ethnically diverse city, racism probably wasn't among them. The racism claim especially bothered the chief, Hugh O'Brodovich, who prided himself on having hired and promoted members of visible minorities during his brief tenure. As the public charge of racism by her lawyers made the rounds, Olivieri became a bit more isolated at the hospital.

The Gang tried to calm the waters. Brenda Gallie told me, "Dr. Olivieri pointed out publicly that the children in her program were non-Caucasian, which was interpreted . . . to mean that we were saying the hospital was racist, which was not what was said." Peter Durie told some of the hematologists and oncologists that he didn't agree that the hospital was racist. One of the hematologists replied, "You can't distance yourself from it. You are absolutely involved in it!" And Helen Chan, who was intimately aware of the variety of colours of the hospital's cancer patients, found that her colleagues were disgusted with her.

The following week, O'Brodovich talked to his division chiefs about the problems they were having in dealing with Olivieri's clinical programs. At a hospital as large as Sick Kids, patients often require care from hematologists, cardiologists, endocrinologists and intensivists at the same time. In the interest of their patients, doctors from different services have to communicate. In addition, patients have a protected right to confidentiality: their cases aren't supposed to be discussed with anyone who isn't involved in their care. O'Brodovich told his staff that Nancy Olivieri had stopped following those rules. She refused to speak with a number of Sick Kids doctors, including her division chief and department chair, unless her lawyer was present. She wouldn't even talk about one of her patients if her lawyer wasn't there.

"How can you run a hospital if every time you go to her, you've got to go through Clayton Ruby?" Hugh O'Brodovich asked rhetorically when I interviewed him. From his point of view, running a hospital that way put patients at risk. In addition, he was violating confidentiality by letting Olivieri's lawyers into the hospital's private sanctum. The doctors he spoke to—his division directors—agreed with him that Olivieri's restrictions on whom she would talk to and under what circumstances made it impossible—or at least dangerous—for her to run a clinical program. Without giving Olivieri a chance to respond, they passed a motion recommending that O'Brodovich assign an acting medical director to run the thalassemia and sickle cell clinics. *The Globe and Mail* later obtained notes from the chief's meeting that revealed that the decision to demote Olivieri was, at least in part, a response to her lawyer's charge that the hospital was racist.

For Olivieri, the frequent use of Ruby and other lawyers meant rising legal bills, which the CMPA was no longer covering. The U of T faculty union took on much of the legal work, while William Graham—from the union's parent organization, the CAUT—readied his group for a long battle. He placed calls to David Nathan and David Weatherall as well as to Alan Schechter, a senior hematologist at the National Institutes of Health, to ask questions and let them know that their help might be needed in Toronto. At the same time, the Gang and other Olivieri supporters formed a fundraising organization that they called Doctors for Research Integrity.

In early January 1999, Olivieri found out about the division chiefs' motion. A letter from O'Brodovich told her she was no longer the clinical program director of the thalassemia and sickle cell clinics, though she would retain her faculty position and her hospital salary. Around the same time, she and her supporters received letters from Strofolino's office reminding them of the hospital's bylaws. No one on staff was supposed to communicate with the media without prior approval. From now on, Olivieri and the Gang were supposed to watch what they said.

These were just the sorts of moves the union had been waiting for. Now Olivieri had lost her job, or at least her title. Though the chiefs may have been focused on patient safety, to the union it looked as if Olivieri was being harassed for her whistleblowing and her supporters were being muzzled—standard intimidation tactics. Graham invited the two Davids, along with Schechter from the NIH and British thalassemia expert John Porter of University College Hospital in London, to come to Toronto to conduct an external investigation.

The four men viewed themselves as emissaries to the university, coming on a fact-finding mission at the request of the Canadian Association of University Teachers. Their idea was also to force the university toward awareness that the Olivieri scandal was receiving international attention. Schechter said in an interview that he and the others "agreed that the only thing that would reverse [Olivieri's demotion] was for the university to realize that this was an international case."

Schechter arrived late on a Sunday evening and received a call in his hotel room at midnight. Arnie Aberman was on the other end of the line. "Why are you here?" the dean wanted to know. "Are you trying to undermine the University of Toronto?" Sometimes with Aberman it was hard to know if he was joking. After chatting, the dean offered to meet the next morning. When Schechter got there, Prichard had joined Aberman. The university president had been speaking regularly with Strofolino and had tried to prevent Olivieri's demotion, saying that due process meant she deserved a chance to explain herself. But he'd failed. When Prichard learned that Weatherall and Nathan were in town to investigate the Olivieri affair, the president decided to take matters into his own hands.

Prichard spoke to Aberman's visitors and made a room available for them to proceed with interviews; then he met with the two

Davids and decided that their roles could not be limited to fact-finding. Weatherall and Nathan soon found themselves acting in a play directed by Rob Prichard, who put his other duties on hold to participate in a bit of shuttle diplomacy at his Rosedale home.

Olivieri and the Gang of Four sat in one room, with their legal counsel. In another room sat Hugh O'Brodovich, Manuel Buchwald, Sick Kids lawyer Bill Carter and a few other hospital leaders. Prichard went back and forth, accompanied by the university lawyer as well as Nathan and Weatherall. Prichard was determined to come up with a pact between the two sides. At one point he asked the hospital administrators, "Is there anything you disagree with?" Hugh O'Brodovich replied, "We're drowning in disagreement."

Later in the day, Prichard had a meeting he couldn't miss and assigned Nathan and Weatherall to take over the mediation effort. Nathan listened to criticisms of Olivieri as if he'd heard them all before. He told the hospital leaders at one point, "We know she's difficult and we know she behaves badly." "That's the understatement of the century," replied a member of the Sick Kids administrative team. But Nathan had a plan for controlling relations between Olivieri and her superiors. He intended to assign the problem to Michael Baker, physician in chief at the Toronto Hospital.

In the evening, Prichard returned and resumed the mediator's role. The key figures stayed on into the late hours of the night. It was past 1 a.m. when they finally reached an agreement that both sides were willing to sign. They'd been negotiating continuously for fifteen hours. Clayton Ruby later told reporters that the three-page agreement was a credit to Rob Prichard, who "kept appealing to everyone's better natures."

Olivieri got her clinical job back; she would be directing the programs responsible for the care of about 450 thalassemia and sickle cell patients at Sick Kids and at the Toronto Hospital. Her line of reporting would be directly to Michael Baker. She agreed not to sue anyone at the hospital or the university over any events that had already happened. She got a mini-sabbatical—six weeks off at some point in the near future. And "all letters of discipline and complaint" in her personnel file were nullified.

The hospital agreed not to sue her and promised to pay up to $150,000 toward her legal expenses. For Ruby and Symes, the dollar figure meant they could be certain of being paid. In addition, the hospital would cover Olivieri's costs if Apotex sued her over her claims about L1. The university tried to deal with her complaints that her program's resources were insufficient. "Dean Aberman will provide an additional $45,000 per year for two years" was how the agreement put it. And the hospital withdrew its letter to Olivieri and the Gang telling them not to speak to the media without prior approval.

Some of those who'd been intensely involved were unhappy with the deal. One member of the Gang of Four claimed to have been "forced to sign," adding, "We'd gone through this hell in order to pay our lawyers."

Prichard hoped he'd sealed not only the hostile letters and damaging reports on Olivieri but the entire case. The U of T president had a strong commitment to Sick Kids, and his skilful negotiating was partly an effort to save its reputation. In 1996, his youngest son had been treated there for a malignant brain tumour. At the age of six, the boy lost his ability to walk and talk. He recovered, but only after months on the oncology service at Sick Kids. "It was miraculous," Prichard told reporters later, a miracle that he and his wife attributed to the hospital and its physicians. Just a few days before Nathan and Weatherall showed up on Prichard's doorstep, Canada's governor general was at Sick Kids to officially open a brand new centre for brain tumour research. The effort mattered intensely to Prichard and his family, yet along with everything else that went on at the hospital, it was being overshadowed in the press by the case of Dr. Nancy Olivieri.

Prichard's other major concern was Olivieri herself. He told reporters that the situation had been "very, very stressful and difficult" for her.

The agreement got Olivieri back in the papers. The *Globe* ran its story of the negotiations next to a large photo of Olivieri standing in front of the Hospital for Sick Children with her mittens on, smiling broadly. But the press corps was growing tired of the story. After the agreement made headlines, an editorial in the *Globe and Mail* asked, "Can we stop now with the squabbling and the threatened lawsuits and get back to work? And that includes you too, Dr. Nancy Olivieri."

Olivieri had won her fight with the hospital, but she hadn't agreed to a truce with anyone. She told reporters, "People are saying, 'Oh, Nancy got her job back. It's over.' But my firing is not the point. The point is still the rights and freedoms of researchers and academic freedom." She said that the faculty union had told her, "The story is not over." And it wasn't.

The two sides read the same words in the negotiated agreement but attached different meanings. The agreement said, "As soon as it is reasonably practicable, Dr. Olivieri will relocate her office to the Toronto Hospital from the Hospital for Sick Children." Sick Kids expected that Olivieri would move her primary office to the Toronto General and become part of the hematology team there. But despite the agreement, Olivieri expected to stay at Sick Kids. Her lawyer said that shortly after the agreement was signed, "the Hospital for Sick Children cut off her telephones, her faxes, her pager, and made it impossible for her to care for her patients or to respond to the inquiries of parents and other physicians." In addition, Olivieri complained that she was taken off the on-call rotation at Sick Kids—implying that she thought she would remain a full member of the Sick Kids heme-onc division.

Baker, who was supposed to be in charge of Olivieri, argued with Sick Kids administrators that she deserved more resources there since she was still in charge of clinical programs at the hospital. "Michael tried till he was blue in the face," said one member of the Gang of Four. But Sick Kids had understood that Olivieri would move to the General and refused to allocate the things Baker or Olivieri thought she deserved, such as an office and a telephone line.

Instead, Sick Kids' Medical Advisory Committee was assessing Arnold Naimark's allegations against Olivieri. The committee spent the early winter of 1999 gathering evidence. That spring it asked Olivieri to respond to a series of questions. "Did you continue to provide L1 to patients after you concluded that it was 'toxic'?" was one. From the questions, Olivieri got a sense of the sort of evidence they'd collected. She figured they'd been talking to Gideon Koren and digging up damaging stories about her. Her lawyer requested the "specifics of the allegations," but Olivieri said the committee didn't reveal what information it had.

As time went on, the feeling among the Gang—and their lawyers—was that the agreement Prichard had brokered wasn't working. Olivieri said that none of the concessions the hospital had agreed upon had "come to fruition." In addition, the agreement didn't compensate Olivieri or the members of the Gang for the harassment they'd suffered. Peter Durie and Helen Chan, for example, were both ranked as average or below average in their hospital evaluations, with the result that they received no bonus or only a very small bonus. The union had filed grievances on behalf of Olivieri, Gallie, Durie and Chan early in 1999 and argued successfully that the evaluations were a form of harassment; each of the doctors received a small bonus. But none of the members of the Gang of Four was serving on committees of hospital departments or the Research Institute. Despite their prominence in their fields and their former high-level committee appointments, Sick Kids had marginalized them.

In the summer of 1999, the Gang began pushing for a new agreement. Arnie Aberman had returned to clinical life in the intensive care unit after serving as dean for five years, and the new dean was David Naylor, a Rhodes Scholar and medical specialist who seemed motivated to try to help. The Gang asked Naylor to mediate, and he tried his hand at shuttle diplomacy, using his suite of offices at the medical school building as a base. He assigned Michael Strofolino, Manuel Buchwald, Hugh O'Brodovich and Michael Baker to one room and Nancy Olivieri, Peter Durie, Brenda Gallie and Helen Chan to another. John Dick was signing off from the efforts because he would soon head to England for a sabbatical.

On several occasions over the course of the summer and fall, the doctors and administrators manned their respective stations. Hugh O'Brodovich told colleagues he was living in the dean's conference room that summer and fall. Dick wrote in an e-mail that he understood that the university was "much more involved" now that there was "a new Dean in place." The hospital administration offered a substantial settlement.

The university was soon scrambling to recover from a related scandal, after university president Rob Prichard was found lobbying the federal government to block legislation that was unfavourable to the generic drug industry. The generics industry was largely based in Toronto, while the brand-name companies were mostly in Quebec. Amid reports that proposed changes to the patent laws would wipe out $40 million in investment by the generic companies, Toronto-based cabinet ministers had written to the prime minister or his deputy to protest the changes as unfair to the generics industry. Prichard followed suit, writing to the prime minister to argue against the legislation. When a campus reporter discovered the letter, Prichard admitted that he'd been encouraged in his lobbying efforts by Apotex CEO Barry Sherman, who had told him that if the proposed law passed, it might become impossible for his company's foundation to move ahead on its promised donations to the university. Prichard apologized publicly for writing the letter, but the incident exposed a coziness between the university administration and Apotex in a way that was impossible to ignore.

In the wake of the scandal, the Gang renewed their efforts to negotiate a new agreement with Sick Kids. "It went on forever," said Peter Durie of their negotiations with David Naylor. "It was a window of opportunity, a new dean with no baggage who might have been able to work something out." But Durie thought the hospital's proposal "was ridiculous." Brenda Gallie described the agreement they'd been asked to sign as "drafted to persecute us," and Nancy Olivieri said it was "a very, very flawed agreement."

They developed a plan, and they wanted the dean to pressure the hospital to accept their proposal. The affiliation agreement between the medical school and Sick Kids was coming up for renewal, and the Gang suggested that the dean could refuse to sign it. The idea was unprecedented. Ending the hospital's affiliation with the university would essentially interrupt training for all budding pediatricians and pediatric specialists at the University of Toronto, Canada's largest medical school. The loss of the residents—even temporarily—could create massive disruptions for patients, because Sick Kids relies heavily on residents to provide front-line care. The Gang called it "the atomic bomb." The dean told them he would "never do that." The medical school and the Hospital for Sick Children renewed their affiliation on schedule, and the window Peter Durie had sensed passed without the two sides reaching an agreement.

To the Sick Kids administration, it looked as if organizations outside the hospital were milking the Olivieri affair for its political value and didn't want an agreement. "Outside forces need this case to push their agenda about drug-industry funding of research," Michael Strofolino said in an interview later. "Their agenda is

'Involvement with private industry is bad; research should be free.'"
There was little question what "outside forces" he was referring to.

At the union, "corporate influence" remained a major issue, and
Nancy Olivieri was the headline case. The U of T Faculty
Association lawyers had a financial stake in extricating themselves
from the case. The time involved was enormous and it was keeping
the union from other essential duties. But neither the local union
nor the CAUT wanted to settle with the hospital without ensuring
that similar problems would be prevented in the future. The scandal
involving Prichard had underscored again how few rules there were
to regulate the university's interactions with private industry. In the
face of that, the union was pushing for an overhaul of the university's
policies. Separately, the harassment the Gang had experienced
showed that whistleblowers lacked protection at the school. The
union was arguing that the answer was to provide medical school
faculty members with formal representation. Specifically, the faculty
union wanted all U of T physicians to become dues-paying members, a notion that Naylor and the hospitals were firmly against.

Yet Strofolino was probably correct that the union had other
incentives for supporting Olivieri. As recently as the mid-1990s, the
union had come under attack by critics in a rival group at the university, who charged that UTFA was bloated and bureaucratic and
didn't support "real" academic freedom. On a separate front, faculty
who disagreed with the union's priorities fought the long-standing
policy of mandatory union dues. The union won its case about dues,
but the fight could re-emerge at any time. Now, with the case of
Nancy Olivieri, the union was proving that it supported academic
freedom and that its support was worth the cost of dues. Graham
emphasized those points when he spoke to professors at a CAUT
conference in 1999. "Attacks on academic freedom . . . will continue
unless consistent and countervailing forces are brought to bear by
university faculty members and their faculty associations," he said.

Olivieri, like her union, had reasons to try to put the negotiations behind her, along with clear incentives to keep them going. She was trying to get back to work on her clinical trials of Novartis's new drug for thalassemia, ICL670. It had proven effective at removing iron in animal studies, and now the company was running a trial to establish the drug's safety in humans; Toronto was one of the study sites. Olivieri was also continuing her work in Sri Lanka with Weatherall, tracking a group of thalassemia patients there, and she had resumed her collaborations with Ontario's provincial genetics lab in Hamilton. But for all that, her negotiations with the hospital remained unresolved, partly because she was dissatisfied with the results. Even with the union's help, she was spending tens of thousands on lawsuits and on legal advice about her fight against L1; she wanted to be sure that any settlement reached with Sick Kids was at a high enough financial level to keep her out of debt.

WARRING BETRAYALS: THE POISON PEN

Gideon Koren's situation at Sick Kids was very different from Nancy Olivieri's. As the hospital's chief of pharmacology, he had a large office and many residents; Olivieri now had to borrow an office. But even before the negotiated agreement put her primary workspace at the Toronto General, she'd had the typical Sick Kids cubbyhole of an office and rarely had more than one or two residents working directly under her. Koren had been a leader at the hospital for years, serving as chief of pharmacology and associate director at the Research Institute. When he stepped down from his Institute position, it was to accept the biggest prize the hospital could bestow on its researchers, an endowed chair. Olivieri said frequently of Koren, "He's on the A-team." She meant it as a snub, but it was true: he was among the doctors that others at Sick Kids—including the hospital's administrators—looked up to.

In his early years on staff, Koren had designed a program to advise pregnant women who were scared that a drug they'd taken could harm a baby. Through the program, he also gathered data about which drugs caused birth defects. Koren published his results in medical and science journals, his program attracted post-doctoral students and residents, and he became widely known.

"He's got fifty people working with him," said one doctor, referring to the large number of post-docs and residents Koren supervised. "They generate ideas and they publish things." Koren's findings were attracting attention, and he was winning contests for grant monies. As a result, he was able to acquire more students and residents than other scientists. They in turn developed projects in his lab, so Koren's name was appearing on scores of papers. Most academic doctors are pleased if they turn out ten or twenty original research papers per year; Koren's publications numbered in the hundreds, and in the publish-or-perish world of academic science, this bred resentment.

Scientists with such long lists of publications could be turning out low-quality science or writing quick and dirty journal articles. By the mid-1980s, universities were even spotlighting the practice and attempting to crack down on it by limiting the number of publications they would consider when a scientist came up for promotion. Koren's jam-packed c.v. raised questions for some of his colleagues.

Those who knew Koren well—his supervisors and the friends who trained with him at Sick Kids—said he was simply an incredibly industrious person. Pharmacologist Stewart MacLeod, Koren's boss at Sick Kids during the 1980s, remarked that he'd never seen anyone as obsessed with writing as Koren. Koren's first language was Hebrew and he'd never totally mastered English, so his efforts to write quickly meant that his work was often rife with grammatical errors. "It's as if a student wrote it up and Gidi never read it," said a scientist who was asked to review Koren's papers for various journals. But Koren wasn't ashamed of that. He thought it was the height of silliness for scientists to waste time perfecting the appearance of a paper. He preferred to dictate his scientific reports and send them to the typing pool in order to get his results into print more quickly.

Outgoing and charismatic, Koren was frequently asked to take on leadership positions at Sick Kids. Said one person who served on a hospital committee with Koren in the 1980s, "I have incredible admiration for his intuition and his ad hoc people skills. He can get people to decide, yes, they can put money here or there . . . He nurtures, or he just gets things rolling." Patients and their parents were equally positive about him. One father said he and his wife had both blamed themselves when one of their children became quite ill. The child was admitted to Sick Kids and assigned to Koren, whose calm concern quickly set the family at ease.

Koren's residents, many of whom were from Israel or the U.S., also lauded him. Several pharmacology residents said their relationships with him were about more than just science. "You could go to him any time and get advice or whatever," said one. Much of the advice was aimed at helping young people move up the ladder.

Koren had once given such advice to Olivieri, and his stature at the hospital had been a help to her. After they became collaborators in the 1980s, she wanted him involved in her projects and wanted others to know he was on board. Then, after he disagreed with her about L1, Olivieri wanted nothing to do with him. In 1997, she spread the word in the scientific community that he was guilty of scientific misconduct, the most serious charge Koren had faced in his academic career. Though she didn't charge him formally (as she had Sher), she did make her allegations against Koren public, telling supporters and colleagues that the abstracts he had co-authored for the meeting in Malta were fraudulent and plagiarized because they contained stolen data, data that she'd already published.

Like many scientists accused of misconduct, he was shattered. If the charge stuck, the consequences for his reputation could be devastating. Olivieri wasn't stopping at misconduct, however. In early 1998, she wrote Manuel Buchwald, alleging that Koren had committed financial improprieties by misappropriating Research Institute funds. It was another grave allegation against a man whose reputation had been unblemished. Buchwald duly assigned his staff to speak to Koren and investigate the missing monies.

A few months later, one of Koren's residents, a young female physician, came to the thalassemia clinic and asked a nurse if she could look at the patients' charts. The way Koren explained it, the resident "had worked on the L1 studies for a year and a half during her fellowship," and "went to the nurse to verify demographic data on a patient" in order to complete a paper. But Olivieri thought Koren's resident was stealing her data. She wrote Aideen Moore, head of the Research Ethics Board, that the resident "took unauthorized access" to a patient's chart, and she informed the head of the hospital's disciplinary committee that the incident involved "illegal access by unauthorized personnel to clinic files." Senior hospital staff held a meeting about the incident, and Koren was called in to explain.

The series of incidents in which he found himself accused of wrongdoing left Koren hurt and frustrated. He'd never been in such a terrible situation. The sorts of accusations he was facing could cost him more than his reputation; if he was found to have stolen money from his employer or data from a colleague, he could lose his job. In May he told Buchwald that he was suing Olivieri for slander and defamation. Even if he was cleared of all of Olivieri's claims against him, he would still be tainted with the brush of scientific misconduct—an accusation with repercussions even for those who are wrongly accused. A 1996 report by the U.S. Office of Research Integrity, based on a survey of scientists accused of misconduct and later exonerated, found that 60 per cent experienced at least one negative consequence of the accusation, including threatened lawsuits, reduced support staff and delays in processing grant applications, and 17 per cent suffered severe consequences, such as the loss of a job or a promotion. Law professor Jesse Goldner of St. Louis University summed up the report's findings in a law journal: "Being accused of misconduct is, even in the best of circumstances, a most unpleasant experience."

For some scientists it could be dreadful. A high-achieving McGill professor—neuropsychologist Justine Sergent—was accused of misconduct in 1994 by an anonymous whistleblower. Sergent directed a laboratory at the Montreal Neurological Institute and published her work in leading journals, including *Science*. She was under investigation by McGill University, but not for misconduct; she had tried to protect her research subjects' confidentiality by not listing their correct telephone numbers on an official research form, and after the university reprimanded her for the practice, she and university administrators began an arbitration about it. McGill and Montreal Neurological Institute officials denied that Sergent had committed misconduct and rejected the anonymous charges, but the letter accusing her was sent to the Montreal *Gazette,* and the paper made the charges public. Three days after the article in the *Gazette*, Sergent and her husband committed suicide. She left a note explaining that the accusation was "a discredit on myself, my work and my career, which I cannot tolerate."

Koren tolerated the accusations against him, but he was angry about them and later described himself as having been "savagely attacked." In that context, he shared what he knew about the L1 trials at Sick Kids with the company and the hospital. As a pharmacologist and an expert on clinical trials, Koren could place L1 in context in a way that few others could have. He'd lived through its early days in Toronto, in the late 1980s, when Olivieri first convinced Canadian authorities to let her test the drug on patients. He had directly supervised many of the residents who worked with her on it and was head of the Research Ethics Board in the early 1990s, when she published her first articles on the drug. As a former close friend and collaborator of Olivieri's, he knew her history from her earliest days on staff at the hospital and knew that her breakup with Apotex could be seen as one of the breakups she'd had with collaborators over the years. He'd been working with Olivieri when she ended her collaboration with Susan Perrine in 1994, and he was still working with her when she split from Graham Sher in 1996.

Koren was also privy to a fact that Olivieri hadn't been open about—that she and Brittenham were both paid consultants to

Apotex while they studied L1. Though it wasn't an unusual situation at the time, it could make Olivieri sound like a hypocrite. She'd been accusing other people of bias because they'd accepted drug company monies, yet she'd kept quiet about her own consultancy contract. David Weatherall seemed unaware of it. He explained in a telephone interview that it disturbed him that scientists would report on L1 at a scientific meeting if they were paid consultants to Apotex. "They've got to really have independence," he said. Bob Phillips also didn't know about it. After reading the confidential report of the misconduct committee that considered Olivieri's charges against Sher, Phillips had written his letter to Buchwald, O'Brodovich, Strofolino and Aberman, and one of the things he asked them was who was a consultant to the company. Even the *New England Journal of Medicine* seemed to have been left in the dark. In 1998, when it published letters disputing Olivieri's claims, the journal was careful to note any Apotex funding. After a letter from Beatrix Wonke and others questioning Olivieri's results, an editor's note appeared stating that Apotex had supported a trainee who worked with them; Alan Cohen's letter, written with research nurse Marie Martin, was followed by a note that he was an investigator in an Apotex-sponsored trial of L1 and that Martin received salary support from the company. But the journal had published Olivieri's 1995 article on L1 without mentioning that the company was supporting her research and the residents who worked on her trials, and her 1998 article without noting that she and Brittenham had been consultants to Apotex until the trials were stopped by the company.

If he wanted to, Koren could say things that could be damaging to Olivieri. In the summer of 1998, I arranged to interview Koren and got my first taste of what he was saying about the drug. When our conversation began, Koren was relaxed and joking, describing himself as a "hyperactive, academic pediatrician," but in his mild-mannered way, he proceeded to raise hard-hitting questions about Olivieri's arguments against L1. Admitting that L1 was less effective than Desferal, he explained why there was a still a need for it. Effectiveness wasn't the only thing to consider, he said. People in Third World countries couldn't afford Desferal. "To put it in perspective, deferiprone appears to be much, much cheaper than Desferal." He said that in some countries where thalassemia was prevalent, the money available for drugs was so limited that "the whole year's worth of what they can put in medication may not buy five capsules of Aspirin." In those countries, "a cheaper version, even if it's not as good as Desferal, may have its validity." He added, "The overall assessment of whether a drug is good or not is not a simple one of whether there are better drugs, but also whether it can be afforded." It sounded logical.

He offered another reason why L1 could prove to be a valuable option. "Many kids on Desferal tell us and the investigators in other places that they will not do Desferal, and indeed, research both from this hospital and others shows that as years of adolescence go by, less and less kids use Desferal." That matched what I'd heard from some of the patients I'd spoken with. No matter how well Desferal worked, some of them wouldn't take it.

Like others who spoke with Nancy Olivieri, I'd walked away from interviewing her believing that she and her collaborators were the only people to have studied this particular drug. Koren explained that it was being studied "in several different countries" and that "there were several protocols" looking into its usefulness. I thought it was available only as an experimental drug; he told me that in some countries, including India, it was already approved. An Indian company called Cipla held the licence for it there, and it was widely used by Indian patients.

He described a hypothetical scenario in which L1 could turn out to be useful, and it was convincing. "For example, how about that a child will take Desferal for one night or two nights and the rest of the time he or she will be able to take the oral drug?" he asked. When I looked into it, I discovered that in India, where the price of Desferal was prohibitive, the practice of combining the two drugs was already common, and I was surprised that Olivieri hadn't mentioned it.

Koren admitted that L1 had some toxicity, but he thought the question of whether it was toxic to the liver was unresolved. "There have been opposing interpretations of the safety of the drug, which is not uncommon in the development of drugs, especially for people who are not very healthy," he said. I thought about it and realized he was probably right. From my clinical background and my work as a medical journalist, I knew of several examples where, despite mixed views of a drug's safety, the drug was eventually accepted as safe. One was Clozaril, an antipsychotic drug used to treat people suffering from schizophrenia. Another was Accutane, a drug used by teenagers and young adults for severe acne.

Clozaril, also known as clozapine, was used to treat schizophrenia in Europe during the 1970s and '80s. After several European patients died, North American doctors and drug agencies shied away from it. Then doctors figured out that the deaths were due to a specific side effect that emerged in a tiny fraction of patients who took it. If they monitored patients closely by checking their blood counts once a week, they could detect the side effect early, before it caused any harm. When Clozaril was eventually marketed in the U.S. and Canada in the early 1990s, any patient who received a prescription for the drug was required to have a weekly blood test. The drug turned out to be safe when controlled that way, and it remains useful for individuals who are very sick with schizophrenia and who don't respond to other drugs.

Accutane caused terrible birth defects when taken by pregnant women, yet people with severe acne often referred to it as the only thing that had ever worked for them. Rather than pull it off the market because of its potential for birth defects, the drug agencies approved it for use on the condition that the possibility of birth defects was underscored to doctors and the public. Doctors who prescribe Accutane have patients sign a form saying that they are aware of its hazards. Female patients must promise to use birth control or to refrain from having sex while taking it, and they submit to monthly pregnancy tests in order to continue their prescriptions. Under that rubric, it remains in wide use.

I figured that if I could think of two examples of drugs that had engendered "opposing interpretations" of their safety, Gideon Koren, who specialized in pharmacology and toxicology, would know of many more. With his clear arguments and professorial manner, Koren persuaded me that there was another side to the story, at least as far as the usefulness of L1 was concerned. He cautioned that the drug wasn't yet approved by drug agencies in Ottawa or Washington. "I believe that by the time it's approved by the regulatory agencies, it will have meant that there's enough data on it," he said. "Before that, we have to be very careful not to guess a verdict of an exercise that has not been completed." I assumed he was implying that Olivieri was guessing at conclusions before all the data were in.

He was circumspect with me, but apparently he said a lot more when he spoke to Olivieri's colleagues. In the spring of 1998, Brenda Gallie had a conversation with him and recalled that he told her, "You know, you really should not defend Nancy. You'll only harm her more."

Koren also talked to Michèle Brill-Edwards, who had known him since the early 1980s, when they were both completing their clinical fellowships in the pharmacology program at Sick Kids. She also knew Michael Spino from that time; he'd been a faculty member in the program. She told me she still felt a "sort of professional

camaraderie and allegiance . . . to Mike and to Gidi." That camaraderie frayed as Koren made allegations to her about Olivieri's
behaviour.

As Olivieri worried about what Koren was saying behind her
back—to other scientists and to the Sick Kids leadership—Peter
Durie glommed onto another issue involving Gideon Koren:
Michael Spino's lab. Spino had a lab at the hospital and his name listed
on Sick Kids' letterhead because he was a consulting member of
Koren's division. Durie thought it was wrong and protested to
Buchwald about it. When Buchwald said the lab wasn't part of the
Research Institute, Durie set out to collect evidence. He staked out
the hospital's eighth floor, making personal observations of who
came and went and conducting interviews with hospital staff whose
labs were nearby. He even had a conversation with Spino. And after
he confirmed that Spino's lab was Spino's lab, he filled three single-
spaced pages with a detailed report to Buchwald describing his "suspicions concerning Dr. Spino's relationship with the Division of
Clinical Pharmacology."

Brenda Gallie speculated to journalists that Koren was beholden
to Apotex because the company was planning to fund a new "drug
trials unit" in Koren's division at Sick Kids. She and other Olivieri
supporters said that the new unit was a huge effort and could be very
expensive. The figures quoted were between $5 and $10 million.

Soon Nancy Olivieri and the Gang had compiled a list of
things they thought Koren had done or might do that were
improper. In the summer of 1998, as reporters began contacting
Olivieri to learn more about her allegations against the hospital
and Apotex and to hear her story of whistleblowing and courage,
she and her supporters shared their list, describing Koren's role
in what had happened in nefarious terms. Olivieri told journalists that the CMPA lawyers who had once represented Koren
dropped him because of unethical behaviour on his part, though

she offered no proof. She mentioned the incident with Koren's resident coming to the thalassemia clinic to check data.

She spoke about the Malta abstracts, saying that Koren had published her research without her name or her approval. She added that while Koren had published with the company and its scientists, the company was blocking her from publishing her opposing views. Then she mentioned to reporters that Koren was still funded by Apotex. She told me, "Dr. Koren is a personal friend of Michael Spino, the senior vice president of Apotex. In addition, when the trials were abruptly terminated by Apotex in May 1996, Dr. Koren continued to receive funding for three fellows. Three research fellows is the equivalent of about $120,000 to $130,000 per year, which is a considerable amount of money . . ." She and her supporters also mentioned that Koren had given Spino a lab at the hospital, so it appeared as if he was going out of his way to befriend company officials, even to the point of misusing hospital resources.

Like Olivieri's close supporters, journalists didn't wonder whether Olivieri was exploiting her standing as a whistleblower to pursue a feud. Instead, reporters allied with her and became her emissaries, carrying multiple accusations from her office to Koren's for his comments. In my interview with Koren that summer, I reviewed the list with him. He declined to comment on some of the allegations but responded to others. He said the CMPA lawyers had told him they didn't think he needed their help because there didn't seem to be any risk of his being sued. Much later, it emerged that Olivieri herself had asked the CMPA lawyers to drop Koren because she wanted separate legal representation.

Koren didn't want to discuss the Malta abstracts per se. He had published data from the L1 trials, and he believed that Olivieri had also published the data. "I don't think any of us perceived that we are not allowed to publish, even if it was against the company's will," he said. When I mentioned the allegation about his resident and the patient charts, he replied, "Again, it's an issue that I don't want to comment on."

He said Apotex paid for his residents' training as part of an agreement to protect the residents. Originally, the residents had been assigned to work on the L1 research, and the company paid for them. When the trials were stopped, there was an agreement hammered out with the company to continue to pay their salaries so that residents in training at Sick Kids wouldn't be harmed in their careers by the debacle of the L1 trials. "It was consensual on everyone that it's unacceptable to not continue to train people who came for that," was how he put it.

But even when Koren responded to Olivieri's charges against him, his calm explanations were no match for the tone she'd used in her comments about him. Her descriptions of Koren made him sound incompetent.

Olivieri's close supporters had the same contempt for Koren as she did. They said he couldn't be trusted and described him as a "con artist," and they were convincing. By the fall of 1998, Olivieri was a media darling as a martyr and heroine, while Koren was barely mentioned in the press. When he was referred to, it was as "Olivieri's co-investigator," or "a friend of Spino's," or "another hospital doctor." In *Maclean's* he became a nameless scientist "who had disagreed with Olivieri publicly over her research findings." The story of his resident approaching the nurse in the thalassemia clinic formed the lead paragraph in the *Maclean's* cover story. In the magazine's version of the events, the nurse was "anxious" when the resident appeared and Olivieri was fearful as soon as she heard about it, "but by the time Olivieri could race down a flight of stairs and into the clinic, the woman had dropped the charts and fled."

Doctors who had worked under Koren were surprised by how he was being portrayed. "He was quoted without all his titles and everything else," said one young doctor. "Like he was nobody, rather than professor and head of the department of pharmacology at the hospital." Koren continued to find the experience horribly difficult, according to his close colleagues. Nationally and internationally, he'd won most of the major honours an academic pharmacologist could collect. He'd published his research in all the leading journals in medicine and pediatrics, and he had extensive medical and scientific connections in Toronto and around the world. Yet the media favoured Olivieri. The attempts Koren and others at Sick Kids made to show that there was another side to the Olivieri-Apotex scandal were failing.

In September, Koren contemplated a lawsuit against Brenda Gallie, claiming that her remarks about him were defamatory. He wrote Gallie to say that he was going to charge her with libel, but he didn't pursue it. Later, he told *Globe and Mail* reporter Krista Foss that he felt as if his hands were tied because of the dictates from the hospital's administration. "We were told not to talk to the media ever, which I religiously regarded," he said.

Secretly, though, someone had been speaking to the press. *Maclean's* revealed that three people had called the magazine to bad-mouth Olivieri, one of whom accused her of stealing from her research grant. When the *National Post* story on Langlois's media advice appeared, Olivieri and the Gang scrambled to figure out who had given the paper access to their private e-mails. They thought someone could have done it by obtaining a master key and using it to get into Peter Durie's office. Once there, that person could have printed out the e-mails. Durie was so convinced of the theft that he got the locks on his office door changed.

Then the Gang learned that someone had sent documents highly critical of Olivieri to the *Globe*'s Michael Valpy. One seemed to be a copy of a letter from the hospital administration to Apotex, but Valpy couldn't tell who had sent it to him because the sender hadn't identified him- or herself. And in late October, Peter Durie got an unusual letter too. Like Valpy's, it was from someone who hadn't bothered to identify him- or herself.

Dated "Oct21, 1998," the letter to Durie was full of misspellings, typos and odd language. It began, "You cannot overestimate the contempt, appaul and mistrust we have towards you,and we were not people that belonged to any camp in this dipute. The damage you have caused HSC is insurmoutable. We do not believe you have done it for higher principles! We are convinced you have your own agenda . . . We all have experienced in one way or another your mesanthropy and a British version of a foul air baloon. It is the right time for you to offer these virtues to a different institution that needs a 'Head of CF.'" It was signed, "All the worse Your appaulled colleagues," and stamped underneath with the funny face of a clown.

Though the letter had no author, Olivieri thought Gideon Koren might have written it because of the odd errors in grammar and syntax. Koren had always been sloppy with word-processing, feeling it wasn't worth his time to correct things. And, as Olivieri knew, in addition to being a scientist he was a playwright, musician and performer. Perhaps he found odd markings such as a clown's face appealing.

A second letter arrived in Durie's office two months later via the hospital's internal mail system. At the time, the Gang was suffering the fallout of their lawyer's racism charge—the claim that Sick Kids failed to provide Olivieri's clinics with greater resources because her patients weren't white. "So Peter, this hospital is not just unethical,it is also racist," the letter began. "And of course every one is racist except for you and Nancy . . . How did you ever get yourself in the middle of this group of pigs?Or did you think that their shit wouldn't touch you?"

This letter, even weirder than the first, continued to a second paragraph. "Olivieri, Chan, Gallie and research integrity???? There are horrendous accounts of their unethical conduct. You, as the only ethical person in this group should run as fast as you can! Many people who respect you for 20 and more years begin to wonder." Again, there was no signature.

Soon after this letter arrived, I heard about it from a person who was close to Olivieri: "There was an anonymous note to Peter warning him to split with Helen, Nancy and Brenda. Someone is desperate and views their career as at risk." Gallie had shown the letters to Michèle Brill-Edwards, who had known Koren longer than any of the rest of Olivieri's supporters. "It's Gidi all over," Brill-Edwards told her friends.

Olivieri, Durie and Gallie had been discussing the correspondence with their lawyers and the police. They knew that from a legal standpoint it didn't meet the definition of hate mail. But it was a form of harassment. "The person doing this is trying to intimidate us," Gallie told me, "trying to get us to be afraid, get us to want to leave, get us to shut up." They had urged the hospital to investigate the anonymous letters, but nothing seemed to be happening.

Then the Naimark Review appeared, with its allegations against Olivieri, and it was clear that Koren had been speaking openly to Arnold Naimark that fall. His claims were damaging to Olivieri, and he'd backed them up by giving Naimark copies of his correspondence. One letter he provided was one he had received from an Israeli friend describing Olivieri's talk at ASH in December 1996. When I interviewed Naimark, he described how persuasive the information was.

"In early December 1996, Dr Olivieri showed slides demonstrating hepatic fibrosis. This was reported to Dr. Koren by a colleague of his," said Naimark. When Naimark searched the files of the ethics board, he discovered that after Olivieri spoke at ASH months passed before she went to the Research Ethics Board. A few years later, the College of Physicians and Surgeons of Ontario would decide that those months weren't crucial, concluding that Olivieri behaved ethically and acted in her patients' best interests, but in 1998, Koren's correspondence led directly to Naimark's conclusion that Olivieri had made serious mistakes.

Naimark hadn't tried to authenticate every document he'd been given, but he intended his materials to become part of a public archive, so he asked the hospital to make the documents accessible to anyone who requested them. For a while, the hospital did. And in her low-profile way, Helen Chan began making a series of trips to the Sick Kids library to look over the multitude of documents that Naimark's team had amassed. She burrowed into them the way she'd previously studied papers that touched on questions in her research. The work was tedious and time-consuming, but Chan was on a mission. She felt she knew Gideon Koren, and she intended to use her knowledge.

Once, she'd worked with him on a cancer research project. In a paper they wrote together, she found errors in his calculations and concluded he was careless. Then she found mistakes in her research account. Koren had signing power over the account, and Chan figured those errors were his fault as well. Now Olivieri thought Koren was one of the primary persons responsible for Naimark's allegations against her, and Brill-Edwards thought he was the one writing the weird letters. Chan sat in the hospital's small library rooms and scanned every document in Naimark's archive, especially the ones Koren was involved in, searching for errors.

Eventually, she found a few letters that worried her. She showed them to Olivieri, who thought they were contrived. Gideon Koren, the two women thought, simply made them up, predated them to make it appear as if they'd been written much earlier, and handed them over to Naimark. The Gang thought Helen Chan had found a gold mine. Olivieri wasn't guilty of any wrong, but the hospital was conspiring to make it look as if she was, they thought. They had to come up with a way to prove it. If they could trace the documents Koren had given Naimark in Koren's computer, they might be able to see when they were originally composed. The computer might also be the repository of the weird anonymous letters that Durie had gotten. Of course, the Gang didn't have access to Koren's computer. Then, all of a sudden, they did.

Koren's office was on the ninth floor of the hospital, down one long hallway from Durie's and up another hallway from Gallie's. In the late spring of 1999, knowing that the chances were high that Koren was the author of the letters, the Gang managed to seize his computer. Afterwards, Gallie said that Durie—who in earlier years had carpeted his home with the treasures he scavenged from Sick Kids—found Koren's old computer in the trash. "One day, since we work on the same floor . . . Nancy and Peter were walking in the corridor," was how Gallie began the story. "And there, sitting beside the blue box, in all the garbage—and everyone throws out old Macintosh computers because nobody wants them any more—was sitting a Macintosh computer, with the printer and the little disk drive, sitting piled like junk in the garbage in the hall.

"And they picked up the box, like everyone does. If you want something out of the garbage, you pick the garbage. It's out in the hall on public property. They picked it up, took it to Peter's office . . . About five minutes later they're standing in Peter's office with the door open and they hear the elevators open. They can't see. Gidi Koren gets out of the elevator, meets his secretary, who is telling him something in Hebrew. He shouts and yells and gets furious and rushes off down the hall to his office."

The next morning, hospital security officers appeared at Peter Durie's office requesting Dr. Koren's computer. "So he threw it out in the garbage, Nancy and Peter picked it up and the hospital seized it from us," Gallie said later. Durie and Olivieri received what was described as a "disciplinary letter" charging them with having stolen

Koren's computer. And the Gang had little to show for their efforts. Gallie explained, "The computer, in fact, is such an old Mac it doesn't have anything in it; it's useless. It doesn't have any documentation or anything."

After the computer episode, the Gang stopped searching garbage. They had already hired a professional detective agency. They wanted to get to the bottom of the anonymous letters, and they thought the hospital wasn't moving on the problem quickly enough. Instead, the hospital was acting on the findings of the Naimark Review by referring its allegations about Nancy Olivieri to a disciplinary committee. The Gang was furious. Olivieri's friends outside Toronto tried to cheer her up by inviting her, once again, to come work at their centres in Oakland, Baltimore and elsewhere.

In January 1999, Brenda Gallie was quoted in the *Toronto Star* as saying Olivieri might leave Toronto because "so many leading institutions" were "clamoring to have her." She described Olivieri as "a scientist of extraordinary honesty" and "a borderline genius." Apparently, no one had told Koren to stop reading the papers. Soon another anonymous letter was wending its way to all Sick Kids doctors through the hospital mail.

This letter began with a feeble attempt at a joke about the idea of a "borderline" genius, quipping that "the minute she produces her first original idea*, Doctors for Scientific Integrity will declare Olivieri a Mainstream Genius.It's just a matter of time." The asterisk referred in a cryptic way to questions surrounding the originality of Olivieri's work. "The L1 was developed and tested first in the UK," the letter said. "Butyric acid was 'adopted' from Susan Perrine, who was one of Olivieri's best friends before the adoption, ect. ect." Below the odd typing, a section of the *Toronto Star* article was attached. Multiple copies of the letter were made, and each copy was folded in three and put into a hospital envelope.

As soon as the Gang received the letter, the detectives they'd hired went into action. They had already investigated around Koren's house and knew the weekly recycling pickup schedule on his street. They now picked up the cache of paper that sat waiting to be recycled at the curb in a familiar Toronto blue box. Gallie described what they found. "In his blue paper box were three copies of this [letter] used as scrap paper, all scribbled on the back. Unfolded." It was at least part of the proof they were looking for that Koren was the author of the anonymous letters.

Next, Clayton Ruby hired two forensic analysts, a documents expert and a linguist. He sent them all of the anonymous letters, along with two letters signed by Koren and filed as appendices to the Naimark report, and another signed document from Koren that the group had a copy of—the letter he'd sent Gallie when he'd threatened to sue her. "It came from Koren himself, typed again on the same computer," Gallie explained.

The linguistics expert was Jack Chambers, a professor at the University of Toronto. The documents man was Brian Lindbloom, a former document examiner for the RCMP. Chambers focused on the spacing and other typing oddities; Lindbloom examined the paper. Both experts compared the anonymous letters side by side with the documents that were signed by Koren.

In an interview, Gallie summed up the analysts' findings. Lindbloom "found on the envelopes where you could see imprints of something having been written on top of the envelope, and you could tell—you could see the writing," said Gallie. "It's just like reading the writing and then analyzing the likely author of that writing, comparing it to other known documents." And Chambers was able to say that the anonymous letters and the signed letters had probably come from the same typist. Months later, Ruby told the press, "Both experts decided that there was strong compelling evidence that Dr. Koren was the author of that mail."

The entire effort, including the detective agency and the experts, had cost the Gang over $200,000. They were covering their costs partly with their personal funds and with donations received via their fundraising group, Doctors for Research Integrity. But the greatest help was coming from the two professors' organizations—the Canadian Association of University Teachers and the U of T Faculty Association. Brenda Gallie acknowledged that those sources of money had been essential: "The CAUT—they've put in a lot of money. We've each put in a huge amount of money. We've mortgaged our houses to fight this battle." Olivieri said later, "The Faculty Association has been unfailingly generous. They've given time, money, and people . . . Those people are unwavering in their support, and they're making all the difference."

In May 1999, lawyers for Olivieri gave the detective's report and the forensic analyses to the university and the hospital, along with a complaint from Olivieri and the Gang that they were being harassed. Peter Durie was away at the time, interviewing for the pediatric chairmanship at the Children's Hospital of Eastern Ontario in Ottawa. When he returned, another anonymous letter was waiting for him, sent through the external mail. It referred to a document hanging on Durie's door.

Things at Sick Kids had gotten so bizarre that Durie and others of Olivieri's supporters at the hospital had begun playing a game usually reserved for university students living in dormitories. They would hang material on their doors—articles, editorials, cartoons and even letters from their superiors. Then they would wait to see if anyone tore the material down. One Sick Kids scientist described how she tacked an op-ed from the *Globe and Mail* on her office door in the winter of 1999. "And it basically said something's rotten at the top. So I made copies and I put one on the outside and I put one on the inside [of the door]. After twenty-four hours it was removed.

I was just curious to know how long it would stay there."

Peter Durie was very involved in this game. Before leaving for Ottawa, he'd hung up a document on his door that described O'Brodovich's new policy of "citizenship scores." Durie thought of the chief's citizenship scores as one more means through which the hospital intended to harass the Gang. They would all be given low scores on citizenship, then their salaries would be docked in accordance with the point system O'Brodovich had put in place.

The anonymous letter said:

Dear Peter

We have read your recent comment attached to your door, regarding the way people are being evaluated at HSC. We absolutely agree with you that HSC is not a good place, only our reasons are somewhat different:

We believe that any normally-functioning hospital would have let people like you go long ago. The very fact that you are still around, contaminating our air and fabric, is a huge sign of weakness of HSC. The way you managed to turn the Division into the most dysfunctional clinical service in the country should have been thoroughly investigated.

We congratulate your sense of humor, which is matched only by your mesanthropy. If we were good citizens, we would have sent a photocopy of this recent masterpiece to CHEO [Children's Hospital of Eastern Ontario], so they can have a better sense of the kind of mesanthrope the candidate Durie is. But in all fairness, we are quite eager to see you leaving, so this is not the right time to be good citizens. Let them have the pleasure of finding themselves who you are.

It was signed, "All the best." But the author hadn't added his name.

About six weeks later, Koren wrote to Michèle Brill-Edwards. Since getting to know Olivieri in the spring of 1998, Brill-Edwards had cast herself as one of Olivieri's supporters and advisers. Yet somehow she remained close to Koren. "Gidi very much saw me as a friend—we were still friends," she said. Koren knew, as few others did, that Brill-Edwards was in a difficult financial situation. She'd left her government position in February 1996, after *the fifth estate* aired a piece on the safety of calcium channel blocker drugs. She'd given the show's producer access to confidential documents to reveal how the decision was made to leave the drugs on the market, blowing the whistle, she hoped, on the way in which her agency was subject to industry influence. A single mother living with her own mother and supporting a teenage daughter, she was doing advocacy work full-time. Koren wrote her in the summer of 1999 in a scratchy long-hand to see if she needed work.

Hello Micheli
I do not have a telephone number for you so I am writing.
There are two potential upcoming option of jobs for a pediatric-pharmacologist here.
I wish to know your availability/interest.
Pl. call me:

He'd given the phone numbers of his two secretaries, and signed it, "With Best Wishes Gidi."

Koren was right that Brill-Edwards needed a salary. She soon took a job staffing the thalassemia clinic at the Toronto General Hospital under Nancy Olivieri, but she filed his letter away.

In the fall of 1999, the hospital hired Barbara Humphrey, a Toronto lawyer with experience in workplace harassment, to investigate the anonymous letters. She reviewed the letters and began conducting interviews. By early November, she had interviewed Olivieri and Durie. Toward the end of that month, she interviewed Koren. But in the view of Olivieri, Gallie, Durie and Chan, Humphrey wasn't moving fast enough. Koren was still denying that he was the author of the anonymous mail, and despite all the evidence they'd produced suggesting that he was probably the author of the letters, the hospital wasn't taking action against him.

Hospital administrators said there was a process that had to be completed before they could act. They claimed they were waiting for Humphrey's investigation to be over, but the Gang experienced the wait as further mistreatment. "It'll be 2004 before they get around to it," Gallie told me in early December 1999. They also feared that the hospital's investigator had been instructed to find a way to clear Koren despite the overwhelming evidence implicating him.

Gallie, who had devoted a huge part of the previous decade to developing genetic tests, now realized that the same technology could offer a foolproof way to finger Koren. They could do DNA testing. As long as the person who sent the letters licked the envelopes shut or licked the stamps that were pasted on them, his or her DNA would be found, since it's contained in saliva. It was an expensive route to take, but it was an incontestable way to identify the letter-writer.

Ruby sent several of the envelopes addressed to Peter Durie to a DNA testing laboratory in British Columbia. The DNA investigation showed that the same person had licked all the envelopes and stamps. Next, they got the hospital's investigator to request a DNA sample from Koren so they could see if it was a match. The sample wasn't forthcoming. But the Gang of Four had an ace in the hole: Brill-Edwards had given them Koren's signed letter offering her a job. When the lab reported that whoever had licked Brill-Edwards's envelope and its stamp was the same person who had licked the other envelopes, the Gang had their man. They turned the information over to the hospital—and to the police.

In early December, Olivieri and her supporters began letting a few journalists know that they'd pinpointed Koren as the author of the anonymous letters. Then they pressed for coverage, calling a *Globe* reporter to say that if the *Globe* didn't run it, another paper would. In mid-December, Barbara Humphrey asked Koren for a sample that she could send for DNA testing. He conceded that he'd written the anonymous letters.

A few days before Christmas 1999, Humphrey tabled the 312-page report she'd compiled on the letters. She met with reporters and said both sides were responsible for the delays she'd encountered. She said Koren had deceived her, but she was also troubled by what Olivieri and her supporters had done. Initially they didn't tell the hospital they suspected Koren, and later they wouldn't provide certain documents for her investigation, such as a letter that had been sent to *Globe* reporter Michael Valpy. In general, she had the impression that Olivieri and the Gang had involved themselves in an escalating series of conflicts. Her report identified specific incidents involving members of the Gang that could have left Koren feeling that he was being attacked, and she recommended mediation between all the parties involved.

But Olivieri and the Gang weren't interested in mediation. The next day the *Globe* and the *National Post* carried the story, referring to the letters as "poison-pen" letters. And Olivieri and her supporters and lawyers held a press conference at the offices of the U of T Faculty Association. Durie said he was worried for his life now that Koren had been exposed as the author of the letters. "He's a trained soldier," Durie told reporters. "He fought in Israel in the Six-Day War." Clayton Ruby, the Gang's lawyer, echoed Durie's sentiments. "Frankly, the doctors were very concerned about their own safety," he said.

The Gang also argued that every article Koren had written needed to be scrutinized in light of the letters. "Everything he's done must be questioned," said Durie. Olivieri stressed that Koren had lied about what he'd done: "At the heart of the matter is the fact that this top researcher in pediatric pharmacology lied repeatedly about issuing anonymous harassing threats." At the time, Koren was president of the Canadian Society for Clinical Pharmacology. Olivieri demanded that he give up that position and all his posts at Sick Kids and the University of Toronto. The faculty association vice-president described Koren as a menace because his conclusions about the drug were the opposite of Olivieri's. "This is the man whose evidence has resulted in the drug's being . . . used today on children, putting children's lives at risk," he said.

But journalists by this time were wondering whether catching Koren would put an end to the scandal. They'd heard Humphrey suggest mediation, and Olivieri and the Gang seemed a long way away from that. At the press conference, the *Globe and Mail*'s Krista Foss asked how the doctors "might be able to move forward from this and recover." Olivieri didn't answer the question. Instead, she went through a litany of things the hospital had done to harass her. "Who promoted Dr. Koren to the position he's in as the chair . . . and the head of a division in the department of pediatrics?" she asked. "Who fired me? Vilified me publicly? Sent e-mails through-out the system . . . that completely misrepresented and falsified the entire series of events?"

Clayton Ruby tried to cast doubt on Humphrey herself. "Ms. Humphrey . . . works for the hospital," he said. "She is not an inde-pendent, impartial third body. She is not like a judge." But the *Toronto Star*'s Rita Daly had the same question as Foss. "So at this point, what can you do to move on and get on with your research?" she asked. Again, Olivieri described how she'd been harassed: "Well, we signed an agreement in January, Rita, that said we'll have a new slate and a clean beginning. And one week after that my bellboys were turned off, I was locked out of my office. You've heard the litany; it's a pathetic litany. I don't remember firing Dr. O'Brodovich. I don't remember evicting Professor Buchwald."

Daly wouldn't let the question drop. "Well, what would it take now to move on?" she said. Gallie responded that they wanted more acknowledgment from the hospital board that there had been "a big problem" and that the board had been misled. And Olivieri said they also wanted one more thing: the hospital's and the university's co-operation with an investigation into the L1 trials that had been commissioned by the CAUT.

Koren resigned as head of the Sick Kids division of clinical pharmacology and as head of the Research Institute's program in population health sciences. He was suspended with pay from his other positions at the university and the hospital while a disciplinary committee considered whether his actions were misconduct and what his punishment should be. To ensure that the committee had all the relevant information, the Gang gave the hospital a binder of documents described as "containing new allegations against Dr. Koren," including the letters Chan had dug up that Olivieri believed were fakes. Ruby said publicly that the doctors suspected Koren of having falsified the evidence he'd given to Naimark. This bordered on forgery, a criminal offence.

The charge of forgery didn't stick. One letter Ruby claimed was falsified was the one Koren had received in 1996 from the physician in Israel who heard Olivieri's talk at ASH that year. After Ruby's claims about it were publicized, the Israeli doctor confirmed that he'd written it, and Ruby apologized for having charged that it was false. But Koren had authored the weird letters to Durie, and that was enough to warrant punishment. In April 2000, the hospital and the university announced that he would relinquish his endowed chair at the hospital and would be suspended for two months without pay. He was also required to pay a fine of $35,000 to partially cover the costs of the hospital's investigation. But he wasn't fired.

Koren received a confidential report of the decision to penalize him in the form of a long letter from Prichard and Strofolino, in which they used the words "gross misconduct" to describe his actions. Olivieri or her supporters managed to get a copy of the letter to a reporter for the *Toronto Star*, and the paper quoted liberally from it in an article about the case. Once again, perhaps unwittingly, Olivieri or her supporters had breached the confidentiality of a scientist accused of misconduct.

The UTFA's William Graham told *Nature Medicine* that the hospital and the university had "damaged themselves by their failure to protect academic freedom and prevent harassment of scholars," but at the university, the head of clinical pharmacology, Neal Shear, refused to accept Koren's resignation from his university position. Shear told reporters, "It takes incredible, incredible frustration to drive people like that to actions so out of character." He said he thought that what drove Koren to it was that the things he cared about most "were being threatened." Others agreed. One doctor at Sick Kids said, "The hospital handled it very, very poorly in not coming forward with a lot of information that they had, and the honest truth is I think that led entirely to these anonymous letters." Humphrey said as much in her report. She discovered that Koren had sought help from the hospital administration more than once to try to counter Olivieri's allegations about him but had been told there was little they could do, a response that left him feeling unsupported and isolated.

Manuel Buchwald was in Europe at a scientific meeting when a colleague asked him what could explain Gideon Koren's behaviour. "Frustration, that's what the lawyer says in her report," Buchwald said. "Oh, so he went crazy too," replied the colleague. Some of the reactions in Toronto were similar. Bob Phillips said of Koren, "He just snapped." Koren himself told a *Globe and Mail* reporter later, "The only way I could express myself was in those letters. It was inappropriate and unbecoming . . . but when you find yourself attacked savagely by five people over three years, you may do these things."

To Olivieri and her supporters, it didn't matter what the explanation was. Koren had committed an academic crime—or several crimes—and deserved to be fired. They saw the poison-pen letters as one more component in Koren's long campaign to discredit Olivieri's work on L1 and damage her reputation. They knew Koren had lied to Humphrey by denying that he'd written the letters, and the Gang suspected that he had previously lied to Arnold Naimark and produced manufactured evidence. Olivieri thought that, even earlier, he'd misinformed the Sick Kids administration, framing her argument with Apotex as a purely scientific dispute.

Michèle Brill-Edwards wrote journalists that Koren's reinstatement was "a betrayal of the public trust." Chan, Durie and Gallie complained to the College of Physicians and Surgeons—the doctors' licensing board—and urged them to investigate Koren for professional misconduct based on the poison-pen letters. Simultaneously, Olivieri accused Koren of misconduct for publishing an article on L1 in 1999, saying that he'd included her data on patients without informing her or seeking her consent. Olivieri saw the decision to keep Koren on at the hospital and the university as further evidence of both institutions' failure to support her.

"You have to understand here that Apotex and Dr. Koren spent a great deal of time and a very, very successful campaign in vilifying me publicly and privately," she explained in an interview. "And of course, some of the public stuff you can counter. But the private innuendo, the sideline glances, the raised shoulders, the mockery, the ridicule—that's not always so easily defensible and they were enormously successful."

Drummond Rennie agreed with her. Rennie's views on whistle-blowers had been steadily reinforced by the misdeeds of the world-wide pharmaceutical industry. Time after time, it seemed, a company misrepresented what had been discovered about a drug and harassed the scientist or scientists who made the unwanted discovery. In several cases, Rennie had moved a contested study— or news about it—onto the pages of *JAMA*. Betty Dong's article on Synthroid appeared there, despite Knoll's attempt to suppress it. In 1999, Rennie learned that a biotechnology firm, Immune Response Corporation, was trying to block publication of data showing that an experimental AIDS therapy didn't work. The lead scientists were AIDS doctors at the University of California who had been sponsored by Immune Response to run a clinical trial. After they reached their negative conclusions, the company refused to provide them with the full data set, and they thought they'd be unable to publish their findings until Rennie and others intervened. Their incomplete results were scheduled to appear in *JAMA* in the fall of 2000.

This was the milieu in which Rennie listened to Olivieri and heard how Gideon Koren and a few of the hospital administrators had undermined her. "They cast doubt, they blackened her . . . and he was the leader in that and that was disgraceful," he said in an interview. Rennie saw Koren as a stereotype: the powerful academic male using his connections to quash a vulnerable female because she'd blown the whistle. "Every case is different, but every case has its Gideon Koren," was his take on the situation. Now that Koren had been caught red-handed over the anonymous letters, Rennie thought he knew what needed to happen. "You get rid of people like that," he said. "You don't have them around in the institution."

Rennie had begun to think that Olivieri was different than other whistleblowers he'd met. "Not everyone's a Nancy," he told her once in 1999. "Not everyone feeds on controversy, not everyone's a Joan of Arc." He remained one of her staunchest supporters.

Koren stayed on at Sick Kids, teaching and doing research. He maintained his large entourage of students, supervising or co-supervising as many as twenty post-doctoral fellows, residents and graduate students at a time, and he continued to issue his usual high volume of scientific papers, "a publication output unmatched in the Faculty," as the dean put it. Some of his papers from 1999 and after had major public health implications, including one on the relationship between vision damage in the newborn and a mother's exposure to organic solvents during pregnancy, and another that showed that pregnant women could safely use the herbal remedy echinacea.

He continued to face censure, however. In September 2000, the university concluded that he had committed misconduct by publishing the 1999 article on L1 without notifying Olivieri. The professors who considered the case said that as a co-investigator he was free to access the data set and write about it but shouldn't have published without consulting Olivieri or Brittenham, since the data also belonged to them. Naylor ordered Koren to retract his article from the journal where it appeared and to apologize to Olivieri and Brittenham.

At the College of Physicians and Surgeons, the complaint that the Gang of Four filed against Koren resulted in a finding that he was unprofessional. He was "cautioned" by the College, but the Gang wasn't satisfied. They appealed, and the decision went to the College's Discipline Committee. Eventually, the committee found Koren guilty of professional misconduct over the weird letters and of research misconduct over the 1999 article. He was formally reprimanded for "conduct unbecoming a physician." Nancy Olivieri and the Gang hadn't moved on after Humphrey's report in late 1999. They kept fighting. And on certain issues that mattered intensely to them, they won.

BATTLE FATIGUE

In the fall of 1999, Nancy Olivieri admitted to a reporter from the *Toronto Star* that she was "awfully distracted." One of the things distracting her was the need to reply to Sick Kids about the questions raised by Arnold Naimark. The hospital and university had promised to support her in 1999, in the agreement hammered out by Prichard and the two Davids, yet at Sick Kids there was still a committee of doctors looking into Naimark's allegations against her. The committee wanted to meet with Olivieri; she refused to meet. Though she responded to their questions, handing in a legal brief and three volumes of documents in October 1999, she felt the whole effort had been a waste of her time. She said the committee's accusations against her had "no basis" and were "completely untrue." Her lawyer requested the "specifics of the allegations," but Olivieri said the committee wouldn't reveal what information it had, so she refused to meet with them.

In the spring of 2000, the case went to the hospital's board of trustees, who referred the questions to the U of T and the College of Physicians and Surgeons of Ontario. The faculty association said the board's decision to involve the College of Physicians and Surgeons—the body with the right to remove a doctor's licence to practise—was part of "a conspiracy to injure Dr. Olivieri's credibility." It wasn't a conspiracy, but it was a long and injurious process for Nancy Olivieri that took her away from more meaningful work.

Olivieri's biggest distraction, though, wasn't the battle she was fighting in Toronto. It was being Nancy Olivieri, Canada's most famous whistleblower. She was winning medals for her courage, and in late 1999, a U.S. publication called *Academe* compared her to the woman she'd emulated at the FDA. "Nancy Olivieri . . . doesn't fancy herself as Frances Oldham Kelsey," the article began. "But for many of the people who hear Olivieri's story, the parallels are unmistakable with the so-called 'heroine of thalidomide.'" Olivieri, like Kelsey, was a Canadian whistleblower, acting to protect the public from a dangerous drug.

Just before Christmas 1999, her whistleblowing role was highlighted on *60 Minutes*. The show landed a small journalistic coup when reporter Lesley Stahl interviewed Barry Sherman of Apotex. Muttering under his breath, Sherman said of Olivieri, "She's nuts." It was too soft for the average television viewer to hear. But Stahl repeated the words several times. "What did you just say to me? You just said to me 'She's nuts.' You just said that to me. You looked at me, and you said, 'She's nuts.'" Sherman's response, "I'll say certain things to you off the record," brought the sharp retort, "We're reporters, we're not your pals." Subsequently, Olivieri sued Sherman for libel for his words on *60 Minutes*.

While her contentions about L1 and Apotex were given a hearing in Toronto-based inquiries and in the worldwide press, the links between the drug industry and medical schools continued to attract attention and grow. In February 2000, the *New York Times* reported that "academic scientists who lack industry ties have become as rare as giant pandas in the wild." Student movements had organized on several American campuses to protest the influence of corporations on university research, and an editorial in the *New England Journal of Medicine* in May 2000 warned that "academic institutions and their clinical faculty members must take care not to be open to the charge that they are for sale."

In her struggle with Apotex, Olivieri had come to stand for all the medical school teachers who weren't for sale. She was an emblem of the fight against corporate villainy in the pharmaceutical industry, a living hero winning awards and honours on an almost monthly basis for her courage. She flew from city to city to accept her honours and speak about her experiences. But all these efforts—to defend her reputation, tell her story and take down her opponents—came at a very high price.

In the spring of 2000, Nancy Olivieri had been battling Apotex and Sick Kids for four years. As the fight dragged on, she was losing ground on all of her professional fronts—her science, her teaching and her clinical work. That spring, I interviewed her for CBC Radio and she acknowledged that her scientific and teaching careers were fizzling out. When we met at the Starbucks in the Sick Kids atrium, she looked fatigued, with shadows under her eyes. She smiled at a senior pediatrician she was friendly with and gave him a warm hello. But when we went up to her office to talk in private, her expression was sour and her words weren't joyful.

She complained that the division chiefs who had recommended her demotion in January 1999 expected her to be friendly to them in 2000. She resented their entreaties and was annoyed that they'd been promoted. "Practically everyone who voted to fire me has gotten an endowed chair," she told me. By contrast, she said, her salary of $138,000 per annum made her the lowest-paid full professor at the hospital. Her bosses at Sick Kids were continuing to harass her, she claimed, and she seemed to view her salary as further evidence of it, though the figure she named was supplemented by a separate salary for her work at the Toronto General.

She was still appointed as a scientist at Sick Kids, but since the 1999 agreement she had not had a lab there. Instead, she worked in

space she'd borrowed from Brenda Gallie. She thought her borrowed space was infected, because the scientist who had used it
before her had been studying a condition called "Q fever." She also
thought she was being spied on. Her brother-in-law, who she said
knew about such things, had told her that her phone lines at the
hospital were tapped. She'd left a grant application with hospital
administrators for a signature and it took several days for them to
return it, she said. She wondered if they were making her wait on
purpose so that her grant wouldn't be approved. Her science was
suffering. Despite having substantial research funds, she told me she
wasn't spending much of her time on research. "I haven't done any
work at all that I could put down in the last eighteen months," she
said. "John Dick—he just spent a week writing a grant. And I think,
'Yes, I used to do that too.'

"Now, my whole life is like this: Who's calling UTFA? Who's
calling this? Who's working on the fundraiser . . . Now it's, come in
the office and there's two calls from two different lawyers, one call
about the grievance, another call about a press release . . . I run into
Elliott [Elliott Vichinsky] and he says, did you read this? And I think,
that's what I should be doing, reading the journals, but the excitement about journal papers and my own papers has had to take a
backseat here."

She said she had "probably twenty-five or thirty papers which
have not seen the light of day . . . They are unprocessed, they are
not at their final stage, they can't be pushed forward." And she
had "no time to direct students." As she saw it, there wasn't anything she could do to change the situation because she was
"embroiled in this fight probably ten or twelve hours a day."
Toward the end of 2000, Olivieri told a reporter for the *Times of
London* that research no longer attracted her. When December
rolled around that year, she didn't even attend the hematology
meetings where she'd spoken from the podium so many times.

Friends and colleagues said she'd almost disappeared from the
scientific arena. Some of the thalassemia patients continued to
complain behind Olivieri's back that she'd almost disappeared
from their clinics as well.

At the Toronto General, Melanie Kirby, the doctor who took
over Graham Sher's clinical duties when he left for the transfusion
service, stayed for about two years. Then she left for the sickle cell
service at Sick Kids and was replaced by Michèle Brill-Edwards, but
the hospital decreased the clinic's hours to a few days a week.

Olivieri was still the program's director and she was based in
Toronto, but patients found her difficult to reach and they rarely saw
her. One patient said, "There's the fear that patients are falling between
the cracks because the clinic director's attention is focused elsewhere
. . . She's too busy fighting for her job . . . What it comes down to is,
the patients aren't being seen." Louisa Tonna's mother, Jan, concurred.
Many of the adult patients, Jan said, "weren't getting to see a doctor
very often; you could go for months without seeing a doctor."

The patients were scared. During 1999 and 2000, three thalassemia patients died, two at home without ever making it to the
hospital. Anxiously, patients chatted about it with each other. Some
wrote to nurse Bev Tyler to ask what was going on. "Two patients
dying in their sleep at home," one patient said. "That's what seems
odd. Why at home and not in the ICU? Why didn't [the doctors]
know they were sick?"

Another adult patient, told that the cause of one of the deaths
was food poisoning, became cynical. As a teenager, living in
Ontario, she had been close to the patient who allegedly had died
of food poisoning. Then she'd moved to the U.K. and begun receiving her care in London. Inquiring about the deaths, she learned that
the thalassemia patients who had died in Ontario weren't seen
as frequently as she was; their doctors didn't seem to be keeping as
close tabs on them, and it disturbed her.

When I spoke with Brill-Edwards in her office in the thalassemia clinic at the Toronto General in the spring of 2000, she was preparing to attend a family meeting about one of the adult thalassemia patients who had recently died. She explained that in that particular case, the patient who died "really fell through the cracks." The patient had gone to the emergency room, but doctors there hadn't figured out why she was having severe headaches. "They knew she was 'thal,'" Brill-Edwards said, "but they didn't connect it." She added, "They didn't call any of the thal people. They didn't call the thal program." I asked if the emergency room physicians would normally phone the thalassemia doctors, and Brill-Edwards was noncommittal. "If they think they know what they're doing, the discretion's theirs to call us or not," she said.

The concerns of adult thalassemia patients and their families were mounting by the spring of 2001, and a meeting was scheduled in an auditorium at the Toronto General Hospital "to kind of clear the air, because people were unhappy," recalled Jan Tonna. "There had been three deaths fairly close together, which is what got people nervous," she added. One young man died in May 2001, and Jan's own daughter, Louisa, had died after being stricken with serious heart disease the previous summer. She'd been twenty-one. At the meeting, Brill-Edwards told Tonna that L1 was a factor in her daughter's death, because Louisa's iron levels had stayed high during the few years that she was taking the drug, but that didn't explain why Louisa wasn't being looked after on a hospital ward, where her heart could be monitored. Instead she died at home in August 2000, apparently from heart failure brought on by iron overload.

In the fall of 2000, while thalassemia patients were worrying about their losses, a seventeen-year-old girl with sickle cell disease entered the Hospital for Sick Children for an operation on her gall bladder. It wasn't an emergency, and the surgery wasn't billed as life-threatening. But while recovering, Sanchia Bulgin bled to death internally. Soon after Sanchia died, her mother called the pediatrician who'd cared for her daughter since she was a small child. The office receptionist took the call, heard what had happened and began weeping. When the doctor spoke to Sanchia's mother, she couldn't believe what she was hearing. What could have happened?

The coroner and the hospital both investigated, and the hospital soon claimed responsibility for the death. An internal report of the hospital's investigation listed a series of errors that had contributed to Sanchia's death. Apparently the various doctors involved hadn't communicated. The sickle cell doctors hadn't been in close touch with Sanchia's surgeons. The nurses and doctors hadn't monitored the patient's hemoglobin level and blood pressure closely after the operation. And the nurses were underinformed about sickle cell disease.

Hearing about Sanchia's death, Manuel Carcao felt personally devastated. It wasn't just that he'd known the young woman from his time on the sickle cell service. It was that he'd spent hundreds of hours on a project aimed at preventing the sorts of errors that had cost Sanchia her life: the guidelines project, with its special section on the best way to care for sickle cell patients undergoing surgery. But the guidelines he worked on in 1998 were never finalized.

At the coroner's inquest, the jurors heard that when Sanchia was admitted for her operation, Sick Kids had guidelines for the care of sickle cell patients in a draft form, but surgical and anesthesiology staff weren't following them. Instead, the draft guidelines had "floated around" the hospital for two years without being formally adopted. The coroner grilled the pediatrician from the sickle cell disease clinic—Melanie Kirby—about the guidelines, but she was reluctant to say very much. "Why the process took so long is not for me to comment on," she told the coroner's jury.

The sickle cell guidelines were finally adopted and distributed at Sick Kids in the late fall of 2000, two months after Sanchia's death.

The lawyer representing the Sickle Cell Association of Ontario told the jurors, "The hospital did nothing after Sanchia's death that it could not have done months before her death."

The inquest jury completed its deliberations in the late spring of 2001 and issued thirty-one recommendations. One was that sickle cell patients should be admitted the day before the operation. Another was that doctors should consider preoperative transfusions for such children undergoing surgical procedures. Both recommendations had been contained in the draft guidelines that had gone on the shelf in 1998. The inquest also found that Sick Kids nurses were overworked and that there was a serious lack of communication by key physicians and surgeons caring for Sanchia Bulgin. In part, the poor communication between the sickle cell program and other programs in the hospital was one of the costs of the hospital's battle with Nancy Olivieri.

23

MOVING ON

In the fall of 2001, the CAUT's three academic inquirers published their analysis. Titled *The Olivieri Report,* it exonerated Olivieri while faulting the university, the hospital, Apotex and Koren. The three professors had conducted their inquiry by examining documents that the CAUT, Olivieri or others provided and by doing interviews. The terms of the inquiry were to investigate what happened, determine whether there were ethical violations or threats to academic freedom, and discover whether Olivieri or her colleagues had been harassed in a way that interfered with their research or clinical work. The three served without compensation, took steps to ensure their independence from the CAUT, and went ahead with their efforts even though administrators from the university, the hospital and the company refused to participate. They explained in their report, "The potential disadvantage of these non-participations was substantially offset by the access the committee obtained to a large quantity of relevant correspondence . . ." They also retained the right to decide "that particular matters [were] not relevant to [the committee's] terms of reference."

In the end, they met with twenty-six people, including Olivieri, Brittenham, Brill-Edwards and the Gang of Four, Nathan and Weatherall, lawyers who had represented Olivieri, and one patient and her family. After completing the report but before publishing it, they let Olivieri and the hospital administrators involved see "a fair summary of the information" on which they'd based their findings, in case an individual wanted to register an objection.

Arnie Aberman wrote them that the material they showed him was "incomplete, incorrect, and misleading" and since he could not review the documents that led to their conclusions, he found it "hardly a reasonable procedure." David Naylor wrote later, "Virtually none of the individuals who are criticized in the report . . . participated in any way with the CAUT Inquiry report." All were consulted on many occasions but refused to participate. The one patient the professors met told them about her experience taking L1; her family described their confusion and worry when she went off of it. But the professors seemed to view the family's concern as falling outside of their terms of reference and they didn't mention it in their report. The professors' decision to let Olivieri and others involved see information prior to publication could have influenced the final product, but very little material was edited out at that point, according to Jocelyn Downie of Dalhousie University in Halifax, one of the report's authors. The published report was a vindication for Nancy Olivieri, with the three professors concluding she deserved to "receive redress" from Sick Kids for the "unfair treatment" she received.

In December 2001, Olivieri received further vindication from the College of Physicians and Surgeons when the College ruled that she had provided her patients with a reasonable standard of care. The College had consulted a panel of experts that essentially dismissed the hospital's questions and allegations. At the medical school, Dean Naylor followed suit and dismissed the charges against Olivieri that the hospital had lodged with the university.

After a mediator became involved, Olivieri and the Gang of Four finally won a new settlement with the hospital and the university in November 2002. Though the terms were confidential, it was described publicly as "generous," and the money was rumoured to be substantial. In exchange, Olivieri essentially agreed to give up her patient care duties for five years and focus solely on her research. She said she felt "pretty terrific" about the agreement. The resolution was fully supported by the faculty union, which had invested so much in it. "We're about a million-dollar organization which has been seized of this issue for almost two years," Rhonda Love explained. The total figure they'd spent fighting the Olivieri case was "almost not calculable."

The settlement with the hospital and the university wasn't the only sign that Nancy Olivieri's supporters had won. The case had also inspired important and lasting changes at the university and its teaching hospitals. "She fought, and with luck, we'll all benefit as a consequence," Drummond Rennie told a documentary producer who interviewed him about Olivieri in 2003. Canadian scientists were already benefiting from the scrutiny her case had brought to bear on a scientist's right to publish and on the university's role in academic-industrial collaborations.

At the university, although the official inquiry into the L1 clinical trials ended in late 1998 when Arnold Naimark tabled his report, the attempts to prevent that sort of fiasco from happening again had continued through 2001, as the medical school and its eight teaching hospitals revamped their policies for dealing with biotech and pharmaceutical companies. They developed a single set of rules that every hospital agreed to. One rule held that research contracts between professors and private companies could "not allow research sponsors to suppress or otherwise censor research results." Another said that faculty members "should be able to submit work for publication within 6 months of sharing the findings with a sponsor"; "delays of up to 12 months" were permitted, but only "in exceptional circumstances." A third rule said that if the sponsoring company disagreed with the contract researcher, the researcher still retained rights "to publish as he or she sees fit" and "to disclose immediately any safety concerns" to study subjects, research ethics boards and regulators.

In addition to accepting the new university rules, Sick Kids administrators revamped their own internal standards, establishing an office to review any deals between the hospital's doctors or scientists and outside companies. At the hospital's Research Ethics Board, the chair's position went from being a voluntary post to a half-time paid slot, mirroring changes that were occurring throughout Canada and the U.S. as boards overseeing research on human subjects started to take their responsibilities more seriously. On a national level, the federal research agency—formerly the Medical Research Council, now the Canadian Institutes of Health Research—began to focus on partnerships between industry and academia. The head of the agency, Olivieri's old flame Alan Bernstein, said that clarifying the role of industry in research was one of his priorities as the nation's top scientific administrator.

The case of Nancy Olivieri even influenced science authorities on an international scale. In September 2001, the editors of some of the world's leading medical journals (including the *Lancet,* the *New England Journal of Medicine, JAMA* and the *British Medical Journal*) established a policy that they would not review or publish work by scientists whose sponsors prevented them from analyzing their data independently or publishing their work freely. Less than one year later, an industry group, the Pharmaceutical Research and Manufacturers Association, committed its members to "not suppress or veto publications" except for a short time to protect intellectual property.

The University of Toronto also began to grapple with the authoritarian procedures of its teaching hospitals, a move that brought the university administration and the hospitals onto a collision course with the faculty association. The UTFA continued to argue that the best solution for medical school faculty was to be represented by the union. The two sides fought for nearly two years, deadlocking repeatedly. Finally, in June 2004, the provost circulated draft policies giving medical school faculty their own dispute resolution mechanisms. The union essentially lost its battle—clinical professors would not become dues-paying members of the UTFA—but it didn't step aside, and intended to represent any member of the medical faculty who sought its assistance.

Even with all these signs of their impact on the world of science, it was a huge relief for the Gang to win a monetary acknowledgment that they'd been in the right. It did more than allow them to pay back outstanding debts. Dick said the financial settlement with the university and the hospital was a "vindication," and Durie described it as "a way to move forward." But after all that had happened, moving forward came more easily to some of them than to others.

Brenda Gallie had already moved her research to the University Health Network, where she continued to work on projects related to the genetic test for retinoblastoma and also embarked on a new career in "cancer informatics," a new field involving the use of computers and Web-based technologies to manipulate the enormous databanks used to analyze genetic data. But she still spent time in the operating suite at Sick Kids, and described herself as "extremely frustrated" with the hospital. In 2003 and 2004, as a featured scientist in a travelling Canadian museum exhibition called "The Geee! in Genome," Gallie said that if she could have a meal with anyone, she would dine with Marie Curie, "a great, determined woman who followed her own ideas."

Helen Chan was still at Sick Kids searching for better chemotherapy for retinoblastoma by collaborating on international clinical trials. Together, the two women continued to win accolades from their patients, including an Ontario man who was blind as a result of tumours in both eyes as a child. Gallie and Chan had saved one of his son's eyes and both of his daughter's. In 2003, when the boy was six and the girl was four, the father told the Terry Fox Foundation, "As the research moved forward, our family moved forward with it."

John Dick went on sabbatical to London's Institute for Cancer Research in the spring of 2000, for a much-needed reprieve. He did science. "I'm at the bench," he said at the time, describing it as "exhilarating." When he returned to Sick Kids, he continued to collaborate widely with colleagues, including the hospital's research director, Manuel Buchwald. In 2002, Dick was awarded an endowed chair, and in 2003, he left Sick Kids for the Toronto General (now part of the University Health Network) to become director of its new stem cell research program. He was a leader in a Canadian dream team with $1 million in federal funds for stem cell research.

Peter Durie was turned down by several universities for the job of chair of pediatrics, and he was sure his role in the Olivieri affair affected his candidacy. He said Michael Strofolino virtually told him as much, and, privately, other gastroenterologists concurred. Prior to the Olivieri issues, they thought, he would have been a strong contender. He remained at Sick Kids as director of research on cystic fibrosis and continued to collaborate with researchers in Toronto and around the world. In 2002, he was a key member of a Sick Kids team that identified the gene responsible for a rare disorder of the pancreas called Shwachman-Diamond syndrome. Predictably, Durie was humble about his role, thanking the families who participated in the study and telling reporters that the work had depended on "patient samples from around the world." The following year he won the major award in his field.

Olivieri turned her battles into a second academic career. She wrote in science journals on academic freedom and went on sabbatical to England in 2001 to study medical ethics and law. When she came back to Toronto, she resumed her research on thalassemia at the Toronto General but once her 2002 settlement was in place she was no longer in charge of patients.

For a time, the changes in her clinical involvement were matched by significant changes in her research. "What a huge hole she's left in the field, by taking herself out and not doing any research worth anything very much during those years," her good friend Drummond Rennie commented in 2003 in the television film *Dying for Drugs*. "It's tremendously sad, and I think her life must be seen at this moment as a tragedy." Olivieri wasn't as downhearted. Mentioning other whistle-blowers she'd met, she said in the film that they had been "destroyed in a way I don't think any of us has been, at least yet." She had continued enrolling her patients in industry-sponsored clinical trials, including a trial of the new Novartis iron-removal drug ICL670 and another of a new, long-acting form of Desferal. In addition, she continued to be well regarded in her field. In 2003, she was the principal investigator in Toronto for an NIH-funded network of investigators known as the Thalassemia Clinical Research Network, and was widely sought-after as a collaborator. She set up a research foundation at the hospital called Hemoglobal, through which she continued her work with Weatherall, Novartis, and the NIH.

But at an early meeting of the NIH network, she warned that the sailing might not be smooth. Her collaborators would include hematologists who disagreed with her about L1 and had accepted Apotex sponsorship for their research. "I have two deletions of the 'forgiveness gene'," one scientist recalls her saying at the meeting, to general laughter. Yet as she'd predicted, she did run into difficulties. In 2004, says David Nathan, "Nancy wrote a letter to the NIH saying that she wanted to do two things simultaneously: run her research in Sri Lanka and continue as Principal Investigator for the NIH Network in Toronto. They refused to allow her to do that." In 2004, the NIH authorities in charge of the network asked her to step down. Nathan says, "I think she probably disagreed with the NIH on the issue of whether she could remain as PI and still be out of the country most of the time. I think that's where the disagreement is."

Gideon Koren survived his disgrace and in 2004 was appointed to an endowed chair at the University of Western Ontario. The dean of medicine praised Koren as "one of very few Canadian physician-scientists whose career is dedicated to drug safety."

Olivieri was still suing Apotex for libel, and the company counter-sued in response, saying that her statements about its employees and products were defamatory. Michael Spino, for one, had hated hearing the things that were said about his company. "I spent the last five years feeling like some sort of scumbag, reading in the newspapers that profits matter more to this company than patients," he told me in 2001. When it came to profits, Barry Sherman of Apotex was an easy target. He joined *Forbes*'s list of the richest men in the world in 2000, and the business press valued his fortune that year at $1.9 billion, a figure that made him the eleventh wealthiest person in Canada. By 2002, he was worth half a billion more. As for his company's new line of brand-name products, Spino and Sherman were proud of L1's success. By 2003, L1 had been approved in twenty-five countries and had earned over $1 million in net profits. "And it is saving lives," said company public affairs officer Elie Betito.

As I write this, L1 is considered a reasonable option for patients who cannot or will not take Desferal—outside of North America. Doctors in the U.K., Italy, India and Taiwan pay their respects to Olivieri's publications, duly noting that L1 has worrying adverse effects that should be watched for. But in practice, many doctors don't view L1 as an exceptionally dangerous drug; patients taking it simply need close monitoring. L1 is the small child hiding in the wings of a bad divorce. Its mother and the company she married to support her work on it are clawing at each other through the courts, but the drug they spawned has a life of its own. It owes its staying power to science.

24

THE SCIENCE OF L1

In 1999, Nancy Olivieri was in Ottawa twice for meetings with Health Canada officials. On both occasions her message was the same: L1 was too dangerous to be approved—and it hasn't been. In Europe, meanwhile, where a score of doctors were studying L1, the scientific issues surrounding the pill had begun to change. In large-scale studies, scientists couldn't reproduce Olivieri's findings. L1 didn't work as well as Desferal, but it worked. It had side effects but it didn't cause liver scarring.

The European drug agency licensed the pill in August 1999. Though the licence was only for emergency use by thalassemia patients, it was a milestone for L1. A delighted Michael Spino said in a press release that the drug had been "thoroughly tested" and "demonstrated . . . to be a safe and effective second line therapy." But Nancy Olivieri was planning expensive and time-consuming litigation to have the licence reversed. As a first step, she applied to the European Court for a judicial review of the drug agency's decision. She said in 2003 that she spent $300,000 fighting L1 in Europe. Ultimately, she was unsuccessful: the European Court gave her a hearing but didn't revoke L1's approval. She told the *British Medical Journal* in January 2004 that she was considering appealing the court ruling.

By 2003, however, L1 was used routinely for thalassemia patients outside of North America. Known as Kelfer in India,

Ferriprox in Europe and Australia and deferiprone in scientific reports, it's officially approved as a second-line treatment for patients who can't use Desferal and it's used widely in combination with Desferal: patients take Desferal injections once every three to four nights and L1 in between. Recent studies in the U.S. show that the combination is working better than either drug alone.

In Canada and the U.S., however, the drug is still experimental. Doctors who want to prescribe it have to contact Apotex and apply to the FDA or Health Canada to use it as an investigational drug. "We get desperate calls on a regular basis from doctors and families around the world inquiring about the availability of this drug," Apotex president Jack Kay said in a press release in 2000. The earliest the drug is likely to be approved in the U.S. or Canada is 2005.

Thalassemia patient groups keep rooting for it. Enough of the precautionary principle; U.S. patient groups want FDA approval of L1 and so do the patient advocates in Europe. George Constantinou, a thalassemia patient and leader in the U.K. Thalassemia Society, is angry at what's happened to L1 in North America. He wrote the editor of the *British Medical Journal* in March 2004 to complain that thousands of patients die annually from iron overload, and that "the Olivieri debate contributes to these deaths by subordinating medical to political issues."

In Constantinou's view, the drug industry giant Novartis seized the ongoing debate to its advantage. Desferal, he noted, "was one of Ciba-Geigy's top earners before it merged into Novartis; a switch to a cheaper chelator, or one not produced by Novartis, will obviously be unwelcome."

Bernadette Modell, the British thalassemia expert, concurs with Constantinou about Novartis. She thinks the company would like to see acceptance of L1 postponed until its own alternative oral drug—ICL670—is ready for market. "It's so terribly disappointing to see these forces operating in one's own little field," she said in an interview. Though Modell gave no clear evidence that the company was attempting to wield influence, Michael Spino did, in a letter to the *New England Journal of Medicine* in 2003.

Spino thinks David Nathan's ties to Novartis represent a conflict of interest that should have prevented him from writing about L1 for the journal. In his letter he pointed out that Nathan's hospital, the Dana-Farber Cancer Institute, had connections to Novartis that Nathan had not disclosed, despite the journal's requirement that authors state all relationships that might bias their work. Nathan was CEO of the hospital when it worked directly with the company to develop Gleevec, the new cancer drug that has made a dramatic difference for patients with certain forms of leukemia. Nathan was also involved in the company's effort to test ICL670. But Nathan argued in the journal that neither of those deals with Novartis constituted genuine conflicts of interest, since he had no financial interest in the company. His long-standing close relationship with Olivieri is a mentorship, but the journal's editors concluded it did not bias him in Olivieri's favour. The journal replied to Spino's complaint with an editor's note that read: "Dr. Olivieri was a fellow with Dr. Nathan in the mid-1980s. Editors consider events that took place more than two years before publication to be immaterial with respect to conflicts of interest."

The FDA is not ready to approve L1 yet, and neither is Canada's Health Protection Branch. The agencies won't discuss L1 since all their information on it is still confidential, but it seems as if they're attending to concerns raised by Nancy Olivieri. However, those concerns are more controversial than ever.

Since 1998, when Olivieri published her *New England Journal of Medicine* article showing that L1 becomes ineffective after long-term use in some patients, a flurry of scientific papers have demonstrated the drug's effectiveness. No doctors have replicated Olivieri's findings that L1 damages the heart by causing scarring, and two separate studies refuted Olivieri and Brittenham's findings that the drug damages the liver. Ian Wanless, an internationally known liver pathologist at the Toronto General Hospital, led one of those efforts.

When Apotex asked Wanless to examine the drug, he recruited two liver pathologists from Europe, and the three doctors evaluated liver biopsies from a large series of Italian patients on L1, publishing their results in September 2002 in *Blood*. "We concluded that deferiprone does not cause liver fibrosis," Wanless said at the time. "We are confident in this result because the study involved a large number of patients and the biopsies were coded and randomized so that no investigator bias was possible." The other study to refute Olivieri was done in Italy, where investigators compared L1 and Desferal in a randomized trial that wasn't sponsored by Apotex. The trial found no difference in progression of liver fibrosis between patients on the two drugs. Doctors in Europe and India have also been convinced by their own clinical experience. With hundreds of patients using L1 continuously for years, there is no sign of patients getting sick or dying as a result of liver fibrosis.

The toxicity trial that Olivieri had convinced Spino to sponsor—her "international trial"—was carried to completion by her former friend at the Children's Hospital of Philadelphia, Alan Cohen, and the results were published in 2000 in the *British Journal of Haematology*. The paper concluded that L1's toxicities are rare and manageable. Of 187 patients, one developed L1's most deadly side effect—the disappearance of all white blood cells—and nine had low numbers of white blood cells. "The study showed that toxicity to white blood cells is a rare side effect of deferiprone, and is not frequent enough to disqualify the drug as a potential treatment for iron overload," Cohen said. He published longer-term results of the same trial in 2003, and the results remained the same: it was extremely rare for a patient to experience the loss of all white cells and rare for patients to develop low numbers of white cells. When those side effects did occur, patients recovered after going off the drug.

In clinical practice, if patients' blood tests show a low white blood cell count, they are supposed to stop taking L1. They're also supposed to go off it if they develop a fever or a sore throat, since those are signs that their white cells aren't working to combat infections. L1's other side effects—nausea, vomiting and joint pains—are more common, and some patients go off the drug as a result of those side effects, while others take standard GI and arthritis medications to cope.

Reporters in Toronto picked up on the new findings as soon as they started to appear. The *National Post* ran a feature article in February 2000 quoting Alan Cohen. The *Toronto Star* also reported on Cohen's work, and in the spring of 2000 CBC Television ran a documentary on its nightly news program, *The National,* covering the scientific disagreement over L1's risks and benefits. The show interviewed British thalassemia specialist Beatrix Wonke, who said she'd been prescribing L1 for several years with good results. She also implied that she doubted the quality of Nancy Olivieri's work, saying that the controversy over the drug was confined to North America. "There is no misunderstanding at all in Europe," she told the CBC's Hana Gartner.

Olivieri and her supporters saw the program as harassment. Winnipeg ethicist Arthur Schafer wrote an op-ed for the *Toronto Star* accusing the CBC of "grave factual errors and innuendo" and explained in an interview that part of what he saw "as objectionable in the CBC's presentation . . . was seeing this as a scientific dispute." He added, "I never saw this as a scientific issue." As far as Schafer was concerned, the scientific questions surrounding Nancy Olivieri's work on L1 weren't worth asking. Schafer was in good company. The Gang of Four saw it the same way, and so did thalassemia's two Davids—Nathan and Weatherall. "What is central to this particular case is the principle of academic freedom," they wrote in the *New England Journal of Medicine* in 2002. "It does not matter whether, in the end, Olivieri was right or wrong in her assessment of the efficacy and safety of deferiprone."

But it matters a lot to Nancy Olivieri whether she's right or wrong about L1, and her opinions about her science matter to officials at Health Canada and the FDA. She charged the CBC with libel for its presentation on *The National*, and the charges themselves brought a hush: the documentary containing Hana Gartner's interview with Beatrix Wonke could not be re-aired or sold to other networks for rebroadcast.

It's not hard to see why the two Davids and Olivieri's supporters closer to home turned blind eyes to the mounting evidence that, when it came to L1, Olivieri was no longer a disinterested observer of the data. Apotex had attacked her, and her hospital was trying to attack her; in that context, it was unconscionable or at least unpopular to question her too closely about her findings. But disinterest and skepticism are essential in science, and in protecting Olivieri, her supporters around the world lost sight of that.

At the conference in Palermo, Sicily, in 2003, an American thal-assemia advocate listened to the papers describing L1's benefits for the heart. Five U.S. patients younger than thirty had died of heart disease in 2002. From what she heard here, they might still be alive if they lived in England. They died largely because they'd stopped taking Desferal, and in England they'd have had access to L1, which could have made a difference. A doctor from the U.S., sitting nearby, concurred. "I'm sure that's true," he said when I asked him about it. He explained that he and his colleagues all had the same experience: some patients simply wouldn't or couldn't use Desferal.

A U.S. survey published in 2002 confirms how difficult patients still find injecting Desferal. Among more than 1,800 patients, nearly half missed at least one dose and most missed five doses in the course of a month, largely because of the drug's adverse effects or because of a patient's negative feelings about it. It's a pattern that will speed a patient's death. In 2000, according to a paper by Bernadette Modell in the *Lancet*, half of British thalassemia patients were dying before thirty-five, mainly because conventional therapy with Desferal was "too burdensome" for them. Three years later, Modell was in Palermo and shared more recent data: British patients were living longer. The mortality rate in the U.K. had fallen to half of what it had been when she put together the 2000 publication. "This is the lowest it's ever been," she told me. The cause could not be pinpointed precisely, but she thought the most "conspicuous change" was that so many patients were using L1, alone or in combination with Desferal.

Scientists who study L1 say it isn't as good as Desferal at taking iron out of the liver, but it is better at removing iron from the heart. Heart disease is a major killer in thalassemia so L1 is playing a crucial role. One of the studies that showed this was conducted at the University of Turin, and its findings kept getting mentioned at Palermo. Comparing fifty-four patients who had been taking L1 for an average of six years with seventy-five patients taking Desferal, the Turin doctors found no deaths in the L1 group but four deaths in the Desferal group. They thought the higher death rate was a result of more cardiac disease: the L1 group had a 4 per cent incidence of serious heart problems, versus 20 per cent in the Desferal group.

Some doctors in England have tested this theory using a novel MRI technique known as T2* (pronounced tee-two-star) that calculates how much iron is deposited in a patient's heart. As the iron deposit increases, the magnetic resonance signal intensity is lost, resulting in black areas on the MRI. As a result, doctors have started prescribing more L1 if a patient's heart appears most affected by iron deposits on T2*, and more Desferal if the liver seems most affected. In a paper about T2* in the *Lancet* in 2002, radiologists at London's Royal Brompton Hospital reported that thalassemia patients on L1 had less iron in their hearts than patients on Desferal, and their hearts pumped more effectively.

In Toronto, only one patient, Corrado, is still taking L1, but others hear about the pill at meetings such as the one in Palermo and read about it on patient websites. Not everyone on L1 is satisfied with the treatment. One Italian woman wrote the Thalassemia

Patients and Friends website that L1 was working for her, but "I must take twelve pills a day to reach this result and my stomach and liver are very upset."

Some patients are taking another Desferal replacement, the Novartis drug called ICL670 that Olivieri, Nathan and others are testing in a clinical trial. It's a powder, not a pill, and has to be mixed in water. "Patients hate it," a Toronto hematologist confided to me. "Ever taken Metamucil?" she asked. "That's what it's like." As a result, some patients discontinue ICL670, but for those who stay on it, it works as well as Desferal, though it can cause abdominal pain and other gastrointestinal side effects. An adult thalassemia patient in Montreal who's been on it for more than a year said she doesn't mind the drug's chalky taste, and her iron level has fallen on the drug. "For me it's much more effective than Desferal," she said. "I haven't missed one dose." Novartis plans to submit the drug for licensing in 2005.

Anita was in Palermo sporting a new smile—she'd finally had plastic surgery on her face. It took her a year and a half to prepare, banking ten bags of her own blood so that surgeons would have a way to treat her if she ran into bleeding problems. For her, the most important session at the conference was the one where Susan Perrine and several other doctors presented their data showing that the various butyrate drugs are working for many patients. Anita still depends on arginine butyrate to survive, as does her brother.

On the last day of the Palermo meeting, a panel of experts discussed the evidence for and against the different treatments, and Chris Gluud, a Danish expert on clinical trials, took the floor with a list of "ten commandments" for doctors running clinical trials. Most trials in thalassemia aren't up to his standards. For example, his commandment number six is that a trial should have adequate blinding, but thalassemia trials typically aren't blinded—as in Olivieri's L1 trials, the doctors usually know what their patients are taking. That bothers Gluud, and he reminded his listeners that in an unblinded trial, no one could be sure of the results. "We know that we are all biased," he said. "We overestimate the effects of our interventions by 40 to 50 per cent."

Some doctors in the audience were muttering that Gluud didn't understand the difficulties of working on thalassemia, but Gluud carried on to his tenth commandment—that researchers have to maintain adequate distance from industry. Otherwise, he said, there's a temptation to interpret their results in favour of the drug they're testing, since unfavourable results could dry up the funding source.

In 2003, Gluud and his colleagues in Copenhagen studied this issue, and their report—on 370 trials published over a period of twenty-nine years—was striking. Fifty-one percent of trials funded by private companies recommended the study drug as the treatment of choice, compared with only sixteen percent of those funded by non-profit organizations. Company-sponsored trials, the group concluded, "may be more positive due to biased interpretation of trial results."

In Palermo, Alan Cohen replied to Gluud's cautionary note about industry: "I would say also, be wary of investigators—they can make mistakes." Someone in the audience asked him to explain. "There's a lot of motives out there besides money," he said. "There's academic advancement, self-promotion, self aggrandizement." Having a drug company as a sponsor isn't the only circumstance that leads to scientists becoming biased about a drug.

Cohen, now physician in chief at the Children's Hospital of Philadelphia, continues to collaborate on Apotex-sponsored trials of L1. His remarks reminded me of my conversation with the American doctor whose patient had said he'd rather die than take Desferal. "I think deep down she was driven by a true concern for her patients. I think that's the only way that an individual would fight to the death," the doctor told me. "She's really fighting to the death and you don't do that unless you truly believe in what you're doing and that you are being wronged and that it is a corporate conspiracy, and that the company is trying to bulldoze the needs of the patients for their corporate interests. You don't tilt against a windmill unless you're damn sure you're right. And at this point, she's so convinced of it, that she's blind. And that happens to scientists. They tend to be obsessive people. Objective people would see that things have changed and you have to reassess."

He asked me not to use his name, saying, "If you quote me, my papers won't get published." He was expressing a common fear among L1 researchers. Olivieri published on L1 in the *New England Journal*, twice, and Nathan and Weatherall have published editorials on L1 there, but other papers on the drug have appeared in less prominent, more specialized journals—*Hemoglobin*, *Haematologica*, the *British Journal of Haematology*, and occasionally, *Blood*. To publish even in those journals has been very difficult, according to L1 researchers in the U.S. and the U.K.

A British doctor cited a specific example in which an influential scientist tried to block publication of the international safety trial of L1 in the *British Journal of Haematology* in 2000. The British doctor said the scientist had argued about it with the journal's editors and was nearly successful in keeping the report out of print. Alan Cohen, the lead author of that paper, has been publishing in science journals for about twenty-five years and says he's never found it so difficult. "Publishing anything about deferiprone [L1] has been unusually hard," he said. Instead of addressing the science of his articles, reviewers question his ethics or attack him with unfounded accusations, saying that he's published the same data multiple times or that he's a consultant to Apotex, without revealing the source of their misinformation. He's accepted Apotex research grants but hasn't ever consulted to the company.

Bernadette Modell has had similar experiences. She sent her paper on the improved survival of thalassemia patients in the U.K.

to the *Lancet* and got back a review that was blatantly hostile. Her paper was rejected. Modell said that she has received "endless letters and correspondence from people [working on L1] who've had trouble getting their work published." The American doctor who asked me not to use his name said he was "having papers rejected right and left," and he was afraid that the situation would worsen if criticisms of Olivieri were traced to him. "It's a small field and Nancy has some powerful allies who are very influential," he said.

This is not a new phenomenon in science. Peer review, the time-honoured system used by medical journals to choose which papers to publish, has been criticized because papers aren't judged on merit alone. Instead, reviewers can use the process to "punish authors they do not like, settle old scores and hold up competitors," wrote the British molecular biologist Peter Lawrence, in an editorial in *Nature* in 2003. Drummond Rennie, of the *Journal of the American Medical Association*, has referred to scientific peer review as "power without accountability," because most journals keep the names of reviewers a secret. According to American and British doctors I've interviewed, in thalassemia research a small group of scientists, including Olivieri, Brittenham, Nathan and Weatherall, have exerted substantial control over publishing and presenting in the field. Scientists who disagree with them about L1 have found it very hard to communicate their findings.

In the past few years, the only positive results about L1 to appear in a top-tier journal were the T2* data from the Royal Brompton Hospital, published in the *Lancet* in 2002. Two years later, the *Lancet*'s editor, Richard Horton, corresponded with me by e-mail about the struggle he and his staff faced over that paper. "When a field is very split like this one, the key point is that the final decision rests with the editors, not the reviewers," he wrote. At the *Lancet*, "a very angry reviewer" felt the editors "had ignored their recommendation" on the paper. "Having heard all sides, we judged that the paper in question had merit," said Horton. "But this one reviewer virtually exploded with anger." The reviewer contested the journal's decision, but the *Lancet* published the paper. In situations like that, Horton said, he turns to his editorial staff. "The fact that you feel part of a very closed community does help to insulate you from the views of even the most well-known individuals."

L1 investigators believe they've seen another chilling effect on their work—their abstracts are less likely to get chosen for presentation at scientific meetings. "Many people in the field have felt that having papers accepted for presentation at national meetings was more difficult," said Alan Cohen.

Thalassemia patients in Toronto aren't complaining about biased peer review—they're worrying about death. "Premature deaths of young adults with thalassemia" was the headline on a press release issued by the Thalassemia Foundation in May 2004—it reported that "fifteen young adults with thalassemia have died in the city in the past two to three years." Most were in their twenties. "Many of these deaths were avoidable," the foundation said in its release. As I was readying this book for publication in the fall of 2004, another patient died, at age twenty-four.

It's not clear why more thalassemia patients are dying in Toronto than in other places. Montreal, for example, has about thirty thalassemia patients followed by Montreal Children's Hospital, compared with Toronto's two hundred. In Montreal, only one patient has died in the past several years. Modell's data show that people with thalassemia are also living longer in the U.K., Cyprus and Italy. The difference from Toronto could be the lack of access to L1. Three Montreal patients were started on it as part of Olivieri's randomized trial, and they remained on it in combination with Desferal after the trial ended. Many British and Italian patients have been on combination therapy with L1 and Desferal. In

Cyprus, according to Paul Telfer of the Royal London Hospital, more than 150 patients have gone on combination therapy since 2000. Yet even in settings where L1 is unavailable, the death rate seems to be lower than in Toronto.

In July 2004, the Thalassemia Foundation and the Toronto-based Anemia Institute held a small meeting in Toronto and invited London physician John Porter to describe his specialized clinic at University College Hospital. Porter sees more than 100 thalassemia patients and doesn't offer L1 or combination therapy, but his program hasn't lost a patient born after 1975. At that meeting, Ian Quirt, the hematologist who currently runs the adult thalassemia program at the Toronto General Hospital, said that Toronto lacks the "very efficient system" that Porter's clinic has established for adult patients. Toronto adult patients only have access to a doctor ten hours a week and Quirt himself is part-time with the clinic.

One clue to the spate of deaths comes from data collected by the Thalassemia Research Network, which shows that many Toronto patients have very high levels of iron in their livers, the result of progressive iron overload. An American hematologist speculates that other patients in Olivieri's L1 trials may have suffered as Louisa Tonna did: after years on L1, switching back to Desferal could have proved too difficult. In London, Modell wonders if Toronto's early deaths could be linked to the crisis around L1 and the breakdown in communication it engendered among physicians. The crisis was profoundly disruptive in the U.K., she says. "Nobody trusts anybody."

Foundation leaders are calling for more physician time and more coordination of thalassemia services between Sick Kids and the Toronto General. Almost all the adult patients I spoke with say that Toronto's adult thalassemia clinic is understaffed. "What we need is a comprehensive care program," Josie said at the July meeting, referring to the sort of five-day-a-week program available to adult thalassemia patients in the United Kingdom. Olivieri also spoke at the same meeting, and criticized Toronto's resources as too limited for clinical services and for research. "There are 53 chairs funded at UHN [University Health Network]," she told those attending the July meeting. "But as I'm sure you all know there's no chair in thalassemia."

Howard, at forty-two, still struggles with Desferal. He isn't part of an ICL670 trial, though he wanted to be. He flew to Boston in 2001 for one of the first tests of the drug, but the Boston doctors found something troubling with his eye and made him stop the drug in case he was suffering a side effect. Then he tried another route for getting off Desferal, volunteering for one of Olivieri's butyrate trials, but butyrate didn't work for him. His hemoglobin dropped to a few points below normal and he became weak from anemia. "I just couldn't function," he said. "I mean I was having trouble walking at that point, trouble walking and talking at the same time." He quit the study.

On his fortieth birthday in 2002, the foundation gave him its Hope Award. He was also the foundation liaison to Canadian Blood Services, and sometimes when he was at the blood services' headquarters in Ottawa, he would see Graham Sher, who rose through the organization's ranks to become its CEO. But Howard is less active with the foundation now. His diabetes persists, his cirrhosis has progressed and he's often tired. He'd like to try combination therapy because he's heard it is helping patients in Europe, but it's not offered in Toronto. Even if it was, he says he wouldn't risk antagonizing Olivieri in order to take it.

"Nancy's got this mentality: either you're with her or you're against her," he explained. "I believe in her." Howard knows she still views L1 as too dangerous for human use, and on that issue—her litmus test for friends and allies since 1996—he won't oppose her. But he wonders about her motivation in a way he never used to in the 1980s and '90s. "I got the impression that her motivation back then was to be the person who found a cure for thalassemia," Howard says. "Now I think her motivation has shifted to her being proven correct and vindicated. Nothing short of wiping this drug off the planet will do it."

PEOPLE

Aberman, Dr. Arnie	ICU doctor; dean of the University of Toronto medical faculty from 1995 to 2000.
Alex	Toronto thalassemia patient and Josie's fiancé.
Ali, Duri-Sadaf	Young Toronto thalassemia patient; part of the L1 trial.
Andrea	Toronto thalassemia patient; part of the L1 trial.
Anita	Thalassemia patient from Guelph, Ontario.
Baines, Dr. Andrew	Scientist; member of the Hospital for Sick Children's board of trustees.
Baird, Dr. Patricia	University of British Columbia geneticist; one of three authors of *The Olivieri Report*.
Baker, Dr. Michael	Hematologist at the Toronto Western Hospital; mentored Nancy Olivieri when she was in training and later became physician-in-chief at the Toronto General Hospital.
Berkovitch, Dr. Mati	Resident in pharmacology at the Hospital for Sick Children during the early 1990s; worked on the L1 trials.
Bernstein, Dr. Alan	Geneticist; became head of the Canadian Institutes of Health Research in the 1990s.
Biagio	Toronto thalassemia patient.
Brill-Edwards, Dr. Michèle	Pediatrician and drug safety advocate; worked for Health Canada's Health Protection Branch as a drug reviewer before resigning to blow the whistle on the agency.

Brittenham, Dr. Gary   American hematologist; collaborated with Olivieri on the L1 trials.

Buchwald, Dr. Manuel   Geneticist at the Hospital for Sick Children; became head of its Research Institute in 1997.

Bulgin, Sanchia   Toronto sickle cell anemia patient whose death was the subject of an inquest in 2000.

Carcao, Dr. Manuel   Hematologist; worked with sickle cell anemia patients as Nancy Olivieri's junior associate.

Chan, Dr. Helen   Hematologist; worked with cancer patients at the Hospital for Sick Children; member of the Gang of Four.

Cohen, Dr. Alan   American hematologist; collaborated with Olivieri on the L1 trials; continued to work on the trials without Olivieri.

Corrado   Toronto thalassemia patient; part of the L1 trial.

Dick, John   Geneticist at the Hospital for Sick Children; member of the Gang of Four.

Dong, Betty   Pharmacist at the University of California whose research was suppressed by a sponsoring drug company.

Dover, Dr. George   American hematologist; collaborated with Olivieri.

Durie, Dr. Peter   Gastroenterologist and cystic fibrosis specialist at the Hospital for Sick Children; member of the Gang of Four.

Fleming, Dr. Kenneth   British liver disease specialist; collaborated with Olivieri.

Fredd, Dr. Stephen   FDA official with jurisdiction over drugs for thalassemia during the 1990s.

Freedman, Dr. Melvin   Hematologist at the Hospital for Sick Children; ran the thalassemia program when Olivieri was in training; later became the hospital's head of hematology.

Friedland, Martin   Former dean of law at the University of Toronto; head of the committee investigating Olivieri's charges concerning Graham Sher.

Friesen, Jim   Former chair of genetics at the University of Toronto;

Kirby, Dr. Melanie — Toronto pediatrician and hematologist; worked with thalassemia and sickle cell patients.

Kontoghiorghes, George — Biochemist who studied L1; member of the University College team, then of the Royal Free team.

Koren, Dr. Gideon — Pediatrician and pharmacologist at the Hospital for Sick Children; collaborated with Olivieri on L1 during the early to mid-1990s.

Langlois, Michael — Toronto-based media handler; advised Olivieri during 1998.

Love, Prof. Rhonda — Member of the executive of the University of Toronto Faculty Association.

MacKinnon, Dr. Janet — Pediatrician and hematologist; worked on the L1 trials as a resident.

Marmorato, Patrizia — Toronto thalassemia patient; part of the L1 trial.

Martin, David — CEO of the Hospital for Sick Children during the early 1990s.

Matsui, Dr. Doreen — Pediatrician and clinical pharmacologist; worked on the L1 trials as a resident.

McClure, Dr. Peter — Head of hematology at the Hospital for Sick Children during the 1960s and '70s.

McLelland, Robert — Chemist at the University of Toronto; made L1 in his lab for use in the L1 trials.

McNeil, John — Business leader; served on the board of the Hospital for Sick Children.

Michael — Toronto thalassemia patient; part of the L1 trial.

Michelson, Dr. Alan — Physician and scientist; collaborated with Olivieri during her research training at Harvard.

Modell, Dr. Bernadette — British pediatrician; ran a thalassemia program in North London in the 1970s; later became an epidemiological expert on thalassemia.

Moore, Dr. Aideen — Neonatologist; served as head of the Hospital for Sick Children Research Ethics Board in the mid- to late 1990s.

Naimark, Dr. Arnold Former president of the University of Manitoba; led the Naimark Review.

Nathan, Dr. David G. American medical leader and authority on thalassemia; head of hematology at Boston Children's Hospital when Nancy Olivieri was working in Boston.

O'Brodovich, Dr. Hugh Chief of pediatrics at the Hospital for Sick Children from 1996.

Olivieri, Dr. Nancy Hematologist; formerly at the Hospital for Sick Children as head of its thalassemia and sickle cell disease programs; leader of the hospital's L1 trials.

Olivieri, Dr. Red Nancy's father, a Hamilton-based pediatrician.

Orkin, Dr. Stuart Hematologist and geneticist at Harvard; ran the lab where Olivieri did research training during the 1980s.

Papageorgiou, Kosta Father of two Greek women with thalassemia.

Paula Toronto thalassemia patient; part of the L1 trial.

Pearson, Dr. Howard Hematologist at Yale; head of its thalassemia program.

Perrine, Dr. Susan Hematologist at Boston University; collaborated with Olivieri on butyrate research.

Phillips, Dr. Robert Former executive director of the National Cancer Institute of Canada; former head of cancer research at the Hospital for Sick Children.

Pitblado, Jim Philanthropist and business leader; chair of the board of the Hospital for Sick Children in 1998.

Prichard, Robert President of the University of Toronto in the 1990s.

Rennie, Dr. Drummond Deputy editor of the *Journal of the American Medical Association* (*JAMA*); a U.S. authority on scientific misconduct and whistleblowing scientists.

Rothstein, Aser Scientist; served as head of the Hospital for Sick Children's Research Institute in the 1970s and '80s.

Rowell, Mary Bioethicist; investigated the Olivieri affair for the hospital's research administration in 1998.

Ruby, Clayton Toronto lawyer; at one point represented Olivieri.

Schafer, Prof. Arthur	Head of the ethics centre at the University of Manitoba.
Schechter, Dr. Alan	Senior scientist at the National Institutes of Health; came to Toronto in January 1999 on a fact-finding mission for the Canadian Association of University Teachers.
Scheuer, Dr. Peter	British liver disease specialist; invited to collaborate with Olivieri.
Shear, Dr. Neal	Head of clinical pharmacology at the University of Toronto during 2000.
Sher, Dr. Graham	Hematologist; trained as a resident under Nancy Olivieri, then served as head of the thalassemia program at the Toronto General Hospital.
Sherman, Barry	Founder and CEO of Apotex.
Shy-Rose	Toronto thalassemia patient; part of the L1 trial.
Siminovitch, Lou	Geneticist; recruited to the Hospital for Sick Children in the 1970s.
Spino, Michael	Pharmacist and pharmacologist; taught at the Hospital for Sick Children, then became an Apotex executive.
Strofolino, Michael	CEO of the Hospital for Sick Children during 1998–2001.
Symes, Beth	Toronto lawyer; at one point represented Nancy Olivieri.
Templeton, Doug	Biochemist at the University of Toronto; collaborated with Olivieri on the L1 research.
Tonna, Louisa	Toronto thalassemia patient; part of the L1 trial.
Tricta, Dr. Fernando	Thalassemia specialist; worked for Apotex on L1.
Tyler, Bev	Thalassemia nurse at the Toronto General Hospital.
Valpy, Michael	Reporter and columnist with the *Globe and Mail*.
Wanless, Dr. Ian	Liver disease specialist in Toronto; studied L1's toxic effects.
Weatherall, Dr. David	British thalassemia expert; collaborated with Nancy Olivieri.

Wonke, Dr. Beatrix   British thalassemia expert; member of the Royal Free team studying L1.

Yip, Cecil   Scientist and vice-dean at the University of Toronto; handled complaints of scientific misconduct.

Zipursky, Dr. Alvin   Hematologist at the Hospital for Sick Children; head of the division when Olivieri was in training there; mentored Olivieri during the 1980s.

Zlotkin, Dr. Stanley   Gastroenterologist at the Hospital for Sick Children; in the spring of 1996 he responded to questions from Olivieri and Spino as head of the hospital's Research Ethics Board.

TIMELINE

1972   Studies provide convincing proof that Desferal saves lives of patients with
        thalassemia.

1976   The FDA approves Desferal.

1977   Desferal is promoted in an editorial in the *New England Journal of Medicine*.

1978   The first Canadians to take Desferal receive it via a Boston-based clinical
        trial that Sick Kids doctors collaborate on.

1980   The Bayh-Dole act, a federal law encouraging collaboration between
        academics and industry, takes effect in the United States.

1982   Toronto's Hospital for Sick Children develops the city's first Desferal program
        for thalassemia patients, directed by hematologist Melvin Freedman. George
        Kontoghiorghes and Robert Hider of Essex University in the U.K. develop
        a series of similar experimental drugs known as L1 through L-7 and patent them.

1985   Kontoghiorghes publishes on L1 in the *Lancet*.

1986   Olivieri and Freedman publish in the *New England Journal of Medicine* that
        high doses of Desferal are toxic to the brain. Nancy Olivieri takes her first
        faculty position at the University of Toronto and the Hospital for Sick Children.

1987   Kontoghiorghes presents short-term evidence at the ASH annual meeting in
        San Antonio, Texas, that L1 works in patients.

1988   Italian doctors document Desferal's adverse side effects on very young
        children: it causes growth retardation. Health Canada's Health Protection
        Branch approves Olivieri's proposal to test L1 in patients with thalassemia,
        and Olivieri begins enrolling patients in a short-term trial.

1989   Biagio dies at age twenty-one from heart failure that developed as a result of his not taking Desferal regularly. First reports of L1 toxicity in animals appear in the *Lancet;* the first human to suffer serious adverse effects of L1 recovers in an intensive care unit in the U.K.; an unsigned editorial in the *Lancet* labels L1 as "too toxic for further development."

1990   Worldwide, more than 130 patients are taking L1 in clinical trials; Olivieri and her group publish the successful results of their pilot study in the *Lancet* and apply to the MRC for funding. Michael Strofolino becomes COO at the Hospital for Sick Children.

1991   An eighteen-year-old dies while taking L1 in India, and his doctors blame the drug, writing in the *Lancet,* "trials of L1 should be halted." Olivieri presents results to the FDA showing that in her patients, L1 works nearly as well as Desferal. Michael Spino leaves the University of Toronto and the Hospital for Sick Children to become an executive at Apotex.

1992   Olivieri and her collaborators document further evidence of Desferal's adverse side effects on very young children (growth retardation) and publish a report in *Blood* showing that L1 is as effective as Desferal and much easier for patients to take; Anita starts taking butyrate as part of Olivieri and Perrine's clinical trial at Sick Kids. As a result of a number of complaints, the department of pediatrics at the Hospital for Sick Children investigates Olivieri's behaviour toward co-workers, but no disciplinary action is taken. Gideon Koren becomes division chief for clinical pharmacology and associate director of the Sick Kids Research Institute.

1992–94   Olivieri and collaborators discover seven new genetic mutations that cause thalassemia.

1993   Ciba-Geigy cancels its plans to test L1 in humans, objecting that the drug is too dangerous. L1 researchers in Bombay accuse Olivieri of inconsistencies and omissions in publications about her L1 research. Olivieri and Perrine publish in the *New England Journal of Medicine* on the effectiveness of butyrate. Apotex signs a contract with Olivieri and Koren to sponsor the trials of L1; Olivieri again presents on L1 to the FDA.

1993–94   Graham Sher works under Olivieri as a research fellow.

1993 or 94   Olivieri first notices that certain patients aren't responding to L1 in the way she expects.

1994   Strofolino becomes Hospital for Sick Children CEO. Olivieri and
              Brittenham become consultants to Apotex; friction develops between
              Olivieri and the company. MacKinnon presents at ASH on the newly
              discovered problem with L1: it stops being effective for some patients.

1995   Olivieri publishes on L1's effectiveness in the *New England Journal of
              Medicine*; she also publishes there, without Perrine, on butyrate's
              ineffectiveness. Sher becomes director of the thalassemia program at the
              Toronto General Hospital; Friesen quits as Sick Kids research head rather
              than relinquish power to Strofolino.

1996   In the spring, Olivieri tells the Research Ethics Board that L1 doesn't work
              for twelve out of eighteen patients in her clinical trial and suggests revising
              her consent forms; she is instructed by the board to do so. Revised forms
              are sent to Spino, who cancels the trials at Sick Kids, orders Olivieri and
              Koren to keep their information on the drug confidential and organizes an
              independent panel to review the trial results. In the fall, Olivieri concludes
              that L1 is toxic to the liver in some patients and presents those findings at
              ASH.

1997   Olivieri writes that L1 is too toxic for human use. Conflicting papers on
              her L1 trial are presented in Malta, including one by Koren and Sher that
              includes data Olivieri considers hers; she replaces Sher as thalassemia
              program director at the Toronto General and accuses him of scientific
              misconduct for using her data in the Malta abstract. The Gang of Four
              begins to support her.

1998   Olivieri publishes in the *New England Journal of Medicine* on L1's
              ineffectiveness and toxicity and speaks publicly about her ordeal. The
              Naimark Review is completed; the faculty union begins to represent
              Olivieri and the Gang of Four; Olivieri stops collaborating with Manuel
              Carcao and he resigns from the sickle cell program.

1999   Olivieri is dismissed as clinical director of the thalassemia clinic by Sick Kids
              then reinstated under the agreement negotiated by Robert Prichard; Koren
              is found guilty of writing the poison-pen letters and later of misconduct.
              L1 is licensed in Europe.

2000   Bernadette Modell writes in the *Lancet* that the main reason for early death
              in thalassemia is that patients won't take their drugs; the unexplained early
              deaths of young adults with thalassemia begin in Toronto; Sick Kids refers
              its questions about Olivieri to the College of Physicians and Surgeons of
              Ontario.

2001   *The Olivieri Report* is published.

2002   Olivieri and the Gang of Four reach a settlement with the hospital. Olivieri's claim that L1 causes liver scarring is refuted by new studies.

2003   L1's use is licensed in twenty-five countries, and the European court rules that Olivieri cannot challenge approval of the drug.

2004   In Ontario, the Thalassemia Foundation questions why more than a dozen young thalassemia patients have died in the past few years; in the U.K., young adults with thalassemia are no longer dying; the *British Medical Journal* reports that Olivieri is continuing her crusade against L1.

ix   *Many of the doctors and scientists who witnessed the events described here*
          Over the long term, I've had access to parties on all sides of this dispute, largely
          because I began covering the story earlier than most journalists. But there are
          gaps in my knowledge. Nancy Olivieri spoke with me on multiple occasions
          from the spring of 1998 through the spring of 2000 but declined my interview
          requests after the summer of 2000, saying that I had not told her I was writing
          a book. Among her collaborators, Gideon Koren agreed to a one-hour interview
          for CBC Radio in the summer of 1998 but declined my subsequent requests;
          Gary Brittenham spoke with me briefly in the summer of 2000 and did not
          agree to a longer interview.

ix   *The administration of the Hospital for Sick Children*
          Olivieri and her supporters received a letter from hospital administrators on
          January 6, 1999, telling them that their conduct was "not acceptable" and remind-
          ing them of hospital bylaws; Apotex threatened Olivieri with legal consequences
          if she divulged information about L1 in May 1996; Olivieri sued Apotex for libel
          over statements made by company officers and the company subsequently coun-
          tersued her in Ontario Superior Court in 2000; Koren wrote Brenda Gallie in
          September 1998 that he would sue her for libel; the UTFA filed grievances against
          hospital and university administrators on behalf of Olivieri and three of her sup-
          porters in January 1999 and filed a separate grievance against the university by the
          same doctors in 2001; Sick Kids administrators sued the univeristy's Grievance
          Review Panel, the UTFA, Olivieri and her supporters in Ontario Superior Court
          in 2001; in the summer of 2001, with the support of the UTFA, Olivieri and three
          of her supporters sought a court injunction to block an agreement about provin-
          cial payments to the Hospital for Sick Children that had been negotiated by the
          hospital, the Ontario Medical Association and the provincial ministry of health;
          Olivieri brought a libel suit against various parties, including CBC television and
          the *National Post* in 2000 and 2001.

x   *Tutu, winner of the Nobel Peace Prize and head of South Africa's famed Truth and Reconciliation Commission, had a simple message*
           See Tutu (1999).

PROLOGUE

2   *In 1998, her hospital sponsored its inquiry to figure out what had happened; two years later, Canada's national organization of university faculty associations conducted its own*
           The hospital's inquiry is the Naimark Review, issued in December 1998 with the official title *Clinical Trials of L1 (Deferiprone) at the Hospital for Sick Children in Toronto: A Review of Facts and Circumstances* (www.sickkids.on.ca/L1trials). The inquiry by Canada's national organization of university faculty associations is Thompson, Baird, and Downie (2001).

2   *John le Carré spoke to Olivieri and spun a fictional account of the events*
           Le Carré's novel is le Carré (2001).

2   *science's moral code*
           For a discussion of the moral codes of science, see Committee on the Conduct of Science (1989) or Macrina (2000). The Tri-Council statement issued by the Canadian research funding councils (the MRC, NSERC and SSHRC) is *The Tri-Council Policy Statement for Ethical Conduct of Research Involving Humans* (1998, updated 1999), www.nserc.ca/programs/ethics/english/policy.htm.

3   *sociologist of science Harriet Zuckerman*
           See Zuckerman et al. (1991), 75.

1: CHILDREN WHOSE BLOOD DOESN'T WORK

7   *Years later, Nathan described how frustrated he'd been*
           See Nathan (1998), 281.

8   *The one that seemed to work best was an injection-only drug called Desferal*
           Ciba chemists introduced hematologists to Desferal in 1968 at a meeting of the International Society of Hematology.

9   *Dr. Bernadette Modell, wanted every child with thalassemia to get the shots*
           See Modell and Beck (1974).

10   *the one from Great Ormond Street showed that the drug protected children with thalassemia from liver damage*
           See Barry et al. (1974).

10   *In Boston, David Nathan jumped on the Desferal bandwagon too*
           See Nathan (1995a), 101.

11   *But Desferal was no longer new, and his editorial left no wiggle room*
        See Weatherall et al. (1977).

2: THE MAKING OF A SCIENTIST

18   *She often told people that it was Red who'd inspired her*
        See Sharon Oosthoek, "Treatment offers hope for blood disorders," *The Hamilton
        Spectator*, January 21, 1993.

19   *It was a strict Roman Catholic girls' school*
        See Lei, Christine (2003). *Academic excellence, devotion to the church and the virtues
        of womanhood: Loretto, Hamilton 1865–1970*. Available from University of Toronto
        Libraries theses collection. See also Doug Foley, "Ties that bind in the world's
        best small city," *The Hamilton Spectator*, December 1, 1999.

20   *Olivieri later accepted a journalist's description of her as "a straight-A nerd"*
        See Jane O'Hara, "Whistleblower: a top researcher says a drug under trial poses
        a risk to patients: the drugmaker threatened legal action against its critic,"
        Maclean's, November 16, 1998.

25   *It came out in September 1987, in the specialty journal*
        See Olivieri et al. (1987).

3: THE ORIGIN OF A DRUG

28   *He applied for funds from the British Technology Group (BTG), an arm's-length agency*
        BTG's effectiveness in promoting industry-university collaborations is described in
        a 1986 study by the consulting firm Arthur D. Little International (*Financial Support
        for Research and Development Provided by Central Government in the United Kingdom, with
        a Detailed Technical Analysis of UK Financial Support for R+D*) and in Young (1987).

29   *Mimosine was isolated in an Australian veterinary laboratory*
        On early uses of mimosine as a defleecing agent in sheep, see, for example, Frenkel
        et al. (1975); Reis, Tunks, and Chapman (1975); Reis, Tunks, and Hegarty (1975).

31   *the patent—a limited one—came through in 1982*
        R. C. Hider, G. J. Kontoghiorghes, and J. Silver, U.K. patent GB-2118176 (1982).

32   *The door was open between academia and industry, said MIT professor Charles Weiner*
        See Weiner (1986). The general atmosphere of the time is discussed in *Lancet*
        (1993).

32   *Al Gore accused Congress of selling the tree of knowledge to Wall Street*
        Gore is quoted in Quinn (2001), 63. Gore refers to his comment in Gore
        (1991).

33   *In a survey, 24 per cent of life scientists at major universities said that they couldn't publish*
        See Blumenthal et al. (1986).

34   *Fifteen years later, doctors from Harvard would argue that universities need to adopt
        explicit safeguards*
        David A. Shaywitz and Dennis A. Ausiello of Harvard, in "A booming partner-
        ship: University and industry: Patients benefit, too, though we all should be vig-
        ilant," *Boston Globe*, September 24, 2000, write of students' vulnerability in
        company-university collaborations: "Universities . . . should adopt explicit safe-
        guards—including full disclosure of industry sponsorship and diligent external
        monitoring—to ensure that students and research fellows (typically the most
        vulnerable and dependent members of the university hierarchy) are able to pub-
        lish their results freely and expeditiously."

36   *"Scientists today don't make discoveries, they publish papers," medical historian Joel Howell
        of the University of Michigan quipped*
        Howell directs the Program in Society and Medicine at the University of
        Michigan Medical School.

37   *Less than six months later, Kontoghiorghes wrote a letter about L1*
        See Kontoghiorghes (1985).

40   *The team measured the amount of iron each patient excreted and published the results*
        See Kontoghiorghes, Aldouri, Sheppard, and Hoffbrand (1987).

41–42   *The paper was published in the* British Medical Journal *that same month*
        See Kontoghiorghes, Aldouri, Hoffbrand, et al. (1987), 1512.

45   *In the spring of 1988, BTG co-sponsored a workshop*
        The workshop was in Crete and is described in Hershko (1988).

4: PUTTING TOGETHER HER TEAM

47   *There had already been reports that the drug caused blindness*
        For that reason, a 1984 editorial in the *Lancet* warned doctors to limit the dose of
        Desferal in order "to limit the risk of acute toxicity to the eye" (see *Lancet* 1984).
        See also Davies, Marcus, et al. (1983) and Borgna-Pignatti, DeStefano, et al. (1984).

47   *the report was published in the* New England Journal of Medicine *in the spring of 1986*
        See Olivieri et al. (1986).

47   *Interviewed by the* Toronto Star *when the study came out, Freedman said*
        See Lillian Newbery, "Drug harms sight, hearing, MDs say," *Toronto Star*,
        April 4, 1986.

50   *Koren had arrived in Toronto to do a pharmacology fellowship just as Sick Kids was emerging*
       from a scandal involving the deaths of more than thirty babies on the cardiac ward
       The scandal of the babies' deaths is described in Spinks (1985).

54   *Olivieri later told the* Globe and Mail *that Ottawa granted permission because*
       See Paul Taylor, "Blood drug passes first test," *The Globe and Mail*, April 6, 1995.

5: RECRUITING THE PATIENTS

56   *He had been started on night-long infusions of Desferal as a baby, but the drug turned*
       out to be harmful if it was given to children under age three
       Olivieri and her colleagues described their young patients whose growth was
       adversely affected by Desferal in Olivieri, Koren, Harris, et al. (1992). Those
       who had gotten the drug before turning two experienced growth failure or
       stunted growth (they were very short compared to other children their age), a
       direct result of early intensive Desferal. See DeVirgiliis et al. (1988) and Piga
       et al. (1988).

56   *Italian researchers who studied Desferal's toxic effects on bones determined*
       See DeVirgiliis et al. (1988) and Piga et al. (1988).

57   *Olivieri referred to the various tests as a "pilot study"*
       See Thompson, Baird, and Downie (2001), 103.

59   *By the spring of 1990, they'd gathered enough data to complete the pilot study and that*
       March
       The pilot study is reported in Olivieri et al. (1990), and the presentation at the
       Cooley's Anemia Symposium is Olivieri, Templeton, Koren et al. (1990).

61   *Later, in presentations and journal articles about her study*
       One presentation was at the Sixth Cooley's Anemia Symposium, March 13–15,
       1990; this led to a paper, Olivieri et al. (1990). Other articles include Olivieri
       N.F., G. Koren, C. Hermann, et al. (1990).

6: A TOXIC DRUG?

64   *They made the discovery public in the* Lancet *in the summer of 1989*
       See Porter et al. (1989).

64   *Some of Hider's mice had a bad physical reaction: severe sweating*
       See Porter et al. (1989).

65   *Hoffbrand and Kontoghiorghes wrote up what had happened and sent it off*
       See Hoffbrand et al. (1989).

65   *his rat studies showed that L1 significantly decreased the number of white blood cells*
       See Kontoghiorghes, Nasseri-Sina, et al. (1989).

66   *In July 1989, he had published a paper advising doctors working on any new drug that
       attached to iron that they needed to experiment on primates*
       See Wolfe et al. (1989).

66   *He wrote of them later that they had "exposed patients to unwarranted dangers"*
       See Nathan (1995a), 118.

67   *In October 1989, the* Lancet *ran an editorial declaring L1 "too toxic"*
       See Lancet (1989).

67   *Researchers were required to file annual reports with their hospital ethics board, but there
       was no active surveillance by the boards*
       The Medical Research Council of Canada had intended for researchers to be
       monitored and had given the nation's research ethics boards explicit power to
       do so, but it wasn't happening. The MRC's 1987 guidelines "contained the
       strongest provisions of any guidelines internationally for active monitoring and
       surveillance of research," writes Paul McNeill (McNeill 1993, 95–96). Yet very
       few ethics boards did any monitoring at all. Researchers were required to file
       annual reports with the boards, but there was no active on-site surveillance of
       research. A few years later, the Law Commission of Canada conducted inter-
       views that confirmed McNeill's findings. "Rarely is there independent monitor-
       ing of the conduct of research," states the Law Commission's report in its exec-
       utive summary. Research ethics board members told the Law Commission
       authors, "I think that research is monitored inadequately probably everywhere"
       (section E-1 189, "Monitoring Effectiveness," #22), and "Right now REBs in
       Canada pretty much just review paper, and then the researcher goes out and
       does God knows what!" (section E-1 189, "Monitoring Effectiveness," #31;
       McDonald 2000).

70   *the Bombay group wrote in the* Lancet *in a report on the boy's death*
       The case of lupus is described in Mehta et al. (1991).

70   *That winter, Hoffbrand's team hospitalized another L1 patient in London for her complete
       loss of white blood cells.*
       See Al-Refaie et al. (1992).

70   *He began telling people that the pill was "finished"*
       See Nathan (1995a).

70   *she wrote a letter to the* Lancet *editors explaining that in her ongoing trial in Toronto,*

twelve patients were taking L1 and none of them had lupus
> See Olivieri et al. (1991).

71   *In the* Lancet, *doctors testing L1 in Bombay and London had been describing joint problems in their patients*
> See Agarwal et al. (1990).

71   *Olivieri had mentioned in her letter to the* Lancet *editors that while joint pains had been seen in Bombay patients on L1*
> See Olivieri et al. (1991).

72   *An American hematologist argued in the* Lancet *that Diamond Blackfan anemia wouldn't cause patients to lose white blood cells*
> See Alter (1990).

73   *That summer, two years after she'd first started working with L1, she went to the FDA's drab headquarters in Rockville, Maryland*
> The meeting at the FDA took place on August 12, 1991, and is documented in Thompson, Baird, and Downie (2001), Section 5A, footnote 8.

73   *Before* AIDS, *the philosophy at the FDA was the one forged in the 1960s by thalidomide*
> The change in the FDA's philosophy is discussed in Brody (1995), chapter 3: "Troubling Ethical Issues in the Approval of New Drugs."

75   *Her team had published a case report about a twenty-nine-year-old thalassemia patient*
> See Olivieri, Koren, Matsui, et al. (1992).

76   *Subsequently, the* Globe and Mail *headlined its article*
> See Paul Taylor, "Pills replace pump ordeal. Drug for blood disorder 'going to save many patients,'" *The Globe and Mail,* May 15, 1992.

76   *One week later, Olivieri attended an NIH-sponsored symposium in Gainesville*
> The symposium was the Third NIH-Sponsored Symposium on the Development of Iron Chelators for Clinical Use, May 20–22, 1992, University of Florida, Gainesville.

76   *Doctors at the NIH had run the pill through a standard toxicity study at a commercial lab*
> See Brittenham (1992).

76   *Scientists in Switzerland at Ciba-Geigy had tested L1 on monkeys*
> See Brittenham (1992).

76   *A summary of the conference concluded there was "a delicate balance between safety and*

efficacy for L1"
See Brittenham (1992).

7: WORKING WITH A RISING STAR

78   *She was looking at other possible uses for L1—others had suggested it could be used as an anti-malaria drug and she was testing it in adults infected with malaria in Africa*
See Thuma et al. (1998).

78   *also giving it to breast cancer patients in Toronto to see if it could block the toxicity of chemotherapy*
Olivieri and Patricia Harper of the Hospital for Sick Children had received a grant for this work from the Canadian Breast Cancer Foundation in 1993; the title of their proposal was "Reduction of anthracycline-induced cardiotoxicity by iron chelators."

79   *"If a medical researcher is not looking for a gene and . . ."*
See Lawrence Surtees, "Market share medication," *The Globe and Mail*, August 14, 1990.

81   *Janet Bickel, a U.S. expert on women in medicine, says that few academic women over forty escape being described as "difficult" by their peers*
Bickel was director of Women in Medicine for the Association of American Medical Colleges in Washington DC and has written extensively on women in academic medicine. She is based in Washington DC and was interviewed by the author.

88   *Doug Templeton said she got "quite pissed off" with him because he refused to add her name as an author*
Templeton's article with his post-doc was Parkes and Templeton (1994).

93   *The research situation was dire. As Howard returned to L1, the study he was taking part in was acutely short on cash*
Olivieri had received an MRC grant to support her work with L1 for 1989–1991 and a second "continuing grant" for July 1991–June 1992, but an application for further funding was unsuccessful. See Thompson, Baird, and Downie (2001), Section 5A, note 3.

8: APOTEX TO THE RESCUE

94   *In the fall of 1991, Olivieri's team at Sick Kids had applied to the Medical Research Council for further backing*
See Thompson, Baird, and Downie (2001), Section 5A, note 3.

95   *Hoping the MRC might still reverse its decision, she contacted David Nathan*

The MRC's reply to Nathan is dated October 8, 1992, and is included in "Olivieri's MRC Application File," cited in Thompson, Baird, and Downie (2001), Section 5A, note 12.

96   *Berkovitch took the lead on writing up and presenting the findings*
His presentation on joint pain at ASH was published in abstract form as Berkovitch et al. (1992) and later published as an article (Berkovitch et al. 1994).

97   *Doctors in Bombay openly accused Olivieri and other L1 researchers of "inconsistencies and omissions"*
The doctors were from the Blood Research Centre in Bombay and reported their concerns in Mehta, Singhal, and Mehta (1993).

97   *Company scientists said one of the biggest problems was that L1 had "no . . . safety margin"*
See Pfannkuch, Bentley, and Schnebli (1993).

100   *Spino wrote and lectured on many of the problems he solved at Sick Kids*
See Sheryl Ubelacker, "Half of Canadians take drugs improperly; New guide to 3,000 medications warns against mixing, skipping, or overdosing," *The Gazette* (Montreal), January 10, 1990; see also Spino M., Sellers E.M., Kaplan H.L., et al. (1978); Kahana L.M., Spino M. (1991); Spino M. (1991).

101   *Sherman was about to embark on the construction*
See Michael McHugh, "Generic drug maker proud of its 'patent buster' label." *Financial Post*, September 4, 1993.

102   *Around that time, Spino and his staff had a novel product for AIDS in the pipeline*
See Rod Mickleburgh, "Wilson rules out paying drug-price compensation," *The Globe and Mail*, January 22, 1993

102   *Hubris aside, though, it wasn't clear how much progress the company was making*
See Rob McKenzie, "A hard pill to swallow," *Canadian Business* 67, February 1994, 44.

103   *"We took on this project to show that Apotex cares, and that money isn't the only thing that motivates the company," he told a reporter for the* Financial Post
See Michael McHugh, "Generic drug maker proud of its 'patent buster' label," *Financial Post*, September 4, 1993.

104   *Brittenham's most unusual claim to fame was an invention called the SQUID*
See Brittenham G.M., Sheth S., et al. (2001)

105   *"When Dr. Olivieri told me about L1, I was happy, oh my God, so happy," Patrizia told a reporter for* Maclean's

See Jane O'Hara, "Whistleblower: A top researcher says a drug under trial poses a risk to patients; the drugmaker threatened legal action against its critic." *Maclean's*, November 16, 1998, 64.

107   *Duri-Sadaf was enrolled in Olivieri's compassionate use trial of L1*
See Allan Thompson, "Sick child will die if she's deported," *Toronto Star*, August 11, 1993.

108   *In 2003, Yale researchers reviewing published studies reported in the* Journal of the American Medical Association (*JAMA*) *that scientists conducting industry-sponsored research often face restrictions*
See Bekelman, Li, and Gross (2003).

108   *Typically, data from clinical trials belong to the sponsoring company, and making them public is the company's decision, as Thomas Bodenheimer explained*
Bodenheimer spoke on "Conflict of Interest in Clinical Drug Trials: A Risk Factor for Scientific Misconduct" on August 15, 2000, at the National Institutes of Health in Bethesda, Maryland.

109   *Michael Spino later described Olivieri and Koren as "scientists pleading for help"*
See Michael McHugh, "Generic drug maker proud of its 'patent buster' label," *Financial Post*, September 4, 1993.

9: UNDOING SUSAN PERRINE

111   *Perrine and his collaborators coined the term "benign sickle-cell anaemia" to describe what they were seeing*
See R. P. Perrine et al. (1972).

111   *Soon, the NIH became interested in the connection between sickle cell disease and fetal hemoglobin*
For more about NIH interest in sickle cell anemia, see Wailoo (2001), 182–84.

112   *It was an intriguing discovery, and in 1985 Perrine published it in the* New England Journal of Medicine
See S.P. Perrine, Green, and Faller (1985).

112   *A group at the Medical College of Georgia had experimented with it during the early 1980s and found that when they added it to cord blood*
See Garbutt and Abraham (1981).

113   *Writing up the experiment, Perrine concluded by saying that butyrate might be used to treat sickle cell anemia or thalassemia*
See S.P. Perrine et al. (1988).

114   *Later, describing herself to a reporter, she said, "My cheekbones are rather large"*
        See Paul Taylor, "New drug seems to halt thalassemia," *The Globe and Mail*,
        January 14, 1993.

114   *Olivieri told a reporter later, "Bone marrow was forming everywhere, including*
        See Sheryl Ubelacker, "Treatment for blood ailment promising: Therapy may
        have saved life of young Guelph woman," *The Canadian Press*, January 15,
        1993.

115   *Perrine took the lead on writing up the results, and when the paper was published (in
        January 1993 in the* New England Journal of Medicine)
        See S.P. Perrine et al. (1993).

119   *The article, co-authored by one of her residents, appeared in* Blood *in the fall of 1994*
        See Sher and Olivieri (1994).

120   *The stark conclusion increased the chance that the paper would be accepted, because the
        journal has a policy of considering a paper even more seriously if its findings are the reverse
        of findings the journal has already published.*
        Dr. Jerome Kassirer, a former editor of the *New England Journal of Medicine*,
        confirmed the policy in an interview.

120   *Her paper came out in June 1995*
        See Sher et al. (1995).

120   *When patients received butyrate steadily for four weeks and went off it for two weeks—a
        form of treatment called "pulse therapy"*
        See Atweh et al. (1999).

121   *Olivieri added hydroxyurea to their regimen and wrote in the* Lancet *in 1997 that their
        "remarkable response" to the two drugs*
        See Olivieri, Rees, et al. (1997).

121   *one of the scientists it funded to do such work was Nancy Olivieri, who planned to treat
        thirty thalassemia patients with sodium phenyl butyrate*
        The NIH lists all funded grants on its CRISP website: http://crisp.cit.nih.gov/
        Olivieri's proposal to combine sodium phenylbutyrate with other drugs was listed
        for fiscal year 2004.

10: THE TRIPLE THREAT

122   *Olivieri's funding from Apotex started in early 1993. Later that spring, she spoke at the
        FDA again*
        Olivieri's 1993 meeting at the FDA took place on October 28. Its purpose was

"to discuss the potential therapeutic use of deferiprone in the U.S.," according to a letter Olivieri wrote to Stephen Fredd in 1997.

128 *Olivieri and other doctors had issued stern warnings of the calamity he faced*
See Joan Breckenridge, "Heart-liver transplant declared success," *The Globe and Mail*, April 21, 1994.

128 *Gino got his new heart and new liver in May 1991 at age twenty-six*
His operation is described in Olivieri, Liu, et al. (1994).

130 *When they learned of the FDA's rules—in June 1995*
See Naimark Review, 24.

130 *The Cleveland Clinic had enforced a ban on consultancies for doctors studying a company's drug and published on it*
See Healy et al. (1989).

131 *The monitors—the company's way of meeting the FDA's and Health Canada's rules—were supposed to visit Sick Kids frequently*
The Apotex practice of using clinical monitors was consistent with federal rules and regulations; in fact, according to a report on clinical trials by the U.S. government Office of the Inspector General 2000, the FDA holds the sponsoring company of a clinical trial "responsible for assuring throughout the clinical investigation that the investigators' obligations, as set forth in applicable regulations, are being fulfilled." To do this, companies use monitors. Companies "oversee investigators, and in turn, the protection of human subjects, almost exclusively through their monitors," who visit the research site frequently and "focus on ensuring the quality of data."

134 *Spino resented the arguments, and at one point in the spring of 1994, he wrote Olivieri and Brittenham, asking them to "recognize that Apotex is not just supplying the drug and paying the bills"*
See Naimark Review, 25.

135 *"You have indicated that there is insufficient time to provide the information*
Spino's letter, dated March 7, 1995, is quoted in Thompson, Baird, and Downie (2001), 127.

11: A NEW PROBLEM WITH L1

141 *The graphs and scatter plots on her slides demonstrated that patients in the compassionate use trial continued to do well*
The 1994 American Society of Hematology meeting took place December 2–6 in Nashville, Tennessee. Olivieri reported that in the Toronto 'compassionate' trial of

L1, in twenty-three patients who had taken L1 for longer than one year, liver iron concentration "has declined significantly" and "magnetic resonance imaging has demonstrated signal changes consistent with reduction of iron within the heart." She concluded, "These data demonstrate the unequivocal long-term effectiveness of L1 in the reduction of body iron stores," and added, "L1 should be offered to patients unwilling, or unable, to use deferoxamine" (see Olivieri, Belluzzo, et al. 1994).

141   *A federal commission assigned to investigate scientific practice—the Commission on Research Integrity—concluded that, in certain cases, a scientist who omitted data was committing misconduct*
See Commission on Research Integrity (1995).

141   *In April 1995, John C. Bailar, a long-time statistical consultant to the* New England Journal of Medicine *and head of statistics at McGill University, addressed the issue in an editorial*
See Bailar (1995).

142   *One such study, published in 1996 by California researchers, showed that in 98 per cent of company-sponsored drug studies published during the 1980s, the results favoured the company's drug*
The California researchers are Mildred Cho and Lisa Bero (see Cho and Bero 1996).

142   *Janet MacKinnon had prepared a scientific abstract on it for a poster session*
The abstract was published as MacKinnon et al. (1994).

144   *the* New England Journal of Medicine *accepted Olivieri's paper describing the L1 trial*
The paper is Olivieri et al. (1995).

145   *The next day, the* Toronto Star *described L1 as "a pill-size reprieve for people with thalassemia."*
See Joseph Hall, "New pill studied for gene disorder," *Toronto Star*, April 6, 1995.

145   *The* Globe and Mail *quoted Olivieri's prediction*
See Paul Taylor, "Blood drug passes first test," *The Globe and Mail*, April 6, 1995.

145   *L1 had proven itself, Olivieri told the Canadian Press*
See "New pill could end pain of gene disorder treatment," *The Hamilton Spectator*, April 6, 1995.

145   *Nathan had been asked to write an editorial about L1 to run in the same issue*
The editorial is Nathan (1995b).

404   NOTES

12: PULLING THE PLUG ON NANCY

149   Spino wrote her in August that Apotex had a legal and moral responsibility
Spino's letter to Olivieri is dated August 14, 1995. See Naimark (1998), 26.

149   She replied by sending him Brittenham's SQUID results showing that in eight of the patients on L1, the iron levels weren't going down
Olivieri provided the data to Apotex on September 18, 1995, with a letter that said, "So that there should be no question as to the occurrence of loss of sustained efficacy of deferiprone in patients . . . and the need to investigate this complication, I have separately enclosed all the data pertinent to the evaluation of efficacy of chelating therapy in every patient who has received deferiprone therapy under my direction in the 'compassionate' cohort of patients. I have also sent this data by fax today."

149   Spino and his staff reviewed the data and thought there was another explanation
Apotex later wrote (in a document entitled "The Deferiprone Contract and Confidentiality"), "When Dr. Olivieri presented her initial view—that there was a sudden and unexpected loss of response—Apotex considered her assessment very carefully. With a detailed analysis, Apotex established that there was no sudden and unexpected change and there was no generalized loss of response." A figure and a bar graph illustrating the individual patient values for liver iron purport to show that there was no net change between the time of Olivieri's 1995 article and the time of her report to Apotex. The document continues, "Because the view held by Dr. Olivieri was scientifically unfounded, we concluded that her assessment was biased." Apotex accepted the assessment of Gideon Koren that "there was a variable response and that, in 3 or 4 patients, there appeared to be an increase in hepatic iron concentrations." Spino wrote Zlotkin on March 1 describing "three patients who are inadequate responders" to L1.

149   This time, she copied her letter to the head of the hospital's Research Ethics Board
Olivieri's letter copied to Stanley Zlotkin of the Human Subjects Review Committee is dated September 15, 1995. It says that ten patients have been "identified as having experienced a loss of sustained efficacy" and also says that the "loss of sustained efficacy" "has now been observed in over 40% of the patients" in that study.

150   "We forwarded her data that she gave us to all the other investigators that we were working with," Spino said
Spino sent the data to one of the L1 investigators in Italy, Dr. Antonio Piga of Torino, on March 15, 1996, with a letter of explanation, and copied his letter to Olivieri.

150   *Koren argued against making a formal report, suggesting that any new concerns about L1*
       could go in their annual report to the ethics board
       Koren's idea that the information could be included in the required annual
       report to the REB is mentioned by Spino in a letter to Zlotkin dated May 2, 1996.

150   *The report—with Koren, Brittenham and Olivieri as authors—went to Apotex and the*
       ethics board in March 1996
       See Naimark Review, 28. The report was titled "Variability in Therapeutic
       Response to Deferiprone."

151   *Olivieri was still an advocate for L1, believing it worked for some thalassemia patients and*
       that it might work in a different way for sickle cell anemia
       See National Heart Lung and Blood Institute Grant Number
       5R01HL057594-03: Deferiprone therapy for sickle cell disease, PI: Nancy F.
       Olivieri. See also Thompson, Baird, and Downie (2001), 321.

151   *And he wrote the ethics board chair, Zlotkin, whom he knew*
       Spino's letter to Zlotkin is dated March 15, 1996. Zlotkin's response to Spino is
       dated March 25, 1996. Spino wrote Zlotkin again on May 2, 1996, "Variable
       response among patients is a common finding in therapy for virtually any disease."

152   *In April 1996, the ethics board issued its directions*
       Zlotkin's letter to Olivieri is dated April 9, 1996.

152   *In a letter Olivieri wrote Apotex about the meeting, she said it "was prompted*
       The letter from Olivieri is addressed to Pat Laplante, APOTEX Research Inc.,
       and dated April 24, 1996.

153   *The day after Olivieri's meeting with the patients, he wrote Zlotkin again*
       The letter from Spino to Zlotkin is dated May 2, 1996, and copied to Olivieri,
       Brittenham and Koren.

154   *Nathan's team decided to stop the experiment. They told the man to discontinue his pills*
       and go back on nightly Desferal
       Nathan's concerns are described in a letter to Olivieri dated March 4, 1996, and
       signed by Beatrice Gee, MD.

154   *Nathan also wrote the FDA. He described what had happened to his patient*
       Nathan's letter to the FDA is dated May 16, 1996, and is signed by Nathan and Gee.

154   *She put all the materials in an envelope and sent them to Zlotkin at the Research Ethics*
       Board
       Olivieri's covering letter to thalassemia patients or parents is dated May 10,

1996, and her letter to Spino enclosing the revised forms and the letter to patients is dated May 20, 1996.

13: FIGHTING BACK

157   *the producer of the British television documentary* Dying for Drugs
The film appeared on Channel 4 in the U.K. in April 2003 and can be found on the channel's website, www.channel4.com/health.

157   *"I wanted to tell the patients there was a problem, but business interests prevented that from happening easily," she told a reporter for* Business Week *two years later*
Joseph Weber was the *Business Week* reporter she spoke to (see Joseph Weber, "The doctor vs. the drugmaker: A dispute over a drug's efficacy turns a partnership into a war," *BusinessWeek*, November 30, 1998).

158   *After that she called the dean of the University of Toronto medical school, Arnold Aberman, and told him she had spoken to a lawyer*
Olivieri described this sequence of events in a letter to Dr. Robert Rivington of the CMPA on September 5, 1997.

160   *Josie wrote later that the clinic staff faced "many pleading, angry, frightened patients"*
Josie's remarks were in an e-mail to Bob McDonald, host of the CBC Radio show *Quirks & Quarks*, sent September 2, 1998.

160   *Olivieri heard about the situation when she got back to town and later described it for a television producer*
Olivieri's remarks are in *Dying for Drugs*.

160   *He said that if the dispute remained unresolved, he would do what he could to obtain the services of the university's lawyers in getting her "proper protection of her intellectual property rights"*
Aberman's remarks were later recalled by Olivieri's lawyer, Steven Mason of McCarthy Tétrault, who documented them in a letter to her dated October 20, 1997.

160   *The medical faculty had an annual research budget of close to $200 million*
See Toronto Board of Trade, Business and Market Guide 1998/99.

161   *They told her, "Be clear about what you want," and she made notes for herself.*
Olivieri's notes are entitled: Briefing Notes, Mediation Session, June 7, 1996.

162   *Others who had started on the pills*
In a letter dated December 2, 1996, Spino wrote Olivieri, "Our records

indicate that we have made more than 80 individual patient shipments for 45 different patients since the studies at HSC were terminated."

163   *The pediatrician spoke to Apotex as well as the hematologists who were testing L1 in Montreal and Philadelphia.*
        Dr. Peter G. Forbath, Corrado's pediatrician, wrote about these contacts in a letter to the Thalassemia Clinic, Toronto Hospital General Division, dated April 16, 1998.

169   *Olivieri later spoke with Corey and determined that the panellists hadn't received all the material she and Brittenham had sent Apotex*
        See Thompson, Baird, and Downie (2001), 174.

170   *"The committee suggests that the words 'unexpectedly' and 'loss of efficacy' be removed from the new consent forms*
        See "REPORT: Expert Advisory Panel on L1 Efficacy," July 12, 1996.

170   *Alan Goldbloom, was also there, and the meeting was held in his office.*
        See Naimark, Knoppers, and Lowy (1998), 33.

171   *Kay wrote that Olivieri was bound by her "contractual obligations" to the company*
        Kay's letter to Joseph Colangelo of McCarthy Tétrault is dated August 23, 1996 and is from firm file no. 11313–012.

171   *In August, Dean Arnie Aberman went alone to a Toronto restaurant to talk to Apotex*
        The dean's meeting is described in the Naimark Review (33) and was confirmed by Apotex.

172–73 *She intended to continue collecting her patients' blood tests and biopsy results*
        The question of whether Olivieri continued her trial and her data collection after Apotex stopped the trial got a lot of attention later. In July 1996, Olivieri wrote, "Both protocols will continue as before," but she said later that she had not continued the trial and had only collected clinical data on her patients, while others claimed that she had continued to gather data for research purposes and therefore was still involved in research on human subjects. The issue was not only a question of semantics: Naimark and others charged that Olivieri should have reported her subsequent findings about L1 to the Research Ethics Board in order to protect patients taking the drug. Her claim that she had not been conducting research was crucial to her ability to defend herself against those charges. Naimark's charges are in the Naimark Review, 89; Thompson, Baird and Downie (2001) accept Olivieri's position and argue for it on pp. 147 and 160.

173   *Olivieri concluded that she was the company's ally*
        Olivieri's description of her meeting at Health Canada is Olivieri (2000).

175   *He wrote up his opinion and filed it as a legal affidavit*
Affidavit of Professor Sir David Weatherall sworn in the City of Oxford in the
County of Oxon, United Kingdom, August 22, 1996.

175   *He followed Weatherall's example, filing an affidavit that described the experts' report*
Affidavit of Dr. David Gordon Nathan sworn in the City of Cambridge,
Commonwealth of Massachussets, August 26, 1996.

14: ON THE WRONG SIDE OF THE FENCE

177   *While looking for an explanation of why the patients had stopped responding to L1*
The study of CP-94 in gerbils is Carthew et al. (1994).

179   *if scientists are too dedicated to finding a particular result, their reports may be biased*
The need for disinterest in one's results and the possibility for self-deception by
scientists is covered in Macrina (2000) and Committee on the Conduct of
Science (1989).

179   *Patricia Huston, a Canadian expert on the ethics of science publishing*
Patricia Huston is based in Ottawa and was president of the Council of Biology
Editors (now called the Council of Science Editors) when I interviewed her in
1998 on the subject of bias in science.

179   *She and Brittenham had a review article on thalassemia that was coming out in February
1997*
See Olivieri and Brittenham (1997).

180   *She got an evening slot and set to work organizing the effort.*
The evening meeting was: Iron Overload in The Haemoglobinopathies, work-
shop sponsored by Elliott Vichinsky and Nancy Olivieri, Children's Hospital
Oakland and The Hospital for Sick Children Toronto, 38th Annual Meeting,
American Society of Hematology, Orlando, Florida, Sunday, 8 December 1996,
21:00–23:00 hours.

180   *he said he would write the* New England Journal of Medicine *to let them know some of
the background of the L1 controversy*
Nathan's intention to contact the journal is referred to in a letter from Joseph
Colangelo of McCarthy Tétrault to Nancy Olivieri dated May 7, 1997. Nathan
had formerly served on the journal's editorial board.

185   *The absence of oversight underscored the teaching hospital administrators' lock on power*
Dr. John Evans, former president of the University of Toronto, in a public letter written in November 1999, called on Toronto's teaching hospitals to: "Put in
place appropriate policies and instruments of conflict resolution recognizing the

special circumstances of clinical faculty members and the inadequacy of labour relations grievance procedures in existence in most hospitals . . ." (see Thompson, Baird, and Downie (2001), 89.

186   *In one letter she said Spino's assistant had said Apotex no longer wanted to provide the drug for the patients*
    Nancy Olivieri's letter to Spino is dated November 25, 1996; he replied to her on December 2, 1996.

186   *Around the same time, the company hired auditors to investigate Olivieri's research accounts at the hospital*
    The auditors, Fazzari & Partners, issued a list of queries for the audit of Olivieri's clinical trial dated December 11, 1996.

187   *Essentially, she delivered a clinical argument in favour of Desferal and against L1*
    The description of Olivieri's presentation at ASH and the responses from Hoffbrand, Spino and others comes from several sources, including handwritten notes taken by individuals who attended the meeting; interviews with individuals who attended; and *Medical Post* reporter Susan Jeffrey's recollections of the meeting, recorded by Susan Prolman of the Union of Concerned Scientists.

187   *Olivieri was to speak at a special evening symposium she'd organized*
    The symposium at ASH 1996 was entitled "Iron Overload in the Haemo-globinopathies," a workshop sponsored by Elliott Vichinsky and Nancy Olivieri. It was held on Sunday night, December 8, 1996, from 9 to 11 p.m.

188   *When he heard from an Israeli friend what she'd reported about liver scarring*
    The Israeli friend was hematologist and internist Michael Lishner of Tel Aviv University's Sackler Faculty of Medicine.

188   *She wasn't an expert in liver pathology, so she had to work with a pathologist*
    The pathologist she worked with was Ross Cameron of the Toronto General Hospital.

189   *It was hours of work, marred by flaws, for the pathologist she worked with was not blinded to the characteristics of the patients whose biopsies they were viewing and, according to some reports, he didn't use an accepted, standard scoring system*
    Ross Cameron's system was described as non-standard by British pathologists that Olivieri subsequently worked with. Cameron himself explained to Olivieri's legal counsel that the system he used for grading the slides was called the Desmet method. His explanation is described in a letter from Joe Colangelo of McCarthy Tétrault to Olivieri on May 7, 1997.

190   *Her lawyers had told her they would have to show her FDA letter to Apotex first, given the
        company's threats*
        Olivieri's letter to the FDA's Stephen Fredd was dated January 22, 1997, and
        signed by Brittenham, Olivieri and Cameron. It was copied to officials at Health
        Canada's Health Protection Branch, to officials in the national health depart-
        ments of Italy and India, and to Spino at Apotex.

191   *Olivieri told her lawyer that when O'Brodovich's secretary reached her, she was given one
        hour's notice to report to the chief's office*
        Olivieri's letter to her lawyer, Steven Mason, describing her meeting with
        O'Brodovich, is dated February 19, 1997.

192   *She wrote in her notes that O'Brodovich was extremely agitated*
        According to Olivieri's typed notes of the meeting, dated February 19, 1997,
        O'Brodovich said "that he believed that there should be no further trials of L1 at
        the Hospital for Sick Children until this [issue of the drug possibly causing liver
        scarring] was resolved. I attempted to explain to him that the trials had been
        stopped but that patients were continuing drug until they could be reasonably
        evaluated. He then claimed he did not want to 'discuss the science.' It was diffi-
        cult to explain to Dr. O'Brodovich as he was extremely agitated and did not want
        to discuss the past history, all of which was relevant to this discussion."

192   *Later, the provincial College of Physicians and Surgeons would determine that Nancy
        Olivieri had acted in the best interests of her patients in informing them of the new risk
        she'd identified with L1*
        Sick Kids referred Olivieri to the College of Physicians and Surgeons of Ontario
        in 2000. The College's Complaints Committee issued its decision on December
        19, 2001, as "Complaints Committee Decisions and Reasons." It was sent to
        Olivieri marked "Private and Confidential" and distributed widely by Doctors for
        Research Integrity.

15: UNDOING GRAHAM SHER

197   *Olivieri was planning to say, at an upcoming thalassemia conference in Malta, that L1 was
        toxic*
        The Malta meeting was the 6th International Conference on Thalassemia,
        April 5–10, 1997.

198   *Certain it was against the rules of science for them to do that, she asked her lawyers to
        request copies of Tricta's abstracts*
        Stikeman Elliott, the law firm representing Apotex, sent copies of Tricta's
        abstracts to Olivieri's lawyers at McCarthy Tétrault on March 17, 1997. The let-
        ter is from firm file no. 11313–012.

200   *After their conversation, Olivieri wrote administrators at the Toronto General, including the*
         hospital's head hematologist, Armand Keating, that Graham Sher had plagiarized her work
         Olivieri's letter to Armand Keating is dated April 4, 1997. She said she had spo-
         ken with authorities at the university and "confirmed that, indeed, as was my
         impression, Graham Sher's actions represent professional research misconduct."

201   *Back in Toronto, she again contacted Keating, the hospital's head of hematology, about*
         Sher's role in the abstract
         Olivieri's second letter to Keating describing her charges against Sher is dated
         April 18, 1997. She enclosed with it the letter that Sher was to sign. She'd hand-
         written on the top of it "Suggested draft."

202   *She wrote Keating at the end of April to say she didn't "wish to wait another two weeks on*
         this issue," and after a few days she wrote Sher herself
         Her next letter to Keating was sent April 25; her letter to Sher was dated May 1.

202   *Sher didn't send his letter. But Olivieri had asked him to reply by a specific deadline, so he*
         wrote to her
         Sher wrote back on May 7; she replied on May 12.

205   *Then he listed the specific figures that he thought proved Olivieri had made an error*
         A verbatim copy of how Sher described the errors in Olivieri's abstract reads as
         follows:

> The issue here is interpretation of the data. Dr. Olivieri present-
> ed an abstract at ASH, December 1996 (authorship NF Olivieri
> for the Iron Chelation Research Group, The Hospital for Sick
> Children, Toronto), in which she claims, among other things, that
> "the hepatic iron concentration increased by 27%, from 14.6 plus
> or minus 5.0 mg/g at last analysis to 18.5 plus or minus 2.5 mg/g
> (p less than 0.025) . . ." I wish to make several comments about
> this abstract. Firstly, the claim of this statistically significant rise in
> hepatic iron concentration is erroneous, since in this cohort of
> 6 patients, the t-statistic is -1.78, and the p-value is 0.105 (and
> not 0.025 as reported) and the 95% confidence interval for the
> difference of the means is -8.96 to 0.99. This forms only part of
> my disagreement with Dr. Olivieri as to her interpretation of the
> data. The abstract presented at ASH was not reviewed by me prior
> to its submission, even though many of the patients were mine, I
> was a collaborator on the study, and a member of this "Iron
> Chelation Research Group." The very allegation being leveled
> against me may thus be made in reverse.

206   *Some of the charges were substantiated, and Folkman submitted corrections*
       The incident and investigation are described in Cooke (2001), 185.

207   *Then, in late August, they interviewed Olivieri*
       Olivieri met with the committee on August 18, 1997.

207   *She told the committee that there was no debate about L1, writing Friedland*
       Olivieri's letter to Friedland is dated August 19, 1997.

207   *Then, in a long and detailed report, they issued their decision*
       The confidential misconduct report on Sher is "Report of the Investigating
       Committee Appointed to Inquire into Allegations of Misconduct against Dr.
       Graham Sher," September 9, 1997.

209   *That was a breach of the university's rules for confidential misconduct proceedings, and the
       dean of the medical school criticized her for that sort of breach later*
       The medical dean's criticism of Olivieri for breaching the confidentiality of mis-
       conduct proceedings is in Naylor (2002c).

209   *In the fall of 1997, [Phillips] wrote a long letter to Buchwald, O'Brodovich and Strofolino
       at Sick Kids and Aberman at the medical school*
       Phillips's letter to Aberman, O'Brodovich and Buchwald is dated September 22,
       1997.

16: THE MAKING OF A WHISTLEBLOWER

212   *"We found what we believe to be very damning evidence of liver toxicity," she once told
       reporters*
       Olivieri's remarks were made at a news conference in Ottawa on October 5,
       1999. See Laura Eggertson, "Test blood disorder drug longer Ottawa urged;
       company accuses maligned MD of aggressive attack on its product," *Toronto Star,*
       October 6, 1999.

212   *David Nathan and David Weatherall later wrote in the* New England Journal of
       Medicine *that Olivieri had discovered L1 was toxic to the liver and that that was what had
       led the company to cancel her study*
       See Nathan and Weatherall (2002).

213   *A reporter for Canada's* Medical Post—*a controlled-circulation newspaper that goes
       primarily to physicians—had attended ASH that year*
       See Susan Jeffrey, "Doctor may be in legal battle after reporting negative findings
       of drug company study," *Medical Post*, January 21, 1997.

213   *Then a long-time medical journalist picked up the story for the* Toronto Star

See Leslie Papp, "Firm axes outspoken scientist's research. Woman went public with concerns about drug's safety." *Toronto Star,* January 26, 1997.

215   *Nearly two decades later, a 1998 analysis by the U.S. Office of Research Integrity would conclude that scientists who blow the whistle on scientific misconduct are primarily males*
See Office of Research Integrity (1998).

216   *The anorexia researcher, Helena Wachslicht-Rodbard, complained to Yale*
See Drummond Rennie's testimony for the Office of Research Integrity, http://ori.dhhs.gov/multimedia/acrobat/sess23.pdf.

216   *though Soman implied that Felig had pressured him to produce results*
This is included in the description of the case given in Broad and Wade (1982).

217   *In JAMA, he wrote of whistleblowers who had been "abused for their courage and persistence"*
See Rennie and Gunsalus (1993).

217   *The Ryan Commission viewed whistleblowers as the underdogs of science*
See Office of Research Integrity (1996).

218   *American medical schools and research universities turned down the idea of a whistle-blowers' bill of rights*
See Kevles (1998) and Goldner (1998).

218   *A series of reports of flagrant misconduct in science had shocked the American public*
See Goldner (1998).

219   *according to one congressman, she lost her house as a result of blowing the whistle*
Ted Weiss, a New York Democrat serving in the U.S. House of Representatives, spoke to O'Toole and wrote about her in the *Chronicle of Higher Education,* June 26, 1991: "Although she followed university procedures exactly, she lost her job and was unable to find another position as a scientist for several years; she even lost her house as a result." O'Toole herself told the Ryan Commission, "I was accused of vindictiveness. I was told that any effort I made to publish a correction would be thwarted, and that any such effort would result in legal actions." (see Burd 1994a).

219   *To some observers it looked as if Imanishi-Kari and Baltimore had been falsely accused; to others it seemed that O'Toole was justified in blowing the whistle but that the system for investigating her charges was broken*
See Kevles (1998).

221   *The report of the company's fight to keep Dong's study out of print appeared on the Wall Street Journal's front page*

Ralph King, "How a drug firm paid for a university study, then undermined it," *Wall Street Journal*, April 25, 1996.

222   *In early 1997, Knoll Pharmaceutical finally capitulated on Betty Dong's paper*
Betty Dong's experience is described in the CBC Radio *Ideas* program "Undue Influence," aired on October 27–28, 1999; transcript available from ideastran@toronto.cbc.ca.

222   *[Rennie] wrote in JAMA that Olivieri, too, had signed a confidentiality agreement*
Rennie's editorial ran on April 16, 1997 (Rennie 1997). Dong's study appeared in the same issue (Dong et al. 1997).

228   *Years later [Strofolino] told the* Toronto Star, *"I came to Sick Kids in 1987 as vice-president, finance*
See Nora McCabe, "Tackling crucial issues," *Toronto Star*, May 28, 1998.

228   *Between 1991 and 1993 the hospital cut 225 jobs*
See Shawn McCarthy, "Insight: Canada's debt," *Toronto Star*, March 21, 1993.

229   *When Strofolino became president and CEO in 1994, the reimbursement package he negotiated*
See Lisa Priest, "Donors to Sick Kids upset over big salary," *Toronto Star*, April 5, 1996.

230   *Strofolino told a reporter that fall that he was trying to run the hospital "like a business"*
See Salem Alaton, "Major surgery: What's the former NHL defenceman Mike Gazdic doing with four hospitals in Toronto? Slashing of course. Meet health care's new breed of player," *Financial Post*, November 1, 1995.

235   *Soon the clinical doctors were hearing that their salaries would be tied to new, supposedly objective measures of their performance*
O'Brodovich later referred to the consultants as "external facilitators" and described the new program as a "career development and compensation program that uses peer review to assess performance in clinical care, education, and research, and directly links an academic physician's performance to compensation" (see Department of Paediatrics, Hospital for Sick Children and Paediatric Consultants, "Career Development and Compensation Programme 2000," 2, and O'Brodovich, Pleinys, and Walker 2000, 94).

238   *Manuel Buchwald was Gallie's boss, and she started meeting with him to fill him in on the LI issues*
As part of his effort to put a new face on the Research Institute, Buchwald had appointed twelve new program heads—one of whom was Brenda Gallie—on January 1, 1998.

239   *Working with Gallie and bench scientist Victor Ling, Chan figured*
           See Chan et al. (1996).

240   *But a science journalist with National Public Radio managed to tell her story*
           Joe Palca's report for NPR aired on *Morning Edition* on May 16, 1997.

240–41   *He also made sure Olivieri was an invited guest at meetings he attended on scientific freedom*
           Olivieri spoke at the meeting "Secrecy and Science" convened by the American Association for the Advancement of Science, September 11, 1997 in Washington, DC.

241   *A researcher at the hospital claimed he had a doctorate*
           See Craig McInnes, "'Superb' researcher is axed over lack of doctorate," *The Globe and Mail*, August 13, 1987.

243   *Convinced that the hospital had been unsupportive and unwilling to help her, she wrote a CMPA official*
           Olivieri wrote Dr. Robert Rivington of the CMPA on September 5, 1997; he wrote her back a letter dated September 25, marked Re: CMPA File 96005157 RNR (ON).

17: PREPARING TO PUBLISH

246   *Part of the problem, as Burt understood it*
           Cameron explained to Olivieri's legal counsel that the system he used for grading the slides was called the Desmet method. See notes for Chapter 14.

249   *Nathan and Weatherall had already written the journal's editors*
           This communication is referred to in a letter from Colangelo to Olivieri dated May 7, 1997.

251   *Gallie, who had tried to help, felt as if things had gotten worse. She spoke to Buchwald again and followed that up with requests in writing*
           Brenda Gallie's letter to Buchwald and Strofolino is dated June 3, 1998.

253–54   *Discouraged, Dick submitted the work to a second-line journal.*
           See Bhatia et al. (1998).

256   *Across the street, at Toronto's Mount Sinai Hospital, researchers occasionally met with board members*
           See Siminovitch (2003), 141.

18: UNDOING MANUEL CARCAO

261   *Toward the end of May she flew to Chicago for an invitation-only conference*

The conference was the 1998 Cantigny Conference on medicine and the media, titled "Ethical Issues in the Publication of Medical Information," sponsored by the Robert R. McCormick Tribune Foundation and held on the grounds of the Cantigny Estate in Wheaton, Illinois, May 12–13, 1998.

19: THE MAKING OF A MEDIA STAR

272   *In 1995, Brill-Edwards had gone on national television in Canada to expose practices she thought led to unsafe drugs staying on the market*
She was interviewed on the CBC network show *The Fifth Estate* on February 27, 1996.

273   *After a while, she felt she wasn't getting anywhere and began sharing confidential information with a reporter*
Brill-Edwards spoke to Montreal *Gazette* reporter Nicholas Regush about Imitrex; he later wrote about her concerns in Regush (1994).

274   *In 1999, the head of Britain's Royal Society rebuked*
See Horton (2003), 316.

275   *CTV producer Andrew Mitrovica (later with the* Globe and Mail) *wrote later that Olivieri struck him that summer as someone who was "transparently motivated*
Mitrovica's description of Olivieri in the summer of 1998 is from his speech accepting an award for his coverage, reprinted by the Canadian Association of Journalists as Andrew Mitrovica, "Whistleblower doctor: Winner of the Open Television (less than five minutes) category, CTV [Canadian Association of Journalists award winners]," *Media*, Summer 1999.

275   *The headline was about the FDA's most famous woman: Frances Kelsey*
See John Schwartz, "A close call over thalidomide," *Washington Post*, July 17, 1998.

280   *The next day, Olivieri's paper came out*
Olivieri's article, written with her collaborators, is Olivieri et al. (1998).

280   *In the same issue, Marshall Kaplan of Tufts wrote an editorial with Kris Kowdley, a doctor from the University of Washington*
See Kowdley and Kaplan (1998).

283   *"If this can happen to Nancy Olivieri"*
Schafer at a press conference on August 27, 1998, as quoted in Rita Daly, "Scientists up ante in Sick Kids fight," *Toronto Star*, August 28, 1998.

284   *Brill-Edwards wrote a letter to the editor of the* Globe and Mail *soon after the story broke, calling for a change in leadership at Sick Kids*

See Michèle Brill-Edwards, "Sick Kids should come clean," *The Globe and Mail*, September 2, 1998.

284   *At one press conference, Brenda Gallie threatened to leave Sick Kids*
Press conference held August 27, 1998.

284–85   *Hospital vice-president Dr. Alan Goldbloom rebutted Olivieri's charges*
See Susan Jeffrey, "Olivieri case prompts Sick Kids review," *Medical Post*, September 22, 1998.

287   *Naimark offered her the chance to assist him, but she turned him down, saying she needed to be assured of being able to add her own separate section to the report if she disagreed*
Baird explains how Naimark invited her to assist him in his "capacity as the Reviewer" and why she declined to be involved in Thompson, Baird, and Downie (2001), 282.

288   *In late October the* Toronto Star *said in an editorial*
See "Sick Kids must set the record straight," *Toronto Star*, October 27, 1998.

289   *She was disturbed that what she heard on the radio didn't match what she knew, and she sent Howard*
Josie sent her e-mail to Howard on August 13, 1998; she sent her e-mail to the CBC on September 2, 1998.

290   *"In a display of the lengths Olivieri's critics will go*
See Jane O'Hara, "Whistleblower: A top researcher says a drug under trial poses a risk to patients: The drug maker threatened legal action against its critic," *Maclean's*, November 16, 1998.

290   Elm Street *had asked Valpy to profile Olivieri*
See Michael Valpy, "Science friction," *Elm Street*, December 1998.

291   *Later, Valpy and Olivieri admitted to seeing each other on a romantic basis*
See Christie Blatchford, "It's not just the kids who are sick: Olivieri's camp goaded hospital poison-letter writer," *National Post*, December 27, 1999.

291   *Gwen Smith, the editor who oversaw the* Elm Street *profile*
See Gwen Smith, "Editor's letter," *Elm Street*, May 2000.

294   *Buchwald and O'Brodovich had written the editor of* Nature Medicine
See Buchwald and O'Brodovich (1999).

295   *there was a controversy over Nancy Olivieri's research that became public in December 1998*

The letters to the editor about Olivieri (1998) are in the *New England Journal of Medicine* 339 (1998): 1710–14. Olivieri's reply is co-authored with Brittenham, Templeton and Fleming.

295   *"Olivieri et al. collected a lot of data during their seven-year study"*
       See Grady and Giardina (1998).

296   *Alan Cohen, who was still testing L1 at the Children's Hospital of Philadelphia, wrote to the journal*
       See Cohen and Martin (1998).

296   *"To our knowledge, the total number of children who are unable to use the standard iron-chelating agent*
       See Brittenham et al. (1998).

296   *Michael Spino also argued with Olivieri*
       See Tricta and Spino (1998).

298   *"We don't usually do cardiac biopsies, but we were concerned*
       Olivieri's comments on CBC Radio aired as "For Profit or for Patients: An Update," CBC Radio, *Quirks and Quarks*, December 12, 1998.

298   *In November she told* Maclean's *that the young man's severe heart problems were "a direct result" of L1*
       See Jane O'Hara; "Whistleblower," *Maclean's*, November 16, 1998.

299   *At ASH she described the case of Michael, the young man in heart failure*
       Michael's case is discussed in Olivieri's abstract for poster number 2184, displayed at ASH on Monday, December 7, 1998, at the Miami Beach Convention Center and appearing on page 237 of the meeting program as "Cardiac Failure and Myocardial Fibrosis in a Patient with Thalassemia Major Treated with Long-term Deferiprone," by N. F. Olivieri, J. Butany, D. M. Templeton, and G. M. Brittenham.

300   *He had written an article in November that L1 "may have been involved in the recent death*
       See Valpy, Michael, "Salvage group tackles Sick Kids' image disaster," *The Globe and Mail*, November 2, 1998. The retraction ran as "Retraction," November 9, 1998.

20: THE WAR OF WORDS

301   *Françoise Baylis wrote in a journal article that Dick was reluctant to hire new staff*
       See Baylis (2004).

302   *He wrote Gallie, "If by some psychological sleight of hand*
       Buchwald's letter to Gallie is dated December 7, 1998.

302–03 *"I am proud to be part of the leadership team at The Hospital for Sick Children*
Gallie's reply is dated December 23, 1998.

303 *His report, titled* A Review of Facts and Circumstances
The Naimark Review's full title is *Clinical Trials of L1 (Deferiprone) at the Hospital for Sick Children in Toronto: A Review of Facts and Circumstances*. Printed copies were distributed to the media, and it is available on the website of the Hospital for Sick Children.

304 *As Michael Valpy wrote in his column*
See Michael Valpy, "Hospital report critical but fails to hit the mark," *The Globe and Mail*, December 10, 1998.

305 *Olivieri said she asked the administration to hire a lawyer*
See Paul Taylor, "A doctor takes on a drug company," *The Globe and Mail*, August 13, 1998.

305 *"A defiant Dr. Nancy Olivieri"*
See Theresa Boyle and Rita Daly, "Olivieri pledges to battle 'bias,'" *Toronto Star*, December 11, 1998.

305 *Olivieri said the review was "fundamentally flawed" and "openly . . . biased."*
See Dick Chapman, "Hospital admits errors," *Toronto Sun*, December 11, 1998, and Boyle and Daly, *Toronto Star*, December 11, 1998.

305 *"Were our children put at risk?" Schafer asked*
See Theresa Boyle and Rita Daly, "Olivieri pledges to battle 'bias'; she gets Sick Kids apology, but seeks new inquiry," *Toronto Star*, December 11, 1998.

306 *according to one Olivieri supporter, Dr. Jeff Smallwood*
Smallwood is quoted in Shuchman (1999), 387.

306 *But Clayton Ruby took it a step further, suggesting that the hospital's unwillingness to hire more staff for Olivieri's clinics was a racist move*
Ruby and Symes wrote a letter on December 10, 1998, to O'Brodovich and Strofolino that said, in part, "Of the 100 thalassemia patients in the hemoglobinopathy program at the Hospital for Sick Children, none of them is of northern European ancestry," and "the clinical coverage is clearly inadequate and places these sick children in jeopardy." Ruby released the letter to the press, and it was described as accusing Sick Kids administrators of "risking the health of 450 poor black, Asian and Mediterranean children" (see Steve Arnold, "Sick Kids neglecting patients, lawyer says," *The Hamilton Spectator*, December 12, 1998).

308   Around the same time, she and her supporters received letters from Strofolino's office reminding them of the hospital's bylaws
> The letter about the hospital bylaws was dated January 6, signed by Buchwald and O'Brodovich, and sent to all four members of the Gang of Four. The Gang circulated it widely with a "Dear Colleagues" letter attached, calling the bylaws letter a "gag order" and "yet another example of why we are compelled to express our views publicly and to seek resolution through a formal grievance process."

309   The university president had been speaking regularly with Strofolino
> See Thompson, Baird, and Downie (2001), 231.

310   Clayton Ruby later told reporters that the three-page agreement was a credit to Rob Prichard
> See Patricia Chisholm, "Calling off the feud: A noted doctor returns to her job at Sick Kids," *Maclean's*, February 8, 1999, 36.

310   Olivieri got her clinical job back; she would be directing the programs responsible for the care of about 450 thalassemia and sickle cell patients
> By 1998, the hemoglobinopathy programs at the Hospital for Sick Children and the University Health Network cared for approximately 450 patients (see Thompson, Baird, and Downie, 2001, 225).

311   "It was miraculous," Prichard told reporters later
> Prichard described his son's recovery to *Globe and Mail* reporter John Allemang (see John Allemang, "I love newspapers," *The Globe and Mail*, June 23, 2001).

312   He told reporters that the situation had been "very, very stressful"
> See Jennifer Quinn and Tanya Talaga, "Blood researcher, hospital agree to end 2 1/2 year battle," *Toronto Star*, January 27, 1999.

312   After the agreement made headlines, an editorial in the Globe and Mail *asked*
> See "Drugs, docs and kids," *The Globe and Mail*, January 28, 1999.

312   She told reporters, "People are saying, 'Oh, Nancy got her job back
> See Shona McKay, "Dr. Nancy Olivieri (Coping with stress and strain on the job)," *Financial Post Magazine*, April 1999, 30.

313   The union had filed grievances
> The UTFA announced the grievances in a statement signed by Rhonda Love dated January 7, 1999.

314   The Gang asked Naylor to mediate, and he tried his hand at shuttle diplomacy

See "Prichard reports on Olivieri's case," *The University of Toronto Bulletin*, October 25, 1999.

314   *Amid reports that proposed changes to the patent laws would wipe out $40 million in investment by the generic companies, Toronto-based cabinet ministers had written to the prime minister*
On the lobbying efforts by the generic industry, see Jane Taber, "Liberals split over new patent laws," *Ottawa Citizen*, November 18, 1999.

314   *Prichard followed suit, writing to the prime minister*
See John Deverell, "U of T appeals to Ottawa to help generic drug firms," *Toronto Star*, September 4, 1999.

315   *"Outside forces need this case to push their agenda about drug-industry funding of research," Michael Strofolino said in an interview later*
Strofolino was interviewed in May 2000 for the CBC Radio program *Ideas*. The complete taped interview is in the author's possession.

21: WARRING BETRAYALS: THE POISON PEN
321   *The way Koren explained it, the resident "had worked on L1 studies*
Koren's explanation of his resident's actions are in a letter he wrote to Olivieri on March 25, 1998.

321   *A 1996 report by the U.S. Office of Research Integrity*
See Office of Research Integrity (1996).

321   *Law professor Jesse Goldner of St. Louis University summed up the report's findings*
See Goldner (1998).

321   *A high-achieving McGill professor—neuropsychologist Justine Sergent—was accused of misconduct in 1994*
The circumstances of Justine Sergent's death were covered extensively in the Montreal *Gazette* and the *McGill Reporter* in the spring of 1994, and the coverage included the full text of her suicide note. See also Ratelle (1994).

322   *and later described himself as having been "savagely attacked*
See Krista Foss, "Sick Kids doctor breaks his silence," *The Globe and Mail*, January 7, 2000.

323   *After a letter from Beatrix Wonke and others questioning Olivieri's results*
See Wonke, Telfer, and Hoffbrand (1998). The editor's note reads: "Apotex recently supported one trainee sponsored by Drs. Wonke and Hoffbrand."

323   *Alan Cohen's letter, written with research nurse Marie Martin*
        See Cohen and Martin (1998).

323   *But the journal had published Olivieri's 1995 article on L1 without mentioning that the*
        company was supporting her research
        See Olivieri et al. (1995). The article refers to a separate study of L1's toxicity
        being conducted under Apotex sponsorship, but doesn't mention that the
        results reported in the 1995 paper were from a study partly sponsored by the
        company.

323   *and her 1998 article without noting that she and Brittenham had been consultants to Apotex*
        See Olivieri et al. (1998). Apotex is included in the list of research sponsors,
        but Olivieri's and Brittenham's consultancies to the company are not
        mentioned.

328   *Much later, it emerged that Olivieri herself had asked the CMPA lawyers to drop Koren*
        See Thompson, Baird, and Downie (2001), 426.

330   *Later, he told* Globe and Mail *reporter Krista Foss that he felt as if his hands were tied*
        See Krista Foss, "Sick Kids doctor breaks his silence," *The Globe and Mail*, January
        7, 2000.

334   *In the late spring of 1999, knowing that the chances were high that Koren was the author*
        of the letters, the Gang managed to seize his computer
        Olivieri and Durie took Koren's computer on June 1, 1999, according to
        Barbara Humphrey's report, as quoted in the *National Post* on December 27, 2000.

335   *In January 1999, Brenda Gallie was quoted in the* Toronto Star *as saying Olivieri might*
        leave Toronto
        See "U of T head should back demoted doctor," *Toronto Star*, January 17, 1999.

336   *Months later, Ruby told the press*
        Ruby spoke at a press conference held at the UTFA offices in Toronto on
        December 21, 1999.

339   *Koren wrote her in the summer of 1999 in a scratchy long-hand to see if she needed work*
        Koren wrote to Brill-Edwards about "upcoming option of jobs" in a letter dated
        July 11, 1999.

341   *The next day the* Globe *and the* National Post *carried the story, referring to the letters as*
        "poison-pen" letters
        See Krista Foss, "Leading doctor now suspended over hate mail," *The Globe and
        Mail*, December 22, 1999; and Marina Jiminez, "'Hate mail' renews credibility

debate: Doctor suspended as 'personal issues' and research overlap," *National Post*, December 22, 1999.

343   *He was suspended with pay from his other positions at the university and the hospital*
Koren was suspended on December 22, 1999, and over the holidays he voluntarily resigned from two of his hospital positions and one of his university posts.

343   *To ensure that the committee had all the relevant information, the Gang gave the hospital a binder of documents*
The Gang delivered its new information to the hospital in the form of a binder with several hundred pages (see Krista Foss, "Another bizarre twist in case of poison-pen MD," *The Globe and Mail*, January 5, 2000).

343   *Ruby said publicly that the doctors suspected Koren of having falsified the evidence*
Ruby's allegations were published in the *Toronto Star*. See Nicholas van Rijn and Scott Simmie, "Widen poison pen probe, lawyers demand; Fresh claims of wrongdoing made on eve of hearing at Sick Kids," *Toronto Star*, January 4, 2000.

343   *After Ruby's claims about it were publicized, the Israeli doctor confirmed that he'd written it*
Dr. Michael Lishner of Tel Aviv University's Sackler Faculty of Medicine confirmed that he had written the letter, and Ruby apologized for his false allegations about it on January 7, 2000. See Nicolaas van Rijn, "Olivieri's lawyer apologizes to Sick Kids doctor; Israeli MD confirms he wrote letter used in disciplinary case," *Toronto Star*, January 8, 2000.

344   *Olivieri or her supporters managed to get a copy of the letter to a reporter for the* Toronto Star, *and the paper quoted liberally from it*
See Harold Levy, "Doctor deemed too good to fire for harassment; many benefit from Koren's expertise, Sick Kids says in its decision," *Toronto Star*, May 4, 2000.

344   *The UTFA's William Graham told* Nature Medicine *that the hospital and the university had "damaged themselves*
See Laura Bonetta, "Hate-mail author trapped by DNA," *Nature Medicine* 6, no. 4 (April 2000): 364.

344   *Shear told reporters, "It takes incredible, incredible frustration*
Neal Shear's comments on Koren are quoted in Krista Foss, "Sick Kids crisis reignites," *The Globe and Mail*, May 5, 2000.

344   *She discovered that Koren had sought help*
Humphrey said that Koren asked the hospital administration for help combatting the campaign against him by Olivieri and others on two separate occasions, in

May and August of 1998 (see Christie Blatchford, "It's not just the kids who are sick: Olivieri's camp goaded hospital poison-letter writer," *National Post*, December 27, 1999).

344   *Koren himself told a* Globe and Mail *reporter later, "The only way I could express myself was in those letters*
See Krista Foss, "Sick Kids doctor breaks his silence," *The Globe and Mail*, January 7, 2000.

22: BATTLE FATIGUE

348   *In the fall of 1999, Nancy Olivieri admitted to a reporter from the* Toronto Star
See Janice Turner, "The price of fame: popularity can be a mixed bag for scientists," *Toronto Star*, October 29, 1999.

348   *She said the committee's accusations against her had "no basis" and were "completely untrue"*
Olivieri's complaints about the Medical Advisory Committee of the Hospital for Sick Children are in her letter to Dr. John M. Bonn of the College of Physicians and Surgeons of Ontario dated April 28, 2000.

349   *in late 1999, a U.S. publication called* Academe *compared her to the woman she'd emulated at the FDA*
See "A drug company's effort to silence a researcher," *Academe—Bulletin of the American Association of University Professors*, November–December 1999.

349   *In February 2000, the* New York Times *reported that "academic scientists*
See Sheryl Gay Stolberg, "Biomedicine is receiving new scrutiny as scientists become entrepreneurs," *New York Times*, February 20, 2000.

349   *an editorial in the* New England Journal of Medicine *in May 2000*
See Angell (2000).

350   *She was an emblem of the fight against corporate villainy in the pharmaceutical industry, a living hero winning awards and honours on an almost monthly basis for her courage*
Olivieri's awards include the first annual Whistleblower Award from the BC Freedom of Information and Privacy Association; the Shadeek Nader Foundation's Callaway Award for Civic Courage; the Ordine al Merito awarded by the National Congress of Italian Canadians; and the Milner Memorial Award from the Canadian Association of University Teachers.

351   *Toward the end of 2000, Olivieri told a reporter for the* Times of London
See Ann Treneman, "Doctors at war," *The Times* (London), Decemeber 14, 2000.

354   *The coroner and the hospital both investigated, and the hospital soon claimed responsibility*

for the death. An internal report of the hospital's investigation listed a series of errors
See Harold Levy, "Hospital takes blame for girl's death; Sickle cell anemia patient 'not adequately prepared' for surgery, according to report," *Toronto Star*, November 10, 2000.

354   *The nurses and doctors hadn't monitored the patient's hemoglobin level and blood pressure closely*
See Jane Gadd, "Hospital felt its probe adequate, inquest told," *The Globe and Mail*, July 6, 2001.

354   *"Why the process took so long is not for me to comment on," she told the coroner's jury*
Kirby's words at the Sanchia Bulgin inquest are quoted in Gay Abbate, "Sickle cell guidelines at Sick Kids delayed for two years," *The Globe and Mail*, May 26, 2001.

23: MOVING ON

356   *Titled* The Olivieri Report, *it exonerated Olivieri*
See Thompson, Baird, and Downie (2001).

357   *Arnie Aberman wrote them that the material they'd shown him was "incomplete, incorrect, and misleading*
See Thompson, Baird, and Downie (2001), 522.

357   *David Naylor wrote later, "Virtually none of the individuals who are criticized in the report . . . participated in any way with the CAUT Inquiry report*
See Naylor (2002b).

357   *Though the terms were confidential, it was described publicly as "generous,"*
See Anne McIlroy, "Olivieri, supporters, win settlement," *The Globe and Mail*, November 13, 2002.

358   *She said she felt "pretty terrific" about the agreement*
See Steve Arnold, "I feel pretty terrific," *The Hamilton Spectator*, December 27, 2002.

358   *"She fought, and with luck, we'll all benefit as a consequence," Drummond Rennie told a television producer who interviewed him about Olivieri in 2003*
Rennie made his remarks in *Dying for Drugs*.

358   *They developed a single set of rules that every hospital agreed to*
The new university rules are described in Naylor (2002a).

359   *In September 2001, the editors of some of the world's leading medical journals*
See Davidoff et al. (2001).

361   *Olivieri turned her battles into a second academic career. She wrote in science journals*
           See Olivieri (2003).

363   *He joined* Forbes's *list of the richest men in the world*
           See "Canada's richest," *Vancouver Sun,* July 25, 2000 and "17 Canucks make bil-
           lionaire list," *Sudbury Star,* June 20, 2000.

24: THE SCIENCE OF L1

364   *She told the* British Medical Journal *in January 2004*
           See Clare Dyer, "Whistleblower vows to fight on," *British Medical Journal*
           328 (January 24, 2004): 187.

365   *It's used widely in combination with Desferal*
           See Mourad et al. (2003).

365   *George Constantinou, a thalassemia patient and leader*
           See Constantinou (2004).

366   *Spino thinks David Nathan's ties to Novartis represent a conflict of interest that should
           have prevented him from writing about L1*
           See Spino et al. (2003).

367   *Ian Wanless, an internationally known liver pathologist at the Toronto General Hospital,
           led one of those efforts*
           See Wanless et al. (2002).

367   *The other study to refute Olivieri was done in Italy, where investigators compared L1 and
           Desferal in a randomized trial*
           See Maggio et al. (2002).

367   *The toxicity trial that Olivieri had convinced Spino to sponsor—her "international
           trial"—was carried to completion by her former friend at the Children's Hospital of
           Philadelphia, Alan Cohen*
           See Cohen et al. (2000).

367   *He published longer-term results of the same trial in 2003*
           See Cohen et al. (2003).

368   *The* National Post *ran a feature article in February 2000*
           See Marina Jimenez, "Whistleblower's claim disputed by some peers," *National
           Post,* February 12, 2000.

368   *The* Toronto Star *also reported on Cohen's work*

See Chris Nuttall-Smith, "Controversial drug is safe, study says; 'Toxicity to white blood cells a rare side effect,'" *Toronto Star*, February 24, 2000.

368   *in the spring of 2000 CBC Television ran a documentary on its nightly news program*
CBC Television's *The National* aired its twenty-five-minute item, titled "When Science Takes Sides . . . Who Do You Believe?" on March 14, 2000.

368   *Arthur Schafer wrote an op-ed for the* Toronto Star *accusing the CBC of "grave factual errors and innuendo"*
See Arthur Schafer, "Smear tactics unfair to Olivieri," *Toronto Star*, April 10, 2000.

368   *The Gang of Four saw it the same way, and so did thalassemia's two Davids*
See Nathan and Weatherall (2002).

EPILOGUE
370   *A U.S. survey published in 2002 confirms how difficult patients still find injecting Desferal*
See Ward, Caro, et al. (2002).

370   *In 2000, according to a paper by Bernadette Modell in the* Lancet
See Modell et al. (2000).

371   *Some doctors in England and the U.S. have tested this theory using a novel MRI technique*
See Anderson et al. (2003).

371   *One of the studies that showed this was conducted at the University of Turin*
The Turin study is Piga et al. (2000).

372   *As a result some patients discontinue ICL670*
See Nisbet-Brown et al. (2003).

373   *In 2003, Gluud and his colleagues in Copenhagen*
See Als-Nielsen et al. (2003).

375   *Instead, reviewers can use the process to "punish authors*
See Lawrence (2003).

375   *Drummond Rennie, of the* Journal of the American Medical Association, *has referred to scientific peer review*
See Martin Enserink, "Peer review and quality: A dubious connection?" *Science*, September 21, 2001, 2187–88.

376   *"Premature deaths of young adults with thalassemia" was the headline*
The press release was date May 4, 2003, and listed contact numbers at the

Thalassemia Foundations and the Anemia Institute for Research and Education, both in Toronto.

377   *In July 2004, the Thalassemia Foundation*
The conference was Best Practices in Thalassemia Care: Canadian and International Perspectives, July 13, 2004, Toronto.

REFERENCES

Agarwal, M. B., C. Viswanathan, J. Ramanathian, et al. 1990. Oral iron chelation with L1. *The Lancet* i, 601.

Al-Refaie F.N., B. Wonke, A.V. Hoffbrand, D.G. Wickens, P. Nortey, G. J. Kontoghiorghes. 1992. Efficacy and possible adverse effects of the oral iron chelator, 1,2-dimethyl-3-hydroxyprrid-4-one (L1) in thalassemia major. *Blood* 80:593.

Als-Nielsen, B., W. Chen, C. Gluud, et al. 2003. Association of funding and conclusions in randomized drug trials: A reflection of treatment effect or adverse events? *Journal of the American Medical Association* 290: 921–28.

Alter, B. P. 1990. Agranulocytosis and thrombocytopenia, Blackfan-Diamond anaemia, and oral chelation. *The Lancet* 335: 970.

Anderson, L. J., B. Wonke, E. Prescott, et al. 2002. Comparison of effects of oral deferiprone and subcutaneous desferrioxamine on myocardial iron concentrations and ventricular function in beta-thalassemia. *The Lancet* 360: 516–20.

Angell, M. 2000. Is academic medicine for sale? *New England Journal of Medicine* 342: 1516–18.

Atweh, George F., Millicent Sutton, Imad Nassif, et al. 1999. Sustained induction of fetal hemoglobin by pulse butyrate therapy in sickle cell disease. *Blood* 93: 1790–97.

Bailar, John C. 1995. The real threats to the integrity of science. *Chronicle of Higher Education,* April 21.

Barry, M., D. M. Flynn, E. A. Letsky, et al. 1974. Long-term chelation therapy in thalassemia major: Effect on liver iron concentration, liver histology and clinical progress. *British Medical Journal* 2 (909): 16–20.

Baylis, F. 2004. The Olivieri debacle: Where were the heroes of bioethics? *Journal of Medical Ethics* 30: 44–49.

Bekelman, J. E., Yan Li and Cary P. Gross. 2003. Scope and impact of financial conflicts of interest in biomedical research: A systematic review. *Journal of the American Medical Association* 289: 454–65.

Berkovitch, M., R. M. Laxer, D. Matsui, et al. 1992. Analysis of adverse rheumatologic effects of iron chelators in patients with homozygous beta thalassemia. [Abstract]. *Blood* 80 (supp. 1): 7A.

Berkovitch, Matitiahu, Ronald M. Laxer, Robert Inman, Gideon Koren, Kenneth P. H.

Pritzker, M. J. Fritzler, and Nancy F. Olivieri. 1994. Arthropathy in thalassaemia patients receiving deferiprone. *The Lancet* 343: 1471–72.

Bhatia, M., D. Bonnet, B. Murdoch, et al. 1998. A newly discovered class of human hematopoietic cells with SCID-repopulating activity. *Nature Medicine* 4: 1038–45.

Blumenthal D., M. Gluck, K. Louis, M. Stoto, and D. Wise. 1986. University-industry research relationships in biotechnology: Implications for the university. *Science* 232: 1361–66.

Bodenheimer, T. 2000. Conflict of interest in clinical drug trials: A risk factor for scientific misconduct. http://ohrp.dhls.gov/coi/bodenheimer.htm.

Borgna-Pignatti C., De Stefano P., Broglia A.M. 1984. Visual loss in patient on high-dose subcutaneous desferrioxamine. *The Lancet*. 1 (8378):681.

Brittenham, G. M. 1992. Development of iron-chelating agents for clinical use. *Blood* 80: 569–74.

Brittenham, G. M., K. A. Fleming, D. M. Templeton, and N. F. Olivieri. 1998. Iron chelation with oral deferiprone in patients with thalassemia. *New England Journal of Medicine* 339: 1713.

Brittenham, G.M., Sheth S., et al. 2001. Noninvasive methods for quantitative assessment of transfusional iron overload in sickle cell disease. *Seminars in Hematology*. 38 (1 Suppl 1): 37–56.

Broad, W., and N. Wade. 1982. *Betrayers of the truth*. New York: Simon & Schuster.

Brody, Baruch. 1995. *Ethical issues in drug testing, approval and pricing: The Clot-Dissolving Drugs*. New York: Oxford University Press.

Buchwald, Manuel, and Hugh O'Brodovich. 1999. HSC clinical trials controversy continues. *Nature Medicine* 5: 2–3.

Burd, Stephen. 1994a. Federal panel weighs a "whistle blower's bill of rights." *Chronicle of Higher Education,* December 14.

Carthew, P., A. G. Smith, R. C. Hider, B. Dorman, et al. 1994. Potentiation of iron accumulation in cardiac myocytes during the treatment of iron overload in gerbils with the hydroxypyridinone iron chelator CP94. *BioMetals* 7: 267–71.

Chan, Helen S., G. DeBoer, J.J. Thiessen, et al. 1996. Combining cyclosporin with chemotherapy controls intraocular retinoblastoma without requiring radiation. *Clinical Cancer Research* 2: 1499–1508.

Cho, Mildred, and Lisa Bero. 1996. The quality of drug studies published in symposium proceedings. *Annals of Internal Medicine* 124: 485–89.

Cohen, A. R., et al. 2000. Safety profile of the oral iron chelator deferiprone: A multi-centre study. *British Journal of Haematology* 108: 305–12.

———. 2003. Safety and effectiveness of long-term therapy with the oral iron chelator deferiprone. *Blood* 102: 1583–87.

Cohen, A. R., and M. B. Martin. 1998. Iron chelation with oral deferiprone in patients with thalassemia. *New England Journal of Medicine* 339: 1713.

Commission on Research Integrity. 1995. *Integrity and misconduct in research.* Washington DC: U.S. Department of Health and Human Services, Public Health Service.

Committee on the Conduct of Science. 1989. *On being a scientist*. Washington DC: National Academy of Sciences.

Constantinou G. March 13, 2004. The disappearing Patient. *BMJ Online*. Rapid responses to: Salvulescu J. 2004. Thalassemia major: the murky story of deferiprone. *British Medical Journal* 328: 358–359.

Constantinou, G., S. Melides, and B. Modell. 2003. The Olivieri case. *New England Journal of Medicine* 348: 860–63.

Cooke, R. 2001. *Dr. Folkman's war: Angiogenesis and the struggle to defeat cancer*. New York: Random House.

Davidoff, F., C. D. DeAngelis, J. M. Drazen, et al. 2001. Sponsorship, authorship and accountability. [Editorial]. *Canadian Medical Association Journal* 165: 786–88.

Davies S.C., Marcus R.E., Hungerford J.L., et al. 1983. Ocular toxicity of high-dose intravenous desferrioxamine. *The Lancet*. 2(8343):181–4.

De Virgiliis, S., M. Congia, F. Frau, et al. 1988. Deferoxamine-induced growth retardation in patients with thalassemia major. *Journal of Pediatrics* 113: 661–69.

Diav-Citrin, O., A. Atanackovick, and G. Koren. 1999. "An investigation into variability of the therapeutic response to deferiprone in patients with thalassemia major. *Therapeutic Drug Monitoring* 21: 74–81.

Dong, B., W. W. Hauck, J. G. Gambertoglio, L. Gee, J. R. White, J. L. Bubp, and F. S. Greenspan. 1997. Bioequivalence of generic and brand-name levothyroxine products in the treatment of hypothyroidism. *Journal of the American Medical Association* 277: 1205–13.

Frenkel, M. J., J. M. Gillespie, and P. J. Reis. 1975. Studies on the inhibition of synthesis of the tyrosine-rich proteins of wool. *Australian Journal of Biological Sciences* 28: 331–38.

Garbutt, G. J., and E. C. Abraham. 1981. Stimulation of minor fetal hemoglobin synthesis in cord blood reticulocytes by butyrate. *Biochemical and Biophysical Research Communications* 98: 1051–56.

Goldner, J. A. 1998. The unending saga of legal controls over scientific misconduct: A clash of cultures needing resolution. *American Journal of Law & Medicine* 24: 293–343.

Gore, A. 1991. Planning a new biotechnology policy. *Harvard Journal of Law and Technology* (Fall).

Grady, Robert W., and Patricia J. Giardina. 1998. Iron chelation with oral deferiprone in patients with thalassemia. *New England Journal of Medicine* 339: 1712–13.

Healy, B., et al. 1989. Conflict-of-interest guidelines for a multicenter trial of treatment after coronary-artery bypass-graft surgery. *New England Journal of Medicine* 320: 949–51.

Hershko, C. 1993. Development of oral iron chelator L1. *The Lancet* 341: 1088–89.

Hershko, C. 1988. Oral iron chelating drugs: coming but not yet ready for clinical use. *British Medical Journal* 296: 1081–82.

Hoffbrand, A. V., A. N. Bartlett, P. A. Veys, N. T. O'Connor, and G. J. Kontoghiorghes. 1989. Agranulocytosis and thrombocytopenia in patient with Blackfan-Diamond anaemia during oral chelator trial. *The Lancet* 2, no. 8660: 457.

Horton, R. 2003. *Health wars: On the global front lines of modern medicine.* New York: New York Review Books.

Kahana L.M., Spino M. 1991. Ciprofloxacin in patients with mycobacterial infections: experience in 15 patients. *DICP* 25: 919024.

Kevles, D. J. 1998. *The Baltimore case.* New York: Norton.

Kontoghiorghes, G. J. 1985. New orally active iron chelators. *The Lancet* 1: 817.

Kontoghiorghes, G. J., M. A. Aldouri, A. V. Hoffbrand, J. Barr, B. Wonke, et al. 1987. Effective chelation of iron in beta-thalassemia with the oral chelator 1,2-dimethyl-3-hydroxypyrid-4-one. *British Medical Journal* 295: 1509–12.

Kontoghiorghes, G. J., M. A. Aldouri, L. Sheppard, and A. V. Hoffbrand. 1987. 1,2-Dimethyl-3-hydroxypyrid-4-one, an orally active chelator for treatment of iron overload. *The Lancet* 1: 1294–95.

Kontoghiorghes, G. J., P. Nasseri-Sina, J. G. Goddard, J. M. Barr, P. Nortley, and L. N. Sheppard. 1989. Safety of oral iron chelator L1. *The Lancet* 2 (no. 8660): 457–58.

Koren, G., D. Farine, D. Muresky, J. Taylor, J. Hayes, S. Soldin, and S. MacLeod. 1984. Significance of the endogenous digoxin-like substance in infants and mothers. *Clinical Pharmacology and Therapeutics* 36: 759–64.

Kowdley, K. V., and M. M. Kaplan. 1998. Iron chelation therapy with oral deferiprone: Toxicity or lack of efficacy? *New England Journal of Medicine* 339: 468–69.

Lancet. 1984. High dose chelation therapy in thalassemia. [Editorial]. *The Lancet* 1 (8373): 373–74.

———. 1989. Oral iron chelators. [Editorial]. *The Lancet* 2: 1016–17.

———. 1993. The patent craze and academia. [Editorial]. *The Lancet* 342: 1435–37.

le Carré, J. 2001. *The constant gardener.* Toronto: Penguin.

MacKinnon, J. A., S. D. Milone, G. M. Brittenham, et al. 1994. Success and failure of iron chelation therapy with the orally active iron chelator L1 in two sisters. *Blood* 84: 258a, abstract no. 1018.

Macrina, F. L. 2000. *Scientific integrity.* 2nd ed. New York: ASM.

Maggio, A., G. D'Amico, et al. 2002. Deferiprone versus deferoxamine in patients with thalassemia major: a randomized clinical trial. *Blood Cells, Molecules, & Diseases* 28: 196–208.

McDonald, M. 2000. *The governance of human research involving human subjects.* Ottawa: Law Commission of Canada.

McNeill, P. 1993. *The ethics and politics of human experimentation.* Cambridge, England: Cambridge University Press.

Mehta, J., S. Singhal, and B. C. Mehta. 1993. Future of oral iron chelator deferiprone (L1) [Comment]. *The Lancet* 341: 1480.

Mehta, J., S. Singhal, R. Revankar, et al. 1991. Fatal systemic lupus erythematosus in patient taking oral iron chelator L1. *The Lancet* 337: 298.

Modell, B., M. Khan, and M. Darlison. 2000. Survival in beta-thalassaemia major in the UK: data from the UK Thalassaemia Register. *The Lancet* 355: 2051–52.

Modell, C. B., and J. Beck. 1974. Long-term desferrioxamine therapy in thalassemia. *Annals of the New York Academy of Sciences* 232: 201–10.

Mourad, F., A. V. Hoffbrand, M. Sheikh-Taha, et al. 2003. Comparison between desferrioxamine and combined therapy with desferrioxamine and deferiprone in iron-overloaded thalassemia patients. *British Journal of Haematology* 121: 187–89.

Naimark A., B. Knoppers, F. Lowy. 1998. Clinical trials of L1 (Deferiprone) at The Hospital for Sick Children in Toronto. A Review of Facts and Circumstances. December 1998.

Nathan, D. G. 1995a. An orally active iron chelator. *Genes, blood and courage: A boy called Immortal Sword*. Cambridge, MA: Belknap Press of Harvard University Press.

———. 1995b. An orally active iron chelator. *New England Journal of Medicine* 332: 953–4.

———. 1998. Pioneers and modern ideas. Prospective on thalassemia. *Pediatrics* 102 (suppl.): 281–83.

Nathan, D. G., and D. Weatherall. 2002. Academic freedom in clinical research. *New England Journal of Medicine* 347: 1368–71.

Naylor, C. D. 2002a. Early Toronto experience with new standards for industry-sponsored clinical research: A progress report. [Editorial]. *Canadian Medical Association Journal* 166: 453–56.

———. 2002b. The deferiprone controversy: Time to move on. *Canadian Medical Association Journal* 166: 452–53.

———. 2002c. I beg to differ. [Letter]. *Canadian Medical Association Journal* 167: 11–12.

Nisbet-Brown, E., N. F. Olivieri, et al. 2003. Effectiveness and safety of ICL670 in iron-loaded patients with thalassaemia: A randomised, double-blind, placebo-controlled, dose-escalation trial. *The Lancet* 361: 1597–1602.

O'Brodovich, Hugh, Ramune Pleinys, and Neil Walker. 2000. Peer-reviewed career development and compensation program for physicians in an academic health-science centre. *Annals of the Royal College of Physicians and Surgeons of Canada* 33: 88–96.

Office of Research Integrity. 1996. *Consequences of being accused of scientific misconduct.* Washington DC: U.S. Department of Health and Human Services, Office of Public Health and Science.

———. 1998. *Scientific misconduct investigations: 1993–1997.* Washington DC: U.S. Department of Health and Human Services, Office of Public Health and Science.

Office of the Inspector General. 2000. *Recruiting human subjects: Pressures in industry-sponsored clinical research.* Washington DC: U.S. Department of Health and Human Services.

Olivieri, N. 2000. When money and truth collide. In *The corporate campus: Commercialization and the dangers to Canada's colleges and universities.* Ed. J. Turk. Toronto: Lorimer.

Olivieri, N. F. 2003. Patients' health or company profits? The commercialisation of academic research. *Science and Engineering Ethics* 9: 29–41.

Olivieri, N. F., N. Belluzzo, M. Muraca, C. C. MacKenzie, S. D. Milone, et al. 1994. Evidence of reduction in hepatic, cardiac and pituitary iron stores in patients with thalassemia major during long-term therapy with the orally active iron chelating agent L1. *Blood* 84:109a, abstract no. 423.

Olivieri, N. F., and G. M. Brittenham. 1997. Iron-chelating therapy and the treatment of thalassemia. *Blood* 89: 739–61.

Olivieri, N. F., G. M. Brittenham, D. Matsui, et al. 1995. Iron-chelation therapy with oral deferiprone in patients with thalassemia major. *New England Journal of Medicine* 332: 918–22.

Olivieri, N. F., G. M. Brittenham, D. M. Templeton, R. G. Cameron, R. A. McClelland, C. E. McLaren, A. D. Burt, and K. A. Fleming. 1998. Long-term safety and effectiveness of iron-chelation therapy with deferiprone for thalassemia major. *New England Journal of Medicine* 339: 417–23.

Olivieri, N. F., J. R. Buncie, E. Chew, T. Gallanti, R. V. Harrison, N. Keenan, W. Logan, et al. 1986. Visual and auditory neurotoxicity in patients receiving subcutaneous desferrioxamine infusions. *New England Journal of Medicine* 314: 869–73.

Olivieri, N. F., L. S. Chang, A. O. Poon, A. M. Michelson, and S. H. Orkin. 1987. An alpha-globin gene initiation codon mutation in a black family with HbH disease. *Blood* 70: 729–32.

Olivieri, N. F., G. Koren, M. H. Freedman, and C. Roifman. 1991. Rarity of systemic lupus erythematosus after oral iron chelator L1. *The Lancet* 337: 924.

Olivieri, N. F., G. Koren, J. Harris, et al. 1992. Growth failure and bony changes induced by deferoxamine. *American Journal of Pediatric Hematology-Oncology* 14: 48–56.

Olivieri, N. F., G. Koren, C. Hermann, et al. 1990. Comparison of oral iron chelator L1 and desferrioxamine in iron-loaded patients. *The Lancet* 336: 1275–79.

Olivieri, N. F., G. Koren, D. Matsui, P. P. Liu, et al. 1992. Reduction of tissue iron stores and normalization of serum ferritin during treatment with the oral iron chelator L1 in thalassemia intermedia. *Blood* 79: 2741–48.

Olivieri, N. F., P. P. Liu, G. D. Sher, P. A. Daly, P. D. Greig, P. J. McCusker, A. F. Collins, W. H. Francombe, D. M. Templeton, and J. Butany. 1994. Brief report: Combined liver and heart transplantation for end-stage iron-induced organ failure in an adult with homozygous beta-thalassemia. *New England Journal of Medicine* 330: 1125–27.

Olivieri, N. F., D. C. Rees, G. D. Ginder, et al. 1997. Treatment of thalassaemia major with phenylbutyrate and hydroxyurea. *The Lancet* 350: 491–92.

Olivieri, N. F., D. M. Templeton, G. Koren, et al. 1990. Evaluation of the oral iron chelator 1,2-dimethyl-3-hydroxypyrid-4-one (L1) in iron over-loaded patients. *Annals of the New York Academy of Sciences* 612: 369–377.

Parkes, J. G., and D. M. Templeton. 1994. Iron transport and subcellular distribution in Hep G2 hepatocarcinoma cells. *Annals of Clinical Laboratory Science* 24: 509–20.

Perrine, R. P., M. J. Brown, J. B. Clegg, D. J. Weatherall, and A. May. 1972. Benign sickle-cell anaemia. *The Lancet* 2: 1163–67.

Perrine, S. P., G. D. Ginder, D. V. Faller, et al. 1993. A short-term trial of butyrate to stimulate fetal-globin-gene expression in the beta-globin disorders. *New England Journal of Medicine* 328: 81–86.

Perrine, S. P., M. F. Green, and D. V. Faller. 1985. Delay in the fetal globin switch in infants of diabetic mothers. *New England Journal of Medicine* 312: 334–338.

Perrine, S. P., A. Rudolph, D. V. Faller, C. Roman, R. A. Cohen, et al. 1988. Butyrate infusions in the ovine fetus delay the biologic clock for globin gene switching. *Proceedings of the National Academy of Sciences* 85: 8540–42.

Pfannkuch, Friedlieb, Phil Bentley, and Hans Peter Schnebli. 1993. Future of oral iron chelator deferiprone (L1) [Comment]. *The Lancet* 341: 1480.

Piga, A., C. Gaglioti, E. Fogliacco et al. 2003. Comparative effects of deferiprone and deferoxamine on survival and cardiac disease in patients with thalassemia major: A retrospective analysis. *Haematologica* 88: 489–96.

Piga, A., L. Luzzatto, P. Capalbo, S. Gambotto, F. Tricta, and V. Gabutti. 1988. High dose desferrioxamine as a cause of growth failure in thalassaemic patients. *European Journal of Haematology* 40: 380–81.

Porter, J. B., K. P. Hoyes, R. Abeysinghe, E. R. Heuhns, and R. C. Hider. 1989. Animal toxicology of iron chelator L1. *The Lancet* 2 no. 8655: 156.

Quinn, Susan. 2001. *Human trials: Scientists, investors and patients in the quest for a cure.* Cambridge, MA.: Perseus.

Ratelle, Louise. 1994. Montreal researcher commits suicide following allegations of fraud. *Chronicle of Higher Education*, April 27.

Regush, Nicholas. 1994. *Safety last: The failure of the consumer health protection system in Canada.* Toronto: Key Porter.

Reis, P. J., D. A. Tunks, and R. E. Chapman. 1975. Effects of mimosine, a potential chemical defleecing agent, on wool growth and the skin of sheep. *Australian Journal of Biological Sciences* 28: 69–84.

Reis, P. J., D. A. Tunks, and M. P. Hegarty. 1975. Fate of mimosine administered orally to sheep and its effectiveness as a defleecing agent. *Australian Journal of Biological Sciences* 28: 495–501.

Rennie, D. 1997. Thyroid storm. [Editorial]. *Journal of the American Medical Association* 277: 1238–43.

Rennie, D., and C. K. Gunsalus. 1993. Scientific misconduct: New definition, procedures, and office—perhaps a new leaf. *Journal of the American Medical Association* 269: 915–17.

Rowell, M. 2004. The Olivieri debacle: Where were the heroes of bioethics? A reply. *Journal of Medical Ethics* 30: 50, http://jme.bmjjournals.com.

Sher, G. D., G. D. Ginder, J. Little, S. Yang, G. J. Dover, and N. F. Olivieri. 1995. Extended therapy with intravenous arginine butyrate in patients with beta-hemoglobinopathies. *New England Journal of Medicine* 322: 1606–12.

Sher, G. D., and N. F. Olivieri. 1994. Rapid healing of chronic leg ulcers during arginine butyrate therapy in patients with sickle cell disease and thalassemia. *Blood* 84: 2378–80.

Shuchman, M. 1998. Legal issues surrounding privately funded research cause furore in Toronto. *Canadian Medical Association Journal* 159: 983–86.

———. 1999. Independent review adds to controversy at Sick Kids. *Canadian Medical Association Journal* 160: 386–88.

Siminovitch, L. 2003. *Reflections on a life in science.* Self-published in Canada.

Spinks, Sarah. 1985. *Cardiac arrest.* Toronto: Doubleday.

Spino M. 1991. Pharmacokinetics of drugs in cystic fibrosis. *Clinical Reviews in Allergy.* 9:169–210.

Spino M., E.M. Sellers, H.L. Kaplan et al. 1978. Adverse biochemical and clinical consequences of furosemide administration. *Canadian Medical Association Journal.* 118:1513–8.

Spino M., D.G. Nathan, D.J. Weatherall. 2003. The Olivieri Case. *New England Journal of Medicine.* 348:860–63.

Thompson, J., P. Baird, and J. Downie. 2001. *The Olivieri report: The complete text of the report of the independent inquiry commissioned by the Canadian Association of University Teachers.* Toronto: Lorimer, http://www.dal.ca/committeeofinquiry.

Thuma, Philip E., Nancy F. Olivieri, et al. 1998. Assessment of the effect of the oral iron chelator deferiprone on asymptomatic plasmodium falciparum parasitemia in humans. *American Journal of Tropical Medicine & Hygiene* 58: 358–64.

Tricta, Fernando, and Michael Spino. 1998. Iron chelation with oral deferiprone in patients with thalassemia. *New England Journal of Medicine* 339: 1710.

Tutu, Desmond M. 1999. *No future without forgiveness.* New York: Doubleday.

Wailoo, Keith. 2001. *Dying in the city of the blues: Sickle cell anemia and the politics of race and health.* Chapel Hill: University of North Carolina Press.

Wanless, I. R., et al. 2002. Lack of progressive hepatic fibrosis during long-term therapy with deferiprone in subjects with transfusion-dependent beta-thalassemia. *Blood* 100: 1566–69.

Ward, A., J. J. Caro, et al. 2002. An international survey of patients with thalassemia major and their views about sustaining life-long desferrioxamine use. *BMC Clinical Pharmacology* 2, no. 3, http://www.biomedcentral.com/1472–6904/2/3.

Weatherall, D. J., M. J. Pippard, and S. T. Callender. 1977. Iron loading and thalassemia: Experimental successes and practical realities. *New England Journal of Medicine* 297: 445–46.

Weiner, Charles. 1986. Universities, professors, and patents: A continuing controversy. *Technology Review* 89: 32–40.

Wolfe, L. C., R. J. Nicolosi, M. M. Renaud, J. Finger, M. Hegsted, H. Peter, and D. G. Nathan. 1989. A non-human primate model for the study of oral iron chelators. *British Journal of Haematology* 72: 456–61.

Wonke, B., P. Telfer, and A. V. Hoffbrand. 1998. Iron chelation with oral deferiprone in patients with thalassemia. *New England Journal of Medicine* 339: 1712.

Young, D. 1987. A British Technology Group success story. *Journal of Medical Engineering & Technology* 11: 247–48.

Zuckerman, H., J. R. Cole, and J. T. Bruer. 1991. *The outer circle: Women in the scientific community.* New York: Norton.

ACKNOWLEDGEMENTS

First and foremost, I thank my sources—the patients and families, doctors, scientists and hospital staff who spoke to me despite their worries about the possible consequences and knowing that I might not see things as they did. I have enormous respect for their courage, and I am truly grateful for their honesty.

I would also like to thank Bernie Lucht of CBC Radio for encouraging me to pursue this story and advising me on how to do it, and two other journalists, Ann Stewart, formerly of CBC, and Pat Sullivan of the *Canadian Medical Association Journal*, for their help as I put together my early features on L1.

For research support, my thanks to medical librarian Edward Leisner of the Erie County Medical Center in Buffalo, New York, for his good humour and his ability to find just about anything. Thanks also to the library's Sharon Klug and Ginny Brennan.

My older brother, Matthew Shuchman, provided phenomenal technology support and advice—without him the text could have been lost in cyberspace.

Three friends were kind enough to read a draft of the book. My sister-in-law, pediatrician Barbara Klock, spent part of her Christmas holidays determining how it would read to her patients and colleagues; medical historian Joel Howell of the University of Michigan offered a historian's crisp analysis; and Linda Pessar, senior psychiatrist at the University of Buffalo, cast her analytic eye on the manuscript.

At Random House Canada, Anne Collins mastered the material and cut to the chase in her indomitable way. Throughout, she could see the story and knew how to tell it, and her steady guidance was a gift. Susan Renouf had the patience and wisdom to figure out what remained unclear and mould it into shape. Thanks also to Pamela Murray. My agent, Helen Heller, shepherded me through the process. Any mistakes in this book are, of course, mine.

My father, Philip Shuchman, and my mother, Hedvah Lang Shuchman, were a terrific sounding board. My dad, who died as I was putting the finishing touches on the manuscript, had been thinking about how scientists do science since he first heard of Maxwell's demons as an undergraduate, but he was also a law professor who cautioned me in my first few months of covering this saga that "cynicism is the beginning of mental health." My mother believes in the value of writing, no matter how long it takes, and her encouragement was always only a phone call away.

I'm also grateful to family and friends who offered a listening ear: Carol Shuchman, Salem Shuchman, Kendall Christiansen, Emily Ets-Hoken, David Kaye, Katy Hanson, Greg Hurray, Philip Hébert, Jim Handman, Bob McDonald, Mort Goldbach, Hazel Ipp, Anthony So, Nancy Zeldis, Sarah Scott, Diane Meschino, Carol Baum, Erin Sigel and Andrew Skolnick.

My parents and my mother-in-law, Theresa Redelmeier, made themselves available to help with our children, sometimes at a moment's notice, as only a grandparent can. During my time with this book, Emma Ortega and Kit Dickenson have showered my family with love and care, and I can't thank them enough.

Don Redelmeier, my husband, is a model for his students, as a doctor and a scientist. Without his commitment to the book and to me, I could not have completed it. Our three children, Daniel, Robbie and Rebecca, were enthusiastic about wanting it finished. Daniel once calculated the number of pages I had to write and the years it would take me—there were a lot of zeroes after the digits but he wasn't that far off the mark. I thank the three of them for their smiles and their patience.

Baker, Michael: as go-between for Sick Kids and Olivieri, 310, 312–13; informed of L1 liver damage issues, 193; and misconduct charges against Sher, 201–2, 204–7; negotiations with Olivieri and Gang, 310, 314; relationship with Olivieri, 21, 25, 48; transfers Sher, 182–84

Baltimore, David, 218–19

BASF, 115–16

Bayh-Dole Act 1980 (U.S.), 31–32, 95, 108

Baylis, Françoise, 301

Belmont Report, 2

Benet, Les, 220–22

Berkovitch, Mati, 81, 90, 92, 96

Bernstein, Alan, 79, 359

Betito, Elie, 363

Biagio (patient), 62–63, 70, 126–27, 296

Bickel, Jane, 81

Black, Conrad, 292

Blanchette, Victor, 249–50

Bloch-Nevitte, Sue, 258

Blood: Olivieri article on thalassemia genetics, 25; Olivieri butyrate article, 119; Olivieri L1 publication, negative, 179–80, 211; Olivieri L1 publication, positive, 76; paper refuting claim of L1 liver damage, 367; recent papers on L1, 374

Bloom, Floyd, 107–8

Blumenthal, David, 33

Bodenheimer, Thomas, 108

Boston Children's Hospital, 25, 111

Boston University, 116

Brigham and Women's Hospital, Boston, 298

Brill-Edwards, Michèle: hired by Toronto General, 339, 352; on importance of publicity for whistleblowers, 284; and Koren's "poison pen" letters, 332–33, 340, 345; questioned by CAUT, 356; relationship with Koren, 326–27, 339; safe drug advocate, 272–74; as whistleblower, 272–73

Britain *see* United Kingdom

British Journal of Haematology, 367, 374

British Medical Journal, 41–42, 198, 359, 364–65

British Technology Group (BTG), 28, 31, 33–35, 38–39, 45, 96, 103

Brittenham, Gary: ASH 1996, 186; consultant to Apotex, 322–23; HBED research, 227; influence, 375; joins Olivieri's research team, 104, 142; and L1 loss of response, 147–50, 152; and

L1 potential for liver damage, 177, 189; L1 research, 129, 131, 134, 138, 198–99, 225, 347, 366; and L1 research cancellation, 158, 161, 168–69; media interviews, 278; presentation to FDA, 122; publications, 179; questioned by CAUT, 356; reports L1 concerns to Health Canada, 173; responds to criticisms of Olivieri's analysis, 295–96; supports Olivieri, 173–74, 189, 198, 223–24, 226–27, 240

BTG *see* British Technology Group

Buchwald, Manuel: agrees to increase Olivieri's resources, 251; agrees to meet with Spino, 251; at hospital forum, 280; becomes chief of Research Institute, 257; collaborates with Dick, 361; criticizes Gallie's performance, 302–3; gets vote of confidence from research heads, 283; good reputation, 241; initiates review of L1 trials, 251, 253; investigates Koren, 320–21, 327; on Koren's "poison pen" letters, 344; and L1 research cancellation, 159, 171; negotiations with Olivieri and Gang, 310; and possible Apotex donation, 259–60; prodded by Olivieri and her supporters, 208–9, 232–34, 236, 238, 241, 249, 251–52, 254, 256, 279, 284; Sher investigation, 323; on Strofolino cuts and changes, 254; writes to *Nature Medicine,* 294

Bulgin, Sanchia, 354–55

Burt, Alastair, 246–47, 249

Business Week, 157, 285

butyrate, 110, 112–21

Cameron, Ross, 246–47, 249

Canada: L1 not approved, 364–66; lack of thalassemia expertise, 10–12; research guidelines, 2–3, 130–31, 359; research and industry, 95; thalassemia mortality, 376; thalassemia prevalence, 11–12

Canadian Association of University Teachers (CAUT): assists with Olivieri's costs, 337; brought in by UTFA, 294; commissions investigation into L1 trials, 2, 343, 356–57; concerned about corporate influence, 316; publishes *The Olivieri Report,* 356–57; supports Olivieri, 294, 308–9, 316

Canadian Blood Services, 378

Canadian Institutes of Health Research: *see also* Medical Research Council, 359

Michelson, Alan, 24, 46

Middle Eastern countries, 6

mimosine, 29–30

Mississauga Hospital, 195

Mitrovica, Andrew, 275

Modell, Bernadette: approached by Hider and Kontoghiorghes, 33–34; on Ciba-Geigy research, 98; on Desferal drawbacks, 370; Desferal prescriptions, 9–10; on difficulty of publishing L1 papers, 374–75; on Novartis research, 365–66; on thalassemia mortality rates, 370–71, 376–77

Mogford, Mary, 257

Montreal Children's Hospital, 123, 150, 162–63, 376

Moore, Aideen, 193, 321

Mount Sinai Hospital, Toronto, 229, 256

MRC *see* Medical Research Council (MRC)

Naimark, Arnold: appointed to investigate Olivieri-Apotex dispute, 285; attempts to meet with Olivieri and Gang, 286, 306; conclusions, 303–4; gets information from Koren, 332–34, 343, 345; investigation, 298–99; offers Baird role in investigation, 287; Olivieri and Gang's attempt to appoint reviewers, 301; Olivieri and Gang's opposition, 294, 298–99, 305–6; raises questions about Olivieri, 303–5, 313, 348; releases report, 303, 332

Nathan, David: appoints committee to review Folkman charges, 206; assists negotiations between Olivieri and Sick Kids, 308–10, 348; concerns about L1, 49, 65–67, 70, 145, 153–54, 196, 226, 245; concerns about Olivieri, 66; Desferal replacement research, 66, 372; disputes CBC TV report, 368–69; expertise and influence, 7, 27, 48, 65–66, 375; frustration with lack of treatment for thalassemia, 7–8; links to Novartis, 366; media interviews, 278; not consulted in Sher misconduct investigation, 207; offers advice to Strofolino and Aberman, 255–56; on Olivieri's character, 154, 300, 310; prescribes Desferal, 10; questioned by CAUT, 356; reputation with staff, 111–12; sides with Hider, 39; supports Olivieri, 25, 48, 95, 175, 180, 198, 211–12, 223, 225–27, 240, 249, 287, 366

National Academy of Sciences, 217–18

National Institutes of Health (NIH): butyrate research, 120; major U.S. research funder, 27; research guidelines, 108, 130, 260; rules for human research, 2; sickle cell research, 78, 111, 151; supports Gallie's and Chan's research, 284; supports Olivieri research, 362; symposium, 76; and whistleblower cases, 215–16, 218–19

National Post, 292, 295, 330, 341, 368

National Public Radio, 240

National Thalassemia Foundation, 184

National, The (TV program), 368–69

Nature, 375

Nature Medicine, 285, 294, 344

Naylor, David, 314–16, 347, 357

New England Journal of Medicine: on corporate influence, 349–50; embargo policy, 214, 261, 275; and errors in published papers, 206; experience with whistleblowers, 215–16; letters criticizing Olivieri's analysis, 295–96; new standards for industry-sponsored scientists, 359; paper on fetal hemogloblin in diabetic mothers, 112; paper on heart-liver transplant, 128; papers on butyrate, 115, 120; publications, negative, on Desferal, 47–48; publications, negative, on L1, 145, 180, 214, 249, 261, 271, 280, 295–96, 366, 374; publications, positive, on Desferal, 11; publications, positive, on L1, 144–45, 154, 323, 374; publications supporting Olivieri, 212, 369; on research ethics, 130; Spino letter about Nathan and Novartis, 366; unaware of Olivieri's consultancy to Apotex, 323

Newsworld, 275

New York Times, 285, 349

NIH *see* National Institutes of Health (NIH)

Novartis, 226, 300, 317, 362, 365–66, 372

Nuremberg Code, 2

O'Brodovich, Hugh: accepts Olivieri's "resignation" and request for leave, 249–50, 266, 276–77, 283, 289; asked by Olivieri for more resources, 159, 240, 249–50, 306; becomes chief of pediatrics at Sick Kids, 159, 257; bothered by racism claim, 307; demotes Olivieri, 307–8; and L1 research cancellation, 159, 170, 190–94; and misconduct charges against Sher, 209, 323; negotiations with Olivieri and Gang, 236, 243, 310, 314; perspectives on Olivieri-